Conquer Your Karmic Relationships

"This book is a deeply insightful guide about relationships on multiple levels, in multiple timeframes, and multiple forms. Karma serves as the *thread* of one's intricate connections to multiple existences, both linearly and laterally. It provides an explanation for an individual to use in resolving major patterns of conflict that prevent the quality of life that one desires. Yet, it includes practical examples throughout the book that one can connect with and gain valuable insights about one's self without becoming mired in complex conceptual ideas. A key element to conflict resolution is the *courage* to confront and resolve an associated fear, commonly experienced over lifetimes, until it loses its power of control. In a sense, this book might be described as a manual for life management—similar to Louise Hays' classic—"You Can Heal Your Life."

William A. Guillory, Ph.D.
Author of The Pleiadian Series:
The Pleiadians; The Hunt for the Billionaire Club;
The Consortium The Aftermath

"A semiautobiographical guide to the dynamics of karma in everyday life.

A Los Angeles–based shaman and "spiritual empath," Dunblazier stays faithful to the spirit of her earlier books, which include Heal Your Soul History (2017). She sees karma as "the accumulation of the energy of all your actions and the responses to them over time and space"—in both your past and present lives—and says that in her past lives, she's been an African tribal leader from around 1000 BCE and a French American from the 1900s. Each of the five parts of her book begins with a parable from one of her past lives and goes on to cover a range of everyday challenges from time management to how to handle feeling attracted to someone already in a relationship. At the end of each section, the author suggests a self-help ritual that can help you achieve a goal, such as "Free Yourself from the Opinion of Others." Dunblazier keeps her message positive, reflecting her belief that "regardless of your circumstances right now, your patterns do not obligate you to continue them if they no longer serve you," and she packs an extensive amount of material into 325 pages. Not everyone will buy her views on subjects like demons or telepathy.... Nevertheless, even readers skeptical of whether they are reading the words of a reincarnated Chief Running Bear may be intrigued by her information on how people make use of concepts like totem animals. For most readers, this book will provide different ways of looking at things. And who wouldn't want to believe, as the author does, that in the end "you are the master of your universe"? A personal view of karma, likely to appeal mainly to readers curious about reincarnation and related topics."

Kirkus Reviews

"I was blown away by the amount of content covered in this life-changing book. From food, money and romantic partners to fear, creativity and spirituality, this comprehensive guide will help you heal your deepest wounds, even those you may not yet be aware of. This should be mandatory reading for anyone who wants to live a more peaceful and joyous life."

Stephanie Chandler
CEO of the Nonfiction Authors Association and
author of *The Nonfiction Book Publishing Plan*

"In a time where so many souls are seeking true guidance and wisdom, Tracee Dunblazier's spiritual gift, Conquer Your Karmic Relationships, offers a powerful and accessible map to cultivate personal responsibility and global empathy. She combines profound metaphysical knowledge with insightful sanity, thus offering the reader tools and techniques to vanquish any karmic relationships. A must read for any truth seeker who wishes to shatter limiting illusions and trumpet their true empowerment."

Austyn Wells
Spiritual Medium & Soul Gardener & author
*Soul Conversations: A Medium Reveals How to
Cultivate Your Intuition, Heal Your Heart,
and Connect with the Divine.*

"Conquer Your Karmic Relationships takes the reader right into the undiscovered territory of healing the energy that you have carried over from your biological or spiritual past. Written in accessible, clear language, you'll be guided through new, life-shifting understandings. This book will change how you perceive yourself and give you the tools needed for a radical transformation and breakthrough. Tracee Dunblazier has shined a light on trauma in a way that makes it safe to heal."

Unicole Unicron
Unicult

"Though science has led us to see the quantum origins of our DNA and has given us a glimpse of the outer Universe, minimal science related to the study of living Life exists. Today, we better understand things and physical matter, but what occurs in the ethereal and spiritual realms remains undeclared.

Tracee Dunblazier took on the task of unveiling some of the unseen realms of the ethereal-spirit-driven world, which, in part, embraces the practice of Holistic Psychology. She addresses those quagmires of communicating with our souls, getting a hold of the realms and the effects of karma, struggling to know our life's purpose and mission, and how individuals coil at the moment needed to confront a situation, which tempts ourselves into denial and apathy.

Exploring the hard-to-believe unseen realities of life gleams excitement for me and serves as the frontiers of a new humanity. Caring for our brothers and sisters, and the planet intrinsically motivate me and my work endeavors. Ms. Dunblazier enables her readership to educate and participate in the ancient quest to achieve answers that the evolution of our consciousness challenges us to discover.

Conquer Your Karmic Relationships serves as an excellent and challenging read for those who desire to break out of their comfort zone and awaken to the prosperities of the Light."

Robert V. Gerard
Holistic Psychologist & Visionary Healer
Author of *Change Your DNA, Change Your Life,*
Handling Verbal Confrontation: Take the Fear Out of Facing Others,
and *Divine Quick Fix Healings*

Copyright ©2020 Tracee Dunblazier

All rights reserved. No part of this book may be used or reproduced in any manner without the written permission of the publisher.

GoTracee Publishing LLC
240 Laurel Street, Suite 101
Baton Rouge, Louisiana, 70801
www.BeASlayer.com

LCCN: 2019919082

ISBN: 978-0-9963907-6-7 print book
ISBN: 978-0-9993623-0-3 ebook
ISBN: 978-0-9993623-2-7, Audio Series Part One
ISBN: 978-0-9993623-3-4, Audio Series Part Two
ISBN: 978-0-9993623-4-1, Audio Series Part Three
ISBN: 978-0-9993623-5-8, Audio Series Part Four
ISBN: 978-0-9993623-6-5, Audio Series Part Five

Editor: Stephen J. Miller at www.FaceBook.com/stephenjmillerediting
Illustrations: Michael J Penn at www.michaeljpenn.com
Cover & interior Design: Nelly Murariu at www.PixBeeDesign.com

Disclaimer: Tracee Dunblazier is neither a medical doctor nor a mental health specialist, and does not offer medical diagnosis or therapy. No information and opinions offered through this title, through GoTracee Publishing LLC., or through any other venue representing Tracee Dunblazier are to be substituted for appropriate mental health or medical help. In no event are Tracee Dunblazier, her agents and/or representatives liable for any damages whatsoever arising out of or in any way connected with any individual's interpretation or use of information contained in this title. By reading this title you recognize and agree to take complete and total responsibility for yourself, your experience, and your actions.

Publisher's Cataloging-In-Publication Data
(Prepared by The Donohue Group, Inc.)

Names: Dunblazier, Tracee, author. | Penn, Michael J., illustrator.

Title: Conquer your karmic relationships : heal spiritual trauma to open your heart and restore your soul / Tracee Dunblazier ; [illustrations: Michael J Penn].

Description: Baton Rouge, Louisiana ; Los Angeles, California : GoTracee Publishing LLC, [2020] | Series: The Demon Slayer's handbook series ; [3] | Includes bibliographical references.

Identifiers: ISBN 9780996390767 (paperback) | ISBN 9780999362303 (ebook)

Subjects: LCSH: Spiritual healing. | Spiritual life. | Dunblazier, Tracee--Religion. | Karma. | Interpersonal relations. | Soul.

Classification: LCC BF1275.S44 D863 2020 (print) | LCC BF1275.S44 (ebook) | DDC 133.9--dc23

Printed in China on FSC paper

THE DEMON SLAYER'S HANDBOOK SERIES

Conquer Your Karmic Relationships

Heal Spiritual Trauma to Open Your Heart and Restore Your Soul

Tracee Dunblazier

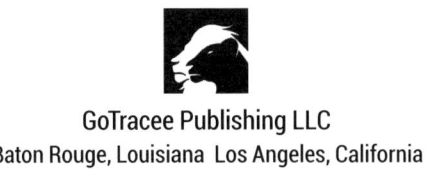

GoTracee Publishing LLC
Baton Rouge, Louisiana Los Angeles, California

Dedication

A friend shared a recurring dream with me, in it she was about to jump off a cliff and was terrified. We began to speak about the metaphor of the cliff as surrender. Learning to flow with the healing energy of grief, and the process of transformation the Creator offers us, it requires our complete surrender. I, then, told her about a recurring dream I had. In it, I was always driving or travelling straight up, in multiple vehicles, over many different surfaces, but always at a ninety-degree angle—hoping that the vehicle I was in had enough torque to get me to the top.

She asked me if I had trouble jumping off the cliff, and I said, "No, evidently my challenge is getting back up the mountain."

I'd like to dedicate this work to my many karmic partners, living and in spirit. You have brought clarity in times of confusion, comfort in times of distress, and love in times of self-loathing. All that I am and all that you are—spirit to spirit—we achieved together.

Thank you for helping me up the mountain.

Acknowledgements

To do this work honestly takes many things, but mostly, many eyes and hands to help with the work and to witness it. They say something watched, changes. I'd like to recognize the team of slayers who put their heart and soul into working with me and supporting my process on all levels. Stephen J. Miller, whose tireless focus kept me on track and made me fight for every em dash. Holly Bush, who spent endless hours over the phone listening to me read passages and offering meaningful insight. My sister Chris, whose endless humor and integrity kept me inspired. Jean Marie Hance, who awakened in me the courage to tell the whole story. Finally, all those living and in spirit who have been my witness and reflected back to me the limitless spiritual matrix that holds all the stories ever told and helped me to remember who I am.

Contents

Foreword by Christian McBride — xv
Preface — xvii
Introduction — xix

PART ONE: PLENTY
Your Karmic Relationship to Food and Money — 1

The Karmic Story: The Art of Remembering What's Important — 5
The Slayer's Path: The Practice of Remembering, Learning, and Having — 11
    Auschwitz: It Is Safe to Remember — 11
    Overcoming Scarcity — 12
    Your Relationship with Food — 14
    Rejection: The Beginning of Self-Mastery — 20
    Your Relationship with Money — 21
The Warrior's Hidden Motto: Need Less — 22
The Slayer's Dilemma: How Much is Enough? — 22
    Complaining: Valuable Waste of Time — 23
    Remembering Your Karma — 23
The Slayer's Motto: I Create My Reality — 24
    Scott's Story — 24
    Addiction is Karma: Targeting Your Addiction at Its Core — 26
The Slayer's Pact: The Choices I Make are an Extension of My Power — 28
    Communication Takes Practice — 28
    The Infinite Connection Between Food, Pleasure, and Hope — 29
    Filling the Void — 31
    Opening to Receive and Retain the New Pattern — 35
    The Universe and Prosperity: Understanding Deficit Driven Choices — 37
    Living With Surplus: Having Too Much Equals Waste? — 40
The Slayer's Altar and Ritual: Living Wealthy — 43

PART TWO: AFFINITY
Your Karmic Relationship to Romantic Love and Your Ancestors — 45

The Karmic Story: The Once and Disappointing King — 49
The Slayer's Path: Leave No Stone Unturned — 54
    What Are the Initial Tell-Tale Signs of a Soulmate? — 54
    What is a Soulmate? — 55
    Are All Relationships Karmic? — 56

The Spiritual Lock and Key	57
Familial Relationship Patterns	58
Ancestral Karma	62
Karmic Romance	68
Incompatibility In A Karmic Relationship	70
The Warrior's Hidden Motto: Trust No One	72
Drama Equals Trauma	72
The Slayer's Dilemma: Blame	74
When Blame Raises It's Ugly Head	74
Anger is the Truth Seeker	76
How Karma is Revealed in a Partnership	76
How to Manage a Karmic Relationship	79
The Slayer's Motto: I Carry on the Traditions that Make Sense	81
Dating Outside of Your Spiritual Patterns	81
Mental Illness and Karma	85
The Slayer's Pact: I Free Myself by Accepting the Truth	90
Using Complete Honesty To Work Through Karmic Patterns	91
Connecting with Power and Presence	99
Mindfulness in All Your Relations	109
The Slayer's Altar and Ritual: Free Yourself from the Opinions of Others	111

PART THREE: UNITY
Your Karmic Relationship to Others and the Environment 115

The Karmic Story: The Place Where All Things Are Possible	119
The Slayer's Path: Harnessing Your Ability to Respond	124
Types of Environmental Soulmates	125
Soulmate Groups	129
The Warrior's Hidden Motto: I Am Invisible	131
Overcoming Invisibility: Namaste	131
Overcoming Blame	132
Accountability	133
Getting in Flow with the Universe	134
The Slayer's Dilemma: Becoming Visible	135
Visibility Exercise	136
The Spiritual Purpose of Self-Pity	137
Overcoming Self-Pity and Other Overwhelming Emotions	137
The Slayer's Motto: I Flow with a Changing World	137
Group Karmic Contracts	139
Changing What I Do Doesn't Change Who I Am	140
Walking Away from a Long Career	141

The Slayer's Pact: Harmony is Inevitable	142
Understanding the Karma of Culture and Tradition	143
Living Multi-Spirited	143
What It Takes to Heal Cultural Wounds	144
Racism and Bigotry	145
Karma of Politics and Religion	147
The Karma of Dignity and Respect	148
The Karma of Leadership	148
The Karma of Corporations and Big Money: Profit at the Expense of Others	149
What Are the Lessons for Disruptors?	150
The Art of Getting What You Want	151
Creating in a Conscious Way	152
Making New Connections	152
Renew and Reset for Love and Peace	156
Trust Yourself and Your World	158
The Slayer's Altar and Ritual: Changing the Way You See Your Environment	160

PART FOUR: MASTERY
Your Karmic Relationship to Authority, Fear, Hate, and Death — 163

The Karmic Story: Building Walls and Bridges	167
The Slayer's Path: Surrender To What Is—The Only Control You Have	172
The Four Walls: Building Spiritual Bridges to Overcome Them	172
Understanding Your Relationship to Authority	173
Understanding Your Relationship to Fear	175
Understanding Your Relationship to Hatred	175
Understanding Your Relationship to Death	176
Soulmates: Your Karmic Authorities	177
The Warrior's Hidden Motto: What I Don't Understand Will Hurt Me	180
The Slayer's Dilemma: Viewing the World with an Open Heart	181
Learning New Things	181
The Slayer's Motto: I Am Stronger than I Know	188
Acknowledging Your Inner Authority	189
Transitioning Conflict and Struggle to Learning and Transforming	189
Fluidity is Strength	191
Trust	192
Dealing with Outer Forces	193
Creating Cooperation and Mutual Aid	194
The Slayer's Pact: Face What's in Front of You	194
Social Justice and Self-Governance: A Global Cry for Healing	195
Communicating About Racism and Bias: Listen, Learn, and Let Go of Shame	195
Patriotism	208

Terrorism from an Energetic Perspective	209
Using Telepathy to Change the Outcome	210
Death, Hauntings, and Karma	217
Suicide and Karma	220
Death and Reincarnation	236
The Slayer's Altar and Ritual: Face or Challenge the Things You Fear	241

PART FIVE: INFINITY
Your Karmic Relationship to Sexuality, Creativity, Spirituality, and the Divine — 245

The Karmic Story: The African Queen No One Remembered	249
The Slayer's Path: The Practice of Forgiveness	253
Ho'oponopono	254
Three Rivers that Lead to the Ocean: Understanding Your Connection to Divinity	255
The Warrior's Hidden Motto: I am Unworthy	260
The Slayer's Dilemma: Building Spiritual Integrity	261
Kundalini Movement in the Body	262
Quantum Spiritual Shifts	262
Healing Crises	263
Building Spiritual Integrity through Honesty: Everyone Lies	264
Karma's Impact: Why People Lie	266
Sexuality and Intimacy: The Birth of Creativity	266
Sexuality and Trauma	270
Sexual Attraction and Karma	271
Understanding Intimacy	275
Hook-ups and Other Sexual Encounters	277
The Slayer's Motto: I Am at Peace with Myself and My History	286
Your Personal Cultural Identity: Finding Your Tribe	286
Magic and Healing	287
Falling in Love with Love	291
The Slayer's Pact: I am Free to Thrive	293
Creativity: Your Connection Between Your Higher and Lower Selves	294
The Spiritual Matrix of Multiple Dimensions	302
Spiritual Patterns and Your Soul	304
Faith Leads to Divinity	312
The Magic of Radical Acceptance	313
The Slayer's Altar and Ritual: Making Your Home a Sacred Space	322
Epilogue	325
Notes	327
Bibliography	329
Other Works by the Author	331
About the Author	333

Foreword
by Christian McBride

Many have said that religion and spirituality are two different things. Some say you can't have one without the other. Some admit that they don't know... or care. I was raised with Christian values, however, my mother was by all accounts at the time "new school." She always taught me that brow-beating someone to attend church every Sunday did not make them more spiritual. She instructed me early on in life that some of the biggest hypocrites were the altruistic bible-thumpers that went to church *religiously*.

I was encouraged to believe in God: that there were other dimensions, larger forces out there greater than humans, and that faith in a higher power and the ability to surrender to this divine knowledge was being spiritual. Whereas, giving practice to these beliefs was being religious. Naturally, I was shown to respect all religions. To consider someone unrighteous because they practiced another religion was about the most unrighteous thing a person could do. With that being said, I find that my longest standing friendships have been with people who are aware of other dimensions and greater forces—spiritual people. They believe in something greater than themselves and are always on a journey to find harmony with it.

I began my professional jazz career at the age of fifteen and played nightclubs and auditoriums from that point on. I was eighteen when I met Tracee in New York City at the now defunct jazz-haven Bradley's, where I played often. What I remember to this day is Tracee's straight-shooting authenticity that made me feel at ease—like a musician playing harmonies with an unseen orchestra. I knew from that moment on that Tracee had a special connection to the world: she was "in tune."

One of the reasons I love playing jazz music is because of the unspoken communication that must happen between the musicians. It's unlike any other style of music, in that the ultimate goal is to emote the joy (and danger) of improvising. You can develop a level of communication with any group of musicians if you play together long enough, but there are times when you just "click" with someone immediately.

Pianist Benny Green is someone I listened to on records with legends like Betty Carter and Art Blakey while I was in high school. When we first met in 1989, I literally felt like I'd met a long-lost brother. I don't know why, but we've remained the best of friends for over thirty years, and we still play together often. I can remember one night performing with Benny at Bradley's, and at some point, I lost my place in the song. That's the absolute worst thing a bass player can do, considering we're responsible for underlining the form of the song and harmonically supporting the melody. In a moment of panic, I opened my eyes, looked over at Benny and murmured out the side of my mouth,

"Where are we? I'm lost." Benny silently mouthed back, "Me too!"

We intuitively just picked a spot in the song to reconnect and it worked! We laughed so loud. I'm sure no one in the audience knew what happened. Then again, if they did know, it was probably that much more entertaining and incredible. That rare connection and telepathy with a person is something that Tracee probes in this amazing book. Soulmate is a term I find all too casually thrown around. It tends to be used in the context of two people in love, but goes far beyond romance. In *Conquer Your Karmic Relationships: Heal Spiritual Trauma to Open your Heart and Restore Your Soul*, Tracee reveals not only the different types of soulmates we encounter in life but also the deeper spiritual connections we have within ourselves that guide our relationship to everything we experience. She explains not only why we connect with the people and things we do but—more importantly—why we endure with them. Much like music, karma is the glue that brings us all together. The few karmic relationships that don't look at the clock, keep score, or hold grudges, but know when to step in and help (or step out and help), are the ones that play through to the next bridge.

When I discovered that Tracee had become the author of the Demon Slayer's Handbook Series, it gave form to the deep spiritual knowledge I'd first witnessed from her those three decades ago, as our lives' paths were rerouting to bigger and better things. The great thing about this book? You don't have to be of any particular religious association to understand where Tracee is coming from. It will put you at ease in contemplating traditionally difficult topics and leave you with a new prospective that will empower you to be the changemaker in your own life. You will come away from reading her latest masterpiece truly comprehending the meaning of soulmates and spirituality.

Tracee is an inspiring, spiritual vessel who can connect with all of us in a soulful way, guiding us to connect with ourselves and the rhythm of the world around us.

So, my friend, let the rhythm move you and your music play on....

Christian McBride
Grammy Award-Winning Jazz Bassist and Composer

Preface

My Spiritual Bounty

The phenomena we call karmic relationships ultimately becomes a profound investigation into the indelible human spirit, which is the through line of each soul that acts as mother, father, teacher, lover, and friend. I was born into a life steeped in the deep karmic patterns invading every aspect of my day and night, controlling all I came across (or so it felt). Even so, I never begrudged them. They kept my beloved spiritual family with me: ancestors from multiple cultures, time periods, and life experiences—the reason for my love affair with history.

After all, if you don't know where you've been, you can't know where you're going.

I can't say, even with all the struggles, that the karmic relationships that I've engaged in have been hard on me, as there was always an incredible feeling of growth, accomplishment, and love that came with each one. I gained knowledge and empowerment from my karmic relationship to sexuality. I gained discipline from my karmic relationship to food and money. I gained true love and compassion from my karmic relationship to men. And I gained leadership from my karmic relationship to my environment and the Creator.

I think what was most difficult to navigate was the judgment of my friends, family, and confidants over the years. The linear cultural traditions of how relationships are *supposed* to go, what a romantic relationship *should* look like, and how a young woman growing up *should* engage the world—all those standards, as people call them, didn't really help a gal like me. They were not the pathways that could lead me to relief, resolution, wisdom, or peace. I was left to find those on my own, which I now understand was my karma.

Yes, it took me decades to comprehend that not everyone is like me, with such a wide berth for connection, acceptance, and compassion for all beings. To tell you the truth, I still don't believe it. I believe humans are fundamentally—underneath all the layers of insecurity, self-doubt, bitterness, and anger—people who want to love and be loved. But also, inherent in the human design is our fundamental desire to grow and expand on every level. This urge to expand, combined with the fear that must be overcome in order to do so (if one is to expand in a way that includes everyone), is the dynamic that leaves us in the position we find ourselves today.

I have always been deeply aware of my spiritual imprints and patterns, even when I didn't have the language to communicate about their presence.

What I came to understand is all our relationships to everything we encounter are because of these subtle karmic patterns that reverberate through our lives. They connect us to the people, places, things, and experiences that will reveal something about us and a bit of our spiritual history. Whether you consider yourself and your life to be simple or complicated—or somewhere in between—your soul calls to you, informing you as to what you need for your growth.

Finally, I have arrived at the end of a very long cycle of soul-to-body healing on every level. Being here also ends the cycle of suffering anonymously with the publishing of my first three books, The Demon Slayer's Handbook Series, which are—among other things—a chronicle of my personal struggles and the road I took to restore my soul. A natural part of that path was chronic depression, anxiety, and multidimensional experiences that have left many days, including birthdays and holidays, often a bit rough. This was most notable since the loss of my father several years ago, which seemed to warrant the end of any real joyous celebration.

Over the years, I have worked hard to overcome the sadness through many different rituals, but the abiding relief did not come over night. It arrived with the reconciling of layer upon layer of spiritual, mental, emotional and physical dynamics that my soul and DNA carried. I hadn't been cognizant to the depth of my own biological shroud of sadness until it was lifted from me.

This led the way to a joyousness of such magnitude and depth I've never felt, and somehow, it seems to be emerging a little more each day. While my suffering may have been anonymous, I certainly was not alone. I have a tremendous amount of gratitude for the many who have walked with me on this road and the ones to forge the path ahead. Doing spiritual work gave me answers to many unanswered questions and returned to me, from time and space, the missing pieces to restore my heart and soul.

It is my wish for you to find comfort, love, wisdom, and courage among these pages—as I have. Drawing on the deep well of forgiveness within your heart, it is my hope that you will share your light with others and own every inch of space you take up, knowing you are seen and loved dearly in this Universe.

10,000 blessings to you,
Tracee

Introduction

Everything in the universe expresses itself through patterns. All beings can be understood by the continual reverberations of energy they emit while moving through the world, attracting similar vibrations to support their momentum. Ultimately, we are all collectors, and what we collect is an expression of the spiritual, mental, and emotional patterns that make up our soul. It is these patterns and the response to them that make up our karma.

Karma is a Sanskrit word that literally translates to mean *action*, or the more comprehensive concept of action and reaction (or cause and effect). It is the fundamental spiritual understanding that all actions send out a ripple in consciousness effecting change long after the original action has been taken. Karma is not necessarily fate, but the spiritual guarantee that we will all get what's coming to us, on all levels. How that happens is up to us and our personal will—we all have multiple options in any given situation. However, once an option has been taken, it begins your path of karma.

Relationships occur with the combining and intersecting of spiritual, mental, emotional, and physical patterns between partners—your partners can be anyone or anything. Much how Mother Earth has the unwavering ability to right the wrongs that have been carelessly or blindly committed against her, our karma—or the weight of our spirit—has the same healing magic. It is this alchemy that will pave the way for your very personal healing path to spiritual redemption, mental reason, emotional transformation, and physical freedom. Regardless of where you start, the chain of events leading to your richness has already begun.

On the human front, the leading factor in how we relate to life and others is through our soul patterns and the frequency they transmit into the world, which connect us to and impact all we come across. It is only through the recognition and mindfulness of these patterns that we begin to unravel who we really are as spiritual beings and the power we hold.

Our connections are the lifeblood of our existence. We have them everywhere we go. Our perception, or lens through which we look at life, is the foundation of all our relations. And these relationships take work, negotiation, and compromise. Now, add to the mix: karma. In our contemporary world, karma describes the spiritual dynamic of the sum of a person's actions in any previous state of existence, as well as the spiritual patterns those actions create and how they impact their fate in future realities. Often, people make the mistake of seeing karma as meaning *an eye for an eye* or *punishment and reward*, but really, it speaks to two patterns of behavior that are created for every experience.

Every notable activity has two sides: the action and the response to it. In relationships, one person carries out an action and the other experiences the impact of it. Karma means we will eventually get to encounter both sides in order to understand the entire dynamic.

Let's say you slap someone in the face. Karma doesn't dictate you will experience a slap in the face necessarily, it says you will experience the pain or impact of the slap you caused. You can experience the shock, degradation, or rejection of that slap in the face—without ever being hit. Any activity happening repeatedly cements into our spirit an energetic fabric we carry with us from lifetime to lifetime, until it is fully expressed and we understand the purpose of its meaning and decide to change the pattern.

Most of all, your karma is your *whole truth*. It can be frustrating to find self-acceptance when our society wants us only to focus on half of our truth: usually the part that is pretty and shiny, which is, very possibly, obscured from our vision—especially in times of distress. In fact, there are people who've lived lifetimes never seeing the beautiful glowing power inherent in their wholeness.

It is a Universal Truth that we're all born with self-loathing. It is the dynamic that occurs the more self-aware we become. It is the spiritual mechanism that inspires us to dig deeply into who we are in our entirety: mind, body, and spirit in a multidimensional life experience.

The less fear we have of acknowledging and honoring our darkness and our light, the more we'll be able to let go of our hang-ups about sex, our attachment to drugs and addiction, the fervor for power and money, and our need to judge and control others.

Take a moment to imagine a world without those things.

Karmic relationships come in all forms and pull from us a profound unconditional love and compassion for ourselves and our soulmates. They feel different, more connected than other unions; we are familiar with their vibration. They are our spiritual family. Like it or not, humans are naturally selfish and self-involved—until they feel safe and connected to our world. Until that point, all we strive for is success towards that end.

Reincarnation and Spiritual Imprints

Everyone carries with them a spiritual history, even those who do not believe in reincarnation. For the non-believers: I don't think how we conceptualize reincarnation matters. Do past-lives equal literal previous incarnations? Or, do spiritual imprints equal metaphorical lives stored like holograms in your spirit? Either way, their presence brings the same knowledge of your personal soul memories—and everyone has them.

I've personally experienced many recollections of past-lives that were as real as I sit here today. It makes perfect sense that I would bring the memories from those spiritual imprints and past-lives into this incarnation to complete the knowledge and hone the wisdom I've cultivated from them. Thinking of them as literal or metaphorical is based on the person needing to understand them and being able to reconcile them with the other *truths* they carry. Both ways tell one's spiritual story.

The soul is eternal, ever-changing, and growing. When trauma occurs, aspects to the spirit and personality can split off or spiritually create another dimension of energy, which will wind up being fed and nurtured by the soul in question or another's life force, becoming a powerful and sometimes dominant influence in the person's perspective and experience of life. So, when the soul's journey fosters the need to retrieve, heal, and balance those aspects of the self, it may spend a lifetime, or several, doing so.

A client asked me if she needed to believe in all this hooey in order to benefit or be impacted by it. My response was definitely *not*. As is with healing, one does not need to believe they can be healed, they must have an undeniable desire to heal. The energy will enact the flow of life force that will inspire and conjure all they need in order to heal and restore balance. Belief is a mechanism to connect you with expanding information. Whatever you believe calls the Universal Truth to you, it does so in stages—for optimum receptivity. Your truth will always lead to the Truth.

The Pathway to Conquer Your Karmic Relationships

This book has been designed in a very specific way. Each part begins with a parable that is one of my personal karmic journeys. Although it is true for me, it can be fiction for you. The purpose is to engage your intuitive brain in finding something within the story with which you can relate or that engages your empathy for the ancestors who've paved the way for our lives today. Certainly, it's not expected that you've had any of these traumatic experiences, as all the stories are of the history, ancient and modern, that blazed the trail for the condition in which we find ourselves and the planet at this time.

The purpose is for you to exercise your compassion by connecting to similar feelings, beliefs, fears, or genuine joys you may have experienced in the accomplishments and trials of your life. Open yourself to empathize with the ancestors and the powerful experiences of their times. Ultimately, acknowledging their stories and offering them the opportunity to grieve through you or receive your authentic gratitude for their wisdom, which can now become your own.

Each part includes eight sections:

The Slayer's Weapons are a set of keywords that are positive or negative dynamics we all experience, such as joy or self-pity. It is through these

Conquer Your Karmic Relationships

dynamics that the slayer is able to witness themselves and others by learning about their deepest spiritual expression—transforming their patterns and environment.

The Karmic Story, as mentioned previously, is from my personal soul history. Its objective is to connect you to your compassion, empathy, and the stories of your own spiritual archive and those of your biological and spiritual ancestors.

The Illustration has been derived from aspects of the spiritual and physical journey of the Karmic Story to help one visualize the magic of the multi-dimensional realm. It personifies how our unresolved past intermingles with present time and creates the future.

The Slayer's Path is the overarching theme a slayer must confront in life by embodying a new way. The concept helps the slayer discover their truth and align with it during the particular phase of development that the path heralds for the slayer.

The Warrior's Hidden Motto is the internal dialogue or the underlying beliefs rooted in insecurity that are the basis of the warrior's conflict to be overcome. At the heart of every warrior is a cause they struggle to resolve. Once dealt with, another will appear—that is the way of the warrior. To become a slayer, one must learn to challenge their need for conflict by releasing themselves from the opinions and actions of others—finding cooperative ways to prosper into the future

The Slayer's Dilemma is the spiritual, mental, or emotional dynamic the slayer must cultivate in order to shift their spiritual patterning. Doing this allows for the reconciliation of discordant or undesired relationships that are no longer necessary to the slayer's growth.

The Slayer's Motto is a tag line or affirmation that a slayer can repeat to remind themselves of their chosen path.

The Slayer's Pact is a unifying idea that all slayers commit to on their journey.

The Slayer's Altar and Ritual is the formula to create a sacred space (altar) and process (ritual) in your home, assisting the slayer in aligning with their highest good and cultivating the mindfulness necessary to recognize the deeper spiritual patterns impacting their lives. It is the physical-world offering that completes and cements the slayer's commitment to overcome any deeply rooted pervasive energy and heal on every level.

The information in the chapters will offer an opportunity to expand your understanding of how you relate to the fundamental building blocks of your life in every way and the spiritual patterns that currently govern them. You will take an in depth look at: your relationship with food and money; your friends, lovers, and family; your environment; the dynamics of authority, fear, hate, and death; and your karmic relationship to sexuality, creativity, spirituality, and the Divine. The purpose of the book's design is for you to access your own stories and self-truths.

Through the process of reading and working the exercises in the book, you will gain insight on how your karma was created. Most importantly, many of the exercises consist of stream-of-consciousness questions—asked in a succinct manner, to be answered quickly and without deliberate thought—to help you recognize your subconscious chatter and your spiritual imprints, which are waiting to reveal what you have and what you will need to transform your karmic relationships. Along with the karmic patterns that are being healed, you'll gain understanding of the personal spiritual tools you've brought into this life.

There are many anecdotes among the pages. Some are actual experiences of clients, friends, and colleagues, written in their own words. Some are stories inspired by real-life accounts where the names and details have been changed to protect privacy and make the spiritual value of the story apparent. I've created them to illustrate, in a defined way, the specific spiritual phenomena at work. Finally, each chapter holds the tales of my life, containing some of the events, past-life visions, and spiritual experiences that illuminated my karmic stories.

I've always been empathic, psychic, and fully aware of my spiritual knowledge, even in the crib. I am not unique in this experience; people across the globe are having quantum spiritual shifts and moving their awareness into the fourth and fifth dimensions of psychic experience (your ability to channel, feel, hear, and see spirit). Sometimes, in the moment, we're not looking for a miracle. We're just looking for an upgrade—an upgrade of our thoughts, feelings, circumstances, and opportunities. Just a minor adjustment in perspective lets in more light on a situation. That light becomes wisdom. And that wisdom, overtime, becomes the resolution we need.

Everywhere, people are opening to their own personal karmic diaries and that of their biological and spiritual ancestry. All, so that together we may begin to heal our many cultural wounds, unwanted karmic patterns, and restore our collective heart and the planet that sustains us all.

> This time of cataclysmic politics, earthly changes, and humanitarian confusion is both powerful and life affirming for those who will accept the challenge of digging deep to unravel and heal their own self-contempt.

PART ONE

PLENTY

*Your Karmic Relationship
to Food and Money*

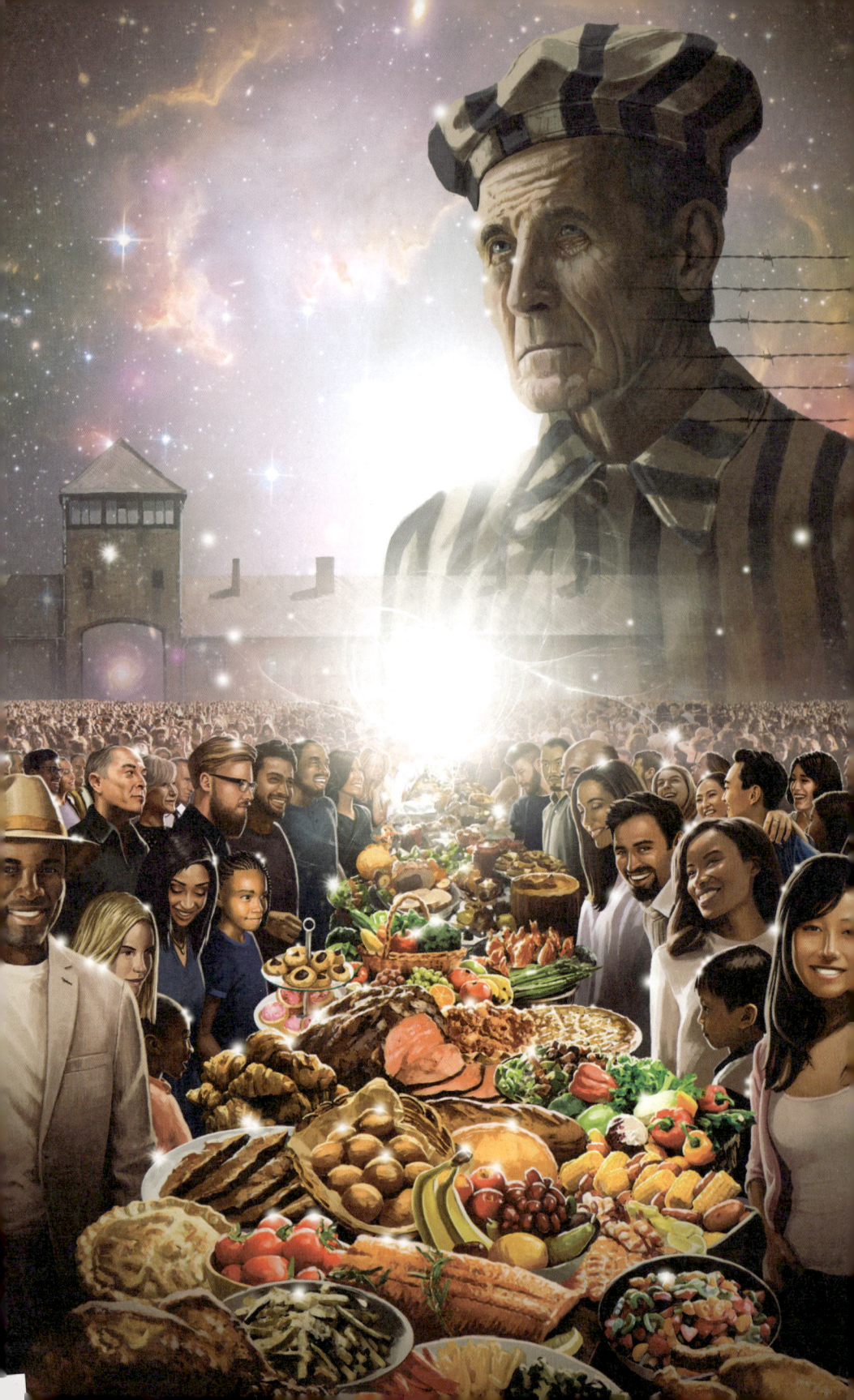

Your Karma Wants You to Believe There is Not Enough—There is Always Enough

The Slayer's Weapons:

Balance, Math, Reason, Abundance, Ebb, Flow, Memory, Consumption, Input, Output

The Karmic Story: The Art of Remembering What's Important

Everything was dark for so long. In fact, I didn't think it would ever be any other way. At the end, there was not much of a transition from life to death; the darkness permeated both. It took decades in this spiritual dimension where my soul exists to recall the slow and steady reduction of my people—first in rumor, then by slander and harassment, next through registration and organization, followed by segregation, and finally via deportation and murder. This was the devastation of the Jewish Holocaust from the early 1930s to May, 1945.

A celebration on the farm was always plentiful. We were a simple family of pig farmers in southeastern Poland, near the Dunajec River. Oh, how my mother loved to set the table with her special dishes lined with gold, resting upon freshly pressed linens. The clanking of the pots and pans in the kitchen signaled the preparation of a feast with at least two different meats, roots with cabbage salad, dumpling soup, and pierogi. But my most favorite part of those dinners was my grandmother's cherry pie at the end. The women would cook all day and let me help.

I had been hunting in the mountains when the Nazis began their invasion of Poland. It wasn't long until they had commandeered our farm, and we were shuttled off to the city of Kraków. Eventually, the Nazis registered what little property we took with us. I, however, was able to keep hidden from them my grandfather's gold pocket watch.

In retrospect, I'm not sure why we hadn't seen the genocide coming, as it had just happened to the Armenians by the Turks of the Ottoman Empire. It was a devilish time we were living in. The memories of those special dinners kept me afloat.

One night, a friend decided to have a secret gathering for his birthday. He lived in the middle of the city, and a small group of us met early in the day so as to make the curfew that had been established. There wasn't much to celebrate with, but it was good to spend time with friends.

I remember trying to get home undetected; it was already past curfew that night and the SS (Nazi police) were out in force. It was colder than usual, and I'd forgotten my gloves. The cobblestone street was dark and silent, and I heard some of the SS men coming down the way. I ducked into a rounded stone entrance to the airshaft of a building to hide myself until they passed, when I was conked on the head by someone waiting for me. They must have been lurking in the shadow.

As it turns out, there was another entrance to the alley on the other side of the building where a little light shown through. They must have seen me from the minute I walked out of my friend's door and were toying with me the whole time—thriving on my fear—waiting to see how long it would take me to realize there was no hope of escape.

I woke up in a building somewhere. I believe it was Altdorf, one of the camps of Auschwitz. It was dirty and the smells were atrocious. I couldn't imagine what was causing them. They had me propped up in a chair, and while they never tended to my injury, they clearly wanted to keep me alive to see what else I was hiding. As fate had it, they'd seen the glimmer of the full moon on my grandfather's gold pocket watch; I'd glanced at it as I stepped out from my friend's flat onto the street. Meanwhile, the hit on the head I had sustained concussed my brain. From that moment on, most of my memory vanished.

The Nazis kept me with them for days, believing I was a spy, or maybe hiding other things. Finally, they transported me to another camp at Auschwitz, and over the coming days and months, I was shuttled from place to place and given odd jobs. I wracked my brain, trying to summon to mind anything before the night I was taken. I couldn't remember who I was or what I did. Was I really a spy? Did I actually have a treasure hidden somewhere? Little did I know, I was just a pig farmer.

It was the fall of 1942. They passed me around from one location to another, doing anything from laundry to office work, until I took ill. I couldn't remember my last decent meal, and the memory of grandmother's cherry pie was gone. I was sickly and holed up in a basement where someone occasionally looked in on me.

Mostly, I was left alone with deafening silence, seeing the faces of people in my head whom I couldn't remember—neither their names nor our relation. In the end, I took comfort in their presence, in the blankness of seeking the understanding of a meaningful life forgotten. We were all victims of this senseless tragedy perpetrated by criminals—vacant of their humanity—disguised as the authority.

I was feeling the sovereignty of my spirit leaving my body more every day, until finally freedom came. Yet still, there was darkness.

Lucas and Me

For years, the subtle presence of father's fourth great-uncle Dornblaser has clung to life within my spirit. From the childhood moment I sat at my mother's feet looking at the book she'd handed me as she worked at her desk, to the current constant gnawing anxiety in my stomach as I sought to uncover the real account of the story I'd read back then (for which there is no lengthy record), I have been haunted by that book. It revealed the story of Lucas Dornblaser and his dismal demise from dysentery at Auschwitz. You have just read his account of what happened, not from any book but from his spirit to mine.

My mother was a wife and a homemaker, but also a genealogist. It was her passion (among many). The perfect fit for the life she and my father had created—a life that revolved around him. One day, as she sat at her desk in the little formal dining room off the kitchen, she sat in awe of something she'd found while tracing the ancestral roots of my father. It was a book that chronicled the many stories from Auschwitz, or World War II in general—I'm not sure exactly. What I do know is the book she handed me, and the paragraph she pointed to, told the story of a man she believed to be the fourth great-uncle of my father.

The words of that seemingly harmless paragraph left an imprint on me and crystallized the one that already existed in my soul. Together, they forged the way I expressed myself in my life in many ways. Not because I was young and impressionable, no. Children are less suggestible then you'd think: they'll receive the energy that their soul already supports.

As the book conveyed, Lucas died a painful death in a concrete basement in Auschwitz in 1942. However, there was no factual accounting of who he was or how he got there. So, for the many months of writing this book, I sought to call down the anecdote of his life from the source.

As an empath, I experience life by allowing the spirit of a person, an event, or an emotion to move through me until I have a complete understanding of every detail I need for the story to make sense. Every day, I gleaned the images of his life: calling on him to speak his truth, anticipating my ancestors to come forth, and waiting for his spiritual guides to offer a morsel of his evolution that could connect the two of us. And every day: nothing. It was a grey blank screen. I began to feel fearful. A little constant anxiety of a pending failure surrounded me. My world was a little darker. My mind became blank and my heart had a shade of apathy I didn't recognize. The once beautiful red roses I'd cut from the garden had slumped and died, and I hadn't noticed.

A trifecta of depression had taken over: weariness, fear, and apathy. This was all that was left of the once creative desire to give voice to an ancestor who deserved his dignity revealed—who deserved to have his story told.

"Why wasn't he speaking to me?!"

I felt so impotent and frustrated. But, as with anything, often the very thing we're looking for is already right in front of us. Finally, it occurred to me that those were the images of his life—at least the ones he could remember. I was experiencing his trauma: the feelings of powerlessness, darkness, and apathy that came from his amnesia.

I reflected back on what I'd been asking: who was he? And as it turned out—*he didn't remember*. It took an enormous amount of time and focus, speaking with him on the subtle levels, bringing his soul out of the darkness. Until, finally, a dream...

> Our beliefs are the inner path to discovering our character, ultimately connecting us to our common spirit.

Welcome Home

Yom HaShoah: Holocaust Remembrance Day

On May 2nd, Yom HaShoah, I was given a dream. The six-million-plus humans who were murdered in the Holocaust are back. They've reincarnated—members of the new global-tribe—here to reawaken hope for the weary.

The Dream:

The doorbell rang. I felt an enormous delight as I approached the large sky-blue glossy-painted wood door to the vast antebellum home I appeared to live in. I looked through the peephole. (Evidently, I still needed security in my dream.) There were endless groupings of people streaming onto the wrap-around porch of this ample home. They were every size, shape, ethnicity, and culture. You couldn't see their religion, or their sexual orientation, or notice even their gender for that matter.

Some were carrying plates, bowls, trays, pots, and casserole dishes full of food. There was a spiritual richness—a wisdom—emanating from this crowd. I could feel authentic character reverberating from each of them. I anticipated an experience akin to sitting for tea with Dorothy Parker at the Algonquin Round Table or conversing with Harriett Tubman under a shady oak. The folk in my dream all brought something, whether or not it was immediately obvious to the eye. Everyone was dressed in colorful, casual elegance, genuinely happy to see one another as if it were just another Thursday night. I think I was the only one new to the party.

Some of them I knew, others I did not; regardless, my heart pounded out such joy as I embraced each of them. And then there was Father's fourth great-uncle Dornblaser, adorned in a fresh linen suit with a straw fedora (classic, yet contemporary). He looked so young, beautiful, glowing—standing with his arms outstretched. I lost my breath.

Next thing I know, I'm walking back into the house, leaving the front door open, and heading towards the kitchen. It was filled with people laughing and chatting while they were preparing and cooking the food. I continued on to the dining room where the long rectangular table was beautifully set with crystal and hints of gold. It appeared to have no end.

As I gazed out over the crowd, every face was unique. They brought a tradition of love, a culture of kindness, and a defiant peace. And it's what I became filled with in their presence: the human values that connected them to one another. Their spirits carried a voracious dignity. They embodied an integrity of knowing the formidable price claiming a title carries. They had gained the understanding that our beliefs are the inner path to discovering our character, ultimately connecting us to our common spirit.

Most of all, their spiritual heritage had shown them that hate was nothing but a faulty alarm system—eventually costing everything. It signals you to what you fear or despise in yourself, not others. Hate is the enmity that keeps you in a low place—vulnerable to the voices that would have you believe this hate is righteous, necessary, and powerful. It deceives you and hides from you the very casualty of wartime weariness—equality. Finally, in the end, hate combined with delusional fantasy, narcissism, and spiritual evil propels a human to do unspeakable things.

Yes, these slayers have reincarnated throughout the decades, but in force (especially now) to recapitulate what may have been overlooked before—so history will not repeat. This time of cataclysmic politics, earthly changes, and humanitarian confusion is both powerful and life affirming for those who will accept the challenge of digging deep to unravel and heal their own self-contempt.

Endless Ripples in Time

The truth is my father's fourth great-uncle had been with me the whole time, telling me his story through the only images he had to offer: the subtle faint impressions left from his amnesia, and the emotional essence of all the ways he'd been led to such a fate.

One of the elements alive in the karmic spiritual patterns of genocide, but often diminished in the collective emotional memory of the subsequent decades following war and tragedy, are the subtleties and seemingly minor decisions made by those alive at the time. It is the collective effects of those minor decisions that create cultural agreements. For example, an individual's decision not to respond to societal issues because they don't appear to affect the individual directly—this creates an unspoken cultural agreement.

You see, he'd been speaking to me about what it feels like to trivialize each right as it is slowly being taken away. He was too tired and fearful to make a stir. The world outside him appeared normal enough, or at least he grew used to the effects of each mental, emotional, or spiritual assault by the governing body until he no longer remembered what it was like before. He put out of his mind what he saw happening to others, until it was happening to him. Circumstances never seem nearly as important or life threatening until they're happening to you; that is how he got there.

Understanding karma means being able to recognize the multiple ripples an event sends out through time and space, and how each of those layers affect each generation, based on their specific vantage point to it. For example, there are several lenses through which we are born into a relationship to a previous tragedy. Here are a few of the current soul groups and the unique vantage from which they process an event like the Holocaust:

- The current living survivors
- The people left to address the geographical space where the event took place and the energy it holds
- The friends and family who have experienced a direct loss from the tragedy
- People who have experienced an indirect loss from the event, i.e., the shame, grief, guilt, anger, depression, fear, anxiety, and dismay that is created in the collective culture as they relate to the event
- Those who have reincarnated with the spiritual memory of the event
- Those in subsequent generations who learn of the event through history books or another person's viewpoint

When speaking of the Holocaust, no matter the position from which you look, there is a subtle yet deeply abiding impact in ways that may appear rational and some that may not. For me, as you will read in the upcoming pages, the direct ancestral-spiritual impact of this event was the foundation of my relationship to food, nutrition, and health. I was constantly monitoring and focusing on how much I had or how much I needed—on every level. May the following pages trigger and reveal your own spiritual patterns regarding food and money, as well as the self-knowledge and acceptance inherently attached and exposed as the unraveling begins.

"AMORAL LEADERS HAVE A WAY OF REVEALING THE CHARACTER OF THOSE AROUND THEM... MR. TRUMP EATS YOUR SOUL IN SMALL BITES."[1]

– JAMES COMEY

Part 1 - Plenty

The Slayer's Path: The Practice of Remembering, Learning, and Having

Uncovering your soul's innate blueprint, discovering new ways of managing or changing those unconscious habits, and making peace with what you have—are powerful challenges. Having a lot is often complicated, having too little can be disheartening, and having just enough makes you wonder if you need more. Cultivating balance is a lifelong pursuit and is dependent on the spiritual imprints of your soul, your subconscious relationship to food and money, and how well you manage the most basic elements of all you possess.

A slayer must:

- Develop self-awareness of their personal and cultural spiritual imprints (or karma)—the practice of remembering the vital elements of the mental, emotional, and physical conditioning and ideology with which they are born, and grieving or celebrating the truth about it.
- Become adept at learning the process of receiving new information that challenges their beliefs.
- Have the processes established to manage emotion, knowledge, and the physical world—all in a balanced way.

Essentially, our spiritual and often unconscious relationship to food and money are the two things that become the foundation of all other connections we will make in our life. Especially if we have *more than*, or *not enough*. For those who find their porridge *just right*—they can celebrate their good fortune with gratitude for the opportunity to experience the foundation of prosperity and build from there.

Auschwitz: It Is Safe to Remember

"Endlösung der Judenfrage" was the Nazi plan to murder Jews living in the territories occupied by the Third Reich. Translated it means: Final Solution to the Jewish Question. You might ask: *It may be safe to remember everything that happened, but why would I want to?* Within the very fabric of your spirit is the essence of every cultural trauma that has occurred—not just the ones connected to your specific heritage but all of them—as they continue to exist today in some way, shape, or form.

We keep the energy of those events woven in our spiritual memory in many ways: via our past-life or soul history, by the energetic imprints in the environment, or through the experiences and beliefs of others that are spoken over us like paint poured on a canvas. They are kept in motion for a few reasons: first, so we don't commit those tragedies again; second, because the people who lived through it in one generation now grieve their pain through us; and third, spiritual pain has a cumulative effect—it is a powerful teacher.

The continual change of perspective leads to an upgrade in ideas that brings about a release of grief and pain until they are definitively transformed into a completely new energetic vibration. We are not free of the memory, but we are imbued with the wisdom to understand and transform what caused the trauma in the first place. This renders the memory powerless.

Remembering means taking an honest look at the cultural climate that cleared the way for such barbaric human behavior. The only way to truly understand what we consider evil from our viewpoint today is to bear witness to it without hate, anger, or fear—in peace—opening your heart to where others went astray. When you break it down to the very slim foundations of any deafening cultural assault, you can always find the illusion of scarcity at its origins—the deep tendrils of lack that inspire in a few vacant souls: gluttony, power mongering, and greed.

The purpose of resurrecting the memory of instances of cultural genocide is to grieve the specific pain left in the collective emotional body of all those affected, to offer perspective, and to release the emotions attached to the response that was given or denied. Finally, we remember to create a moratorium in similar present day behavior. Karma means understanding the journey leading up to an event, the processing of all the elements of emotional expression caused by the event, and then applying that new conscientiousness to your choices today.

Overcoming Scarcity

Forgiveness is a way of life. It is a perspective that allows for bitterness to seep into the ground and become useful for the seeds of inclusivity to grow. It is important to begin by using your deeply held beliefs to uncover and reveal the Truth. *Your truth leads to the Truth*—the convictions we hold that are true for us and become the basis of our separation from others. Ultimately, they make way to what universally connects us and includes everyone.

We all carry a bit of social bias and bigotry. And all bias is anchored in scarcity in some way: what you can't have, what you don't have, what others are keeping from you—anything you believe implies there just isn't enough for you. Now is a good opportunity to admit these subtle or obvious beliefs exist. Explore what they are. Recognize them. Find out why they live in you—then grieve.

Cry, explain, and wonder your way to forgiveness—giving compassion to yourself and your ancient broken heart—through letting go. The first step to overcoming scarcity is to evaluate your relationship to food and money.

War Equals Money

As long as there have been humans on Earth, there have been wars. Albeit, in simpler times there were simpler skirmishes, but conflict is always about the search for a better life or protecting life itself. In less populated centuries, battles were initiated over land and food, human and geographical resources, and then opportunity and commerce. But ultimately, wars have been—and still are—instigated over the illusion of ownership and money. No matter the wartime facade (whether it be freedom, independence, anger, entitlement, retaliation, or human rights), war equals money.

Spiritually speaking, after the mask is lifted from the wartime machine meant to garner forces and generate the flow of cash to the few who benefit from it, what is left for decades to come? What is left are the waves of breaking down and building back up of the human condition on all levels. The mental, emotional, physical, and spiritual effects of war will endure for lifetimes and are imbedded in our culture today. If you look deeply, you will see the subtle reverberations of war-based scarcity impacting your current relationship to money, with very few degrees of separation if any.

Food Equals Life

Yes, this is the general rule. However, it may not be the truth for some: there are accounts and scientifically noted claims of yogis abstaining from food and water for up to 70 years[2], hunger strikes for over 70 days, and a man addressing his obesity by fasting for over a year to lose more than half his body weight. I, myself, have gone over four months without solid food. The truth about food and water, for each individual, is where they put their attention and belief.

When you focus on the spiritual elements of yourself, your world opens up to another level of need and self-awareness. This allows for a wider array of opportunities that meet all your needs. Whereas, when you focus on your physical experience, you become centered on fulfilling all your needs through your body—which isn't possible.

Your Relationship with Food

Your relationship with food isn't only your connection to the multiple kinds of foods, recipes, and meals you will traverse in a lifetime, but it speaks to the very essence of how you relate to your ability to have sustenance, nurturing, safety, and life.

I have always had a fairly common relationship with food; that is, I've always needed to have a little extra of everything, just in case. Emptiness was akin to vulnerability, in my mind. I've never hoarded, per se. I just wanted to be sure I wouldn't run out of anything—certain household goods, for example. When shopping for toilet paper, I'd buy 36 rolls even though there was only room for six. I'd buy 12 cans of tuna, just in case of an unexpected event. Other canned goods would sit in my cabinets for years, never to be eaten.

Food is a type of currency, but it is also a lens by which we see all other currencies in our lives. The way we handle money, the way we process love, the way we feel secure—all are a result of our original relationship to food. It is also how we gage whether there is enough for us in all our relationships, and the value of our ability to receive all that we want or need.

Understanding how we value currency, then, is the obstacle each of us must resolve within ourselves in order to survive. Ultimately, we must match the magnificent, regenerative, restorative abilities of the physical body with the limitlessness of our spiritual connection to light. When you open and expand your understanding of how you relate to food, a whole new world of receiving opens-up—all the way to the cellular level.

When your body becomes fluid, any stagnation or *dis-ease* that exists becomes obvious. What else becomes obvious are the finer patterns of where the stagnation began. On every level—mentally, emotionally, spiritually—you will see the thoughts and events that formed the energy of that broken leg when you were five, or that cancer you are fighting so hard to overcome. You'll be able to see and understand why things happened the way they did and what you gained from them, giving you the ability to release yourself from the spiritual trauma left behind. This will allow you to view yourself, and all of your encounters, in a way that most serves you today.

That's not to imply that any suffering we experience doesn't serve us and that we shouldn't choose it, it's exactly the opposite. Suffering is an opportunity for us to be clear about what we're doing and why we're doing it—to see the historic patterns, understand them, and embrace the entirety of the experience.

A little refresher from the previous Demon Slayer's Handbook volumes: grieving for ten minutes or more actually changes the neurons in the brain, essentially transforming the information being grieved, and leaving room to repopulate the brain with a new concept, idea, or reality. Grieving allows us to recognize the shadow (or unknown parts of ourselves). It is the real honey in the hive—the rich karmic patterns that sustain us through time and space.

We rediscover each recurring spiritual design of our soul and its purpose, knowing we can be released to another vibration of patterns that deeply express and transform all we are capable of. This, in turn, leads us to an inexhaustible sense of self-dignity and a more genuine compassion for others far and wide—from all who reside on this planet to galaxies across our solar system.

The Relationship Between Grief and Food

The indelible connection between food and grief is powerful. People naturally attempt to over feed or starve the grief they feel instead of expressing it. Our desire to eat comes from signals sent from the amygdala, the primal emotional center of the body found in the brain. These emotions also are responsible for interpreting our level of safety. When someone is feeling unsafe, regardless of the threat—physical, mental, emotional, or spiritual—they will seek to counter that lack of safety.

Those of us who have a deeper awareness of (or more exposure to) the subtle vibrations that connect us to the feelings and psychic terrain of others will often receive those psychic signals as an unconscious threat, from which they must protect themselves. The actual threat is the taking on of others' emotions that consolidate our own into an impending wave of grief that is at best uncomfortable, and at worst, overwhelming. The real antidote to this psychic threat is grief; regardless, depending on how one feels about it, eating can create a false sense of comfort.

It's common for anyone who has deep empathy or is in the helping business, or who has experienced abuse and been victimized in some way, to use food as a tool of comfort in times of stress. Any extra pounds the body carries serves as a layer of protection to the intuitive frequencies around us. In my experience, it doesn't work for long and puts off the inevitable grief for another time—or even a different lifetime.

Cinnamon's Story

One such account is that of a longtime client I met over a decade ago. For the purpose of this book and anonymity's sake, I asked her what her pseudonym should be.

"I've always wanted to be named Cinnamon," she replied.

It made perfect sense: she's spicy and sweet and leaves a lasting impact anywhere she goes. I'd like to share with you Cinnamon's story.

Cinnamon spent her life feeling too big for the world. By kindergarten she was the largest, tallest kid on the playground, even amongst the boys. The youngest of five children, and as a member of an ultra-thin family (rail thin by her memory), she always felt different. With the sudden loss of her father at the age of two, tragically, this young family was left in emotional ruins. Her mother confessed many years later that Cinnamon would sit and watch her cry way too often, and that always, her daughter's response was to say that she would make it better. Cinnamon became the empath of the family, taking on the grief, anger, and frustration from which the other family members found it easier to look away.

As a teen, and on into adulthood, she became an emotional eater. Like a binge drinker, it soothed and quieted the demons inside—for a time. As her weight exploded and health deteriorated, an overwhelming feeling of hopelessness took root. There was no way out—no way to lose the more than 100 pounds needed to come off in order to assuage her many anxieties and physical issues. She told me she would've sold her soul to lose that weight. Deep inside there was a constant desire to be happier and to find some peace. Soon, she began therapy with an eating disorder specialist. She had some success, but not the relief she needed.

"By the time I met Tracee I was on a path to heal," she reported, "but still searching for what I knew was missing: the piece that would fill that deeply lingering void. Our first session surprised and startled me—I was astonished that my soul was so willing and eager to help me."

I remember meeting Cinnamon for the first time. She was majestically stunning, with a hero's laugh. We were in the heart of the Bible Belt. I had a lot of respect for all my clients who had the courage to step forward, addressing their deep-seated spiritual patterns and the entities they carried, outside of a religious context. It's one thing to face the scary, hidden parts of yourself and another to do it while moving against the cultural norm of your family and friends.

As Cinnamon and I began to dig into her relationship to eating, it became clear that her connection to the extra weight wasn't related to food. It was connected to her desire to ground the additional emotional energy she took on from everyone in her environment. Not only did she receive energy from those she knew and loved, she was also a magnet for other spiritual entities. She recalled the following experience from one of our sessions.

"I remember sitting with Tracee; I think it was our second session. She had spoken of the difference between ghosts and other entities in our first session. In fact, I think I originally went to see her about my haunted century-old house. We were talking about my body consciousness, and she asked if I was happy with myself. I said, in general, I was, but that I'd been frustrated that my new weight loss program was not progressing at all. Tracee suggested that we try an intuitive exercise and asked me to close my eyes."

I guided Cinnamon's attention to the place in her body that was holding her resistance to losing weight. She immediately identified her belly. When I asked her to acknowledge the energy in that area, she laughed out loud and said, "They told me to fuck-off."

"Oh, I see. How many critters are there?"

Cinnamon laughed again and said, "Too many to count: a horde. A horde?! Terrifying!"

This time we both laughed uproariously. It's common, during a shamanic healing, to have an experience you can't possibly imagine having until you have it—and often, laughter is the best response. Once the guffaws subsided, we went through a visualization process to remove the spiritual energies from her body, and she immediately felt the energy shift. We visually filled that hidden space with the energy of hope and a golden-yellow light.

Later she recalled:

"It was profound. It gave me the emotional expansion I needed to accept myself fully and for my soul to heal. A new space opened up in me that was filled with hope and peace. After that, I made the decision to have weight loss surgery and have lost 135 pounds. The surgery itself was just a tool, a tool that I am able to use to this day—exactly four years later. I don't believe it would have worked if I'd not rid myself of those spiritual entities, which I affectionately call *The Horde.*"

Releasing the horde of entities allowed Cinnamon's energy to shift completely and to change her resonance—no longer feeling an obligation to take on the grief and pain of others. It was just the lift she needed to change and sustain her detrimental relationship to food to one based on actually feeding her body the nutrients it needed to remain in balance. Cinnamon has since opened her own art studio and has dedicated her life to creating art that helps others expand their perspectives on life.

> A little refresher from the previous Demon Slayer's Handbook volumes: grieving for ten minutes or more actually changes the neurons in the brain, essentially transforming the information being grieved, and leaving room to repopulate the brain with a new concept, idea, or reality.

Food Intake and Output: A Child's First Opportunity to Control

If you've ever spent time around a willful child, it's common for food to become a negotiation tactic to get them to follow instructions or behave. Essentially, a child's first ability to control themselves or others is to refuse or embrace food, and at times, dictate at what point they release waste by peeing during a temper tantrum—ramping up the emphasis on their willpower.

Not for nothing, but your irritating little human is beginning the art of self-mastery. The most profound job of a parent is to define and enforce boundaries under all circumstances, and when it comes to food, naturally, their habits can easily become the habits of their children. Every morning my father would drink a six-ounce glass of orange juice and raise his pinky finger as he drank it. These days, I don't drink juice too often. When I do, it brings pleasant feelings—and you can bet I'm flying that pinky every time without thought.

The first five years of life can reveal a child's spiritual predisposition towards food (their food karma) and can inevitably dictate their eating behaviors and patterns in conjunction with cultural traditions, familial beliefs, and food availability. The combination of these factors and a child's rapid growth ultimately builds their connection to their physical bodies, sense of safety, environmental mastery, and self-control.

It's been proven that we eat for multiple reasons other than being hungry; in fact, we may feel hungry when we are sad, thirsty, anxious, bored, or dealing with any other conditioned response we have connected to a snack. If we were children who were rewarded with food in our early development, it can be expected that we will reward ourselves with food as adults. So, how do we go about recognizing the mental, emotional, and spiritual connection to the what, why, and when of our eating dynamic?

Take a moment now, to jot down some notes on your childhood experience with food to include in the ritual at the end of the chapter.

Self-Loathing and Food

In American culture today, we make great strides to honor all shapes and sizes, but the focus is still superficial. The fact that someone is or isn't overweight is not the issue. The issue is the individual's relationship to food and their behavioral eating dynamic. The spiritual root of the way we acknowledge our physical body is understood through the concept of self-loathing.

Human beings take in millions of pieces of information at all times. The goal is to access, metabolize, and interpret as much of that information as we need, based on our evolution. Imagine for a moment you are your bodiless soul, floating around the universe free and unencumbered by physical matter; your vision, awareness, and feelings—as they are today—are all intact. The only things missing are the physical responses to those feelings.

Now imagine being injected into a little infant body—a little fatty blob of flesh generated for you by your parents—no access to the soul memory of who you are. Feel the brief moment of devastation the spirit feels entrapped by that body's inability to express the spirit's vast information and experience. That is self-loathing.

In this context, self-loathing is the initial lens by which we perceive all the ways we relate to our physical needs, getting them met, and often the way we make efforts to interpret, ground, or ignore our emotions. It's important as you contemplate self-loathing to be mindful of the true meaning of its presence. All those things you don't like about yourself or others are the hidden, powerful aspects of your spiritual and emotional knowledge. Once uncovered, they will reveal your unique skillsets in life. Start by taking a moment to review your connection between emotions and food.

How many times have you used food as a bridge to:
- Celebration?
- Comfort?
- Boredom?
- Distraction?
- Quelling anxiety or grief?
- Making friends?
- Contemplating a decision?

These are only some examples. There may be others that come to mind for you.

Rejection: The Beginning of Self-Mastery

We all have a baseline of rejection—how we are conditioned to receive it and use it. Whether we are rejecting ourselves or others, things or ideas, food flavors or consistencies—it is a pathway to meeting our own needs. In this life, it begins with the body's processing of food.

If you eat something that isn't right for you, your body will reject it in some way, shape, or form. Whether a subtle or obvious response, your body's intelligence knows what is right for you at any given time during your life cycle and its changing needs. Learning to listen to your inner voice and your subtle physical responses—outside of any fear-based conditioning—is the key. As a child, I would break out in hives any time I ate a tomato product. My memory of this faded, but my antipathy toward them remained. It wasn't until the last decade I started to question why I disliked tomatoes. My sister, in a conversation, revealed to me that in my early years I had an allergy to them—the experience of which I had no memory. I decided to give tomatoes a go again, and to my surprise, I enjoyed the taste and no longer broke out in hives.

Physical and emotional pain or irritation is the first obvious physical response to something that doesn't serve us. But before pain comes, there are the subtle impulses of rejection. The glimmering thoughts of *I don't like that* or *I don't want that* are the initial messages often drummed out of our realm of authority early on in life. This happens when a parent insists their child eat the brussels sprouts or drink the milk, in spite of their objection. This can be based on anything from socio-economic status, as we learn to like what we can afford, to a controlling, fearful, or delusional parent. A person can only educate another with what they have or know—the best or worst of their experiences.

We had several rules at the dinner table in my family: dinner was served every night at 5:30 sharp, no elbows on the table (or you'd squish the invisible fairies), and you had to eat all the food you served yourself. One of the most potent memories I have of childhood dinnertime was chatting while passing around the food dishes, as we each served ourselves a portion from each bowl. Not paying attention, I served myself a half plate of lima beans—my most despised food. You can imagine the response of horror I had when remembering the finish-everything-on-your-plate rule while looking at my nearly full plate of limas. I burst into tears and begged to put them back. For a five-year-old, it was pure terror.

Even though my mother compromised and let me return half the limas, it took dressing them with a quarter stick of butter to get them down. In spite of it all, I occasionally enjoy them today. I do believe, however, it was the beginning of my love affair with butter.

Today, as I sit down at the table for a relaxing meal and nonchalantly plant my elbows on the table, my body reels back with a brief pang of guilt for the possible murder of my beloved fairies. And then I think: *fairies can't die that way!*

Your Relationship with Money

The connections we make between food and money are indelibly linked. Often, the food options and habits you have are a direct result of your access to money. Money affects everything from what you eat, when you eat it, and how much of it you waste. If money has been free-flowing in your life, then you are more apt to have a relaxed physical connection with food. It most likely has always been available to you anytime you wanted it. Conversely, if at any point you have genuinely hungered for a meal, you are more likely than not to focus on every meal that comes your way.

Similarly, learning to have money is just as much of an acquired skill as learning how to go without. Our karmic, familial, cultural, and experiential beliefs—for a time—dictate how we feel about and use money. The illusion of my solidly middle-class upbringing immediately hollowed out with the death of my father. Although we had practically paid off our nice house in a stable neighborhood, it was only because of my mother's ability to fiercely wield a budget that the bills were settled every month. We went from eating many fresh foods to more canned options, and we used dry milk to supplement the whole milk we had been used to drinking.

Interestingly, my older sister remembers using powdered milk before my father passed, as a lower fat option. My direct memory is starting the dried milk after my father died, as a money saving option. Both of those memories could have some truth to them. But importantly, they reveal the underlying, differing spiritual relationship to having enough that was unique to each of us.

It is these subtle perceptions that make us individuals. Distinct in our special combination of imprints, we hold different truths based on our perspective and experiences. Those subtle personal truths will lead us to the overarching spiritual Truth we all have in common. It is these subtle personal beliefs that garner our social biases, not only dictating our relationship to ourselves but also our relationship to others.

Today, there is no situation where we don't need the influence or connection of another to access food or money. Think about that, everything we do, on some level, includes others; understanding this will help make clear to you your foundational relationship to food and money. This comprises any inherent conflicts or solutions you hold on any level: mentally, emotionally, physically, spiritually, or etherically (the etheric body is the first layer of the energy body that governs physical habits). Go forth, reassured that anything you learn—good, bad, or indifferent—is certainly better known as opposed to hidden. What is within our conscious perspective, we are empowered to choose or change.

The Warrior's Hidden Motto: Need Less

The warrior's path is always one of conflict and struggle. A warrior seeks out conflict in order to find its path to resolution. Once resolved, he will move on to the next conflict. The warrior's hidden motto is the underlying belief or emotion that drives their mission. When we are struggling with the dynamic of having enough or more than we require, we must overcome the sneaky fear of being a burden to others. I've heard at least a thousand people in my career negotiate prosperity by trying to need less, so that their needs don't impact others. Counter-intuitive as it may seem, we tend to draw back, diminish ourselves, or reduce our needs in times of conflict.

Unfortunately, one cannot create more by needing less. We create more, first, by needing more. When you set your lowest common denominator of expectation to meet your needs, you eventually will create a life that meets all your requirements. Prosperity is born by surpassing your necessities and setting your sights on fulfilling your desires, contentment, love, and happiness. As you make the shift from the physical realm to your emotional wellness, your physical stability, wealth, and health will follow suit.

The Slayer's Dilemma: How Much is Enough?

Imagine your whole life you've gone without. There's not been much, and what you had, you had to share with others. One day, you are brought to a remote island with a cave deep in its volcanic matrix. The door to the cave is opened for you. In it is everything you've ever wanted, whether it's gold and jewels (riches beyond your comprehension), a banquet of food that replenishes itself, a group of people to love and serve you, or time to do, see, and express all that you are effortlessly.

The slayer's fear is that he will be escorted out as quickly as he was brought in, or that soon after her arrival, the many people with whom she must share will appear. Because, how do you believe in enough when there has never been enough? As we learned from Cinnamon's story, her life turned around the minute she made the decision to put herself first. Her prosperity gained traction the moment she gave herself permission to be the artist she'd always been but had been afraid to reveal to others. Now she makes a living through her art studio and gallery, and her entire family thrives. Once you acknowledge your fear and allow yourself to learn a new way of life, you will find ways to receive and manage more of everything.

"Pain is the breaking of the shell that encloses your understanding."[3]

– Kahlil Gibran

Complaining: Valuable Waste of Time

Complaining is a lazy way to avoid asking for what you want. When we complain, it is our intellectual way of accessing the pain, frustration, disappointment, or trauma that we are dealing with regarding the topic of our grievance. Unfortunately, if your protestation continues on into days and weeks, the next order of business is most likely grief. Emotionally releasing what bothers you first, allows for your objection to lead to a conceptual resolution of the problem. It frees you up to go to work on it, ultimately finding a way to figure out and then communicate what you want.

Remembering Your Karma

Becoming aware of your silent karmic patterns isn't as difficult as you'd think. But there are two things required: a deep desire to know the truth, and a complete willingness to be honest with yourself every step of the way. The spiritual patterns that govern your decisions are like a next-door neighbor, in that they've been there as long as you can remember. You may never speak, but you recognize the pattern of their footsteps or the jingle of their keys as they make their way to the front door.

You must now become aware of your own personal self-talk about food and money. Often, we can look at the things we are surrounded by to give us an indication of the beliefs we may be secretly harboring. One of the ways we do this is by paying attention to the biases we hold about others.

Take a few moments to contemplate what those biases are. Start with politics, weight, religion, healthcare, fashion, or immigration. No matter where you stand on the issues, there's a hotbed of information about you and your relationship to food and money that's dying to, unashamedly, spill out. But this time, instead of focusing on what others are doing, ask yourself:

What am I doing to help myself? What am I afraid of? Why? Remember, the point of this game is complete honesty—no judgment—just the opportunity to investigate the current beliefs and feelings you have.

The Slayer's Motto: I Create My Reality

We are always emboldened to create our own reality, even when it feels as if our destiny is set in stone. Believing our success is controlled by others or an outside force, and then overcoming it, is a stop on the path to prosperity. Its true lesson is teaching that we never really do anything by ourselves—even when we are independent. Our lives are made up of a series of things we are given and those we purchase, both connecting us to others. If we grow our own food, where did the original seed come from? In order for you to create the reality you want for yourself, you must get on board with collaborating with others for your success.

Doing that requires two things: letting go of money or resources being an obstacle to your fortune and accepting that your true collaborator is the Creator and Universe. Your intention and choices drive your spiritual energy to send signals to the collective energy source, informing it of what or who to send to you to amass what is necessary in achieving the result you're expecting.

Yes, the result you expect. The reality you have is based on the way you perceive your circumstances. The karmic connection governs the circumstances you are born into and the patterns you recreate over and over—until you don't. Whatever the state of your affairs, what's valuable is whether or not you perceive you are empowered within them.

Scott's Story

Many years ago, I counseled a man whose business was failing. It had been in the family for decades and survived three generations. Since his early twenties, the trade had been very successful, but at the point we met, every day was a struggle. He was thousands of dollars in debt and behind in payments. Not only that, the work had lost its luster for him. Every week we spoke of what his life might be like doing something else, and every week he was sure things were going to turn around.

It wasn't until he was about to lose the house and his wife threatened to leave that he was willing to have an honest conversation about what came next. The resistance he had at considering closing the door on this way of life didn't match what he had to lose. Of course, there were feelings of failure, disappointment, and grief at letting down everyone in his family who'd worked so hard to build the entity that had sustained them all. Still, there was something else that was blocking him from letting go.

I decided to take him on a shamanic journey to meet face to face the obstacle that was holding him back. We called on the spirit guides that would join him in the endeavor, and at first sight, he burst into tears. It was his father who had passed several years back. He was overwhelmed at the idea his father wasn't angry with him for losing the business. In fact, the first thing his father said was:

"Son, that business is no longer necessary for everyone; that's why it's not doing well. It's not your fault. It was the trade of my father and his father, not yours. I am grateful you held on to it until I could let go, but now it's your time to find what suits you and your generation. Do something you enjoy and maybe something that serves others."

As he quieted himself from this completely unexpected message, we continued our visualization and walked through the door to meet what was truly holding him back. As he passed through, he absolutely fell into his grief, crying uncontrollably. Encouraging him to continue crying until there was nothing left, I waited. It was about twenty minutes later when we spoke.

I asked, "Who's in the room waiting for you?"

He said, "It's the man I killed."

Many years prior, he had been in a car accident and had hit a man on a bicycle. His name was Aaron. He did his best to help Aaron until the ambulance arrived, but the biker died on arrival to the hospital. Although the police deemed it an accident, Scott never forgave himself. Some years after the accident, he met with the family, and they offered their forgiveness; still, he couldn't forgive himself. He couldn't tolerate receiving compassion from everyone around him, so he began, in many ways, to punish himself. He pulled away from his wife, stopped spending time with friends, and began spending all his time at the business—which, despite all of his attention, was slowly losing steam.

Scott continued: "Aaron is telling me I have to forgive him. He says he's happy, and that it was his time. I don't understand. He wants me to know that he'd known of his pending death. Somehow he'd known, and he was at peace with it. He's asking *me* to forgive *him*!" Scott cried, covering his face with his hands.

"Scott," I said, "I think he's asking you to let him go."

About a week later, Scott announced the liquidation of his business. For the final month, he decorated a wall with photos of every family member and person who'd contributed to its life—including Aaron. He figured, without Aaron the business would have diminished years before. Shortly after the liquidation was done, he learned how to install solar panels and got on a crew with a local company that was rapidly expanding. Today, he's a project manager. His family is happy. And most of all, Scott is at ease with himself and his life.

Addiction is Karma: Targeting Your Addiction at Its Core

Addiction is your longtime not-so-friendly companion. If you're going to win the war, you've got to know your enemy. Right? It's the most common approach people take when battling their dependency. But what happens when your problem is your friend?

Addictive patterns exist on every level of human experience: behavioral, physiological, emotional, and spiritual. That's why the suffering and disappointment continue even after the substance has been overcome. You can be addicted to work, a feeling, a behavior, or the attachment to an event—not just a substance, an action, or an activity.

So how do you address your recurring spiritual patterns that anchor your addictive choices—the ungrieved traumas from lives or centuries past—the ones you've lived with since birth? The first step is to recognize that the repetitive patterns you experience, at one time, had great purpose.

They were your champions, companions, and friends. They served you and even saved you from continuing harm. They are the revered elders of your soul's tribe, whose mission is to carry forward your power and spiritual history for generations to come. Doesn't that sound like something that deserves your respect?

Everything we do has purpose. The point at which we are ready to transition from the thought, emotion, or behavior of our once righteous, now outdated and inappropriate great warrior, is the moment we must take stock of his accomplishments. Through research and consideration, we must either give her a new job or our unfettered gratitude and retirement.

When it comes to our addictions, we must look for their place of origin. We have the power, knowledge, discipline, and love to transmute and transition all of them—at the time of our choosing.

The Karma of Eating Disorders

Many people suffer from deep-seated eating disorders like anorexia and bulimia. An eating disorder on the spiritual patterning level often has nothing to do with food and more to do with life, death, and control. I've worked with many clients who suffer with lifelong addictive patterns. Often, included in their spiritual imprints, is the soul memory of a death at the hands of another. Entering into the new life with spiritual memory of loss and death, manifests in the current incarnation as self-controlling behaviors.

One such client who recalled a past life memory of being gassed at Auschwitz-Birkenau had come into this life with the compulsion to help others in a holistic way. As a young man he suffered from anorexia. This peaked in his second year of college, weighing approximately 130 pounds with his 6'2" frame. Soon, he learned through therapy that he needed to replace the impulse to control his life through his eating dynamic with another eating habit that didn't threaten his existence. Embarking on a holistic path, he chose a vegan diet, worked as a colon hydro-therapist, and has devoted every day since college to helping others. He supports them in understanding and retraining their relationships to their bodies, eating patterns, and digestion.

Even so, he suffered greatly from nightmares, fear, and an irrational anger at having to waste so much time on food. The horrors of one of his nightmares led him to me. During our session, we regressed him back to the karmic point of origin of his conflict with food. As it turned out, the issue wasn't about food at all. The prevailing memory was the moment his frail body collapsed in the gas chamber of Birkenau.

After the past life imprint-recall, he grieved for seven days. He didn't work. He didn't see anyone. He stayed, for the most part, in bed and mourned. Today, he's now chosen the Flexitarian diet (occasionally adding meat or fish to a predominantly plant-based diet), still runs his holistic care business, and is in a satisfying relationship. These are things he believed he could never have while constantly under assault from his nightmares.

The Slayer's Pact: The Choices I Make are an Extension of My Power

A slayer must eventually accept their choices are theirs alone. No matter the inspiration or influence, a slayer knows that she is the one accountable for her actions. There comes a time in any situation or condition that we no longer want to continue—where we decide that things can be different. Once we've made that decision, the Creator can conspire with the Universe on our behalf to show us a new path forward.

Communication Takes Practice

The place to start is to accept exactly where you are: your feelings, your physical condition, your environment, and your beliefs. Next, if you're ready, state fully and completely what you want. What will be the end result of the change? It's almost impossible for anyone to give us what we need if we are unable to ask directly for it. Consider that communicating your needs and desires takes practice, even ones that are simple common sense.

When I was eighteen, I moved to New York City. After two weeks I landed a job as the cashier at Tom's Diner on 113th and Broadway. *Pete the Greek* was the boss. (That's what everyone called him.) Pete was thirty-six years old, about 6'2", and—of course—Greek. His pale skin (the kind you get from working 20 hours a day) distracted from his beautifully chiseled face. He had a handle-bar mustache that was big enough to take away the focus from his good looks, and was blessed with a charming *I am here to serve you* attitude. Pete made everyone who walked through the door feel welcome.

I was grateful for the work and the little money it brought. But soon, as all my circumstances began to change, I came to understand that NYC was my new home, or rather, it was the home I'd always wanted. And so, I was going to need a new place to live that I could afford and a job that would produce the amount of money needed to support my new life.

I'd worked as a waitress in my hometown—at the Souper Salad; surely, the skill would translate. Pete gave me a Sunday night table-serving shift to see how I'd work out, and I was off and running (to what quickly appeared to be the end of my waitressing career). As it turned out, the drink-serving skills I'd acquired from my previous job didn't translate to the fast pace of a New York City diner, particularly at dinner hour.

Pete the Greek was spinning me like a top. His everything-is-beautiful attitude soon gave way to another disposition. He was a yeller and enjoyed screaming about everything, whereas I was non-confrontational and very uncomfortable with loud talking. There weren't more than twenty tables in the place and there were two of us servers working, plus Pete. But the number of dishes, side dishes, soups, salads, breads, drinks, and condiments per person was unreal. I was overwhelmed at the sheer quantity of details to remember, not to mention the momentum of the activity.

I asked Pete to make an ice cream sundae for table twelve—twice. They'd been waiting for almost fifteen minutes since I'd cleared their dinner plates. At this point in my life, I had never raised my voice to anyone. It was difficult for me to ask for something once, let alone repeat it twice. Finally, table twelve complained to Pete about the wait for their ice cream. Immediately, he called me over and began to yell.

I'm not sure if it was the pressure-cooker effects of the diner (I was stressed and exhausted) or because it was midnight and I didn't care anymore, but all of a sudden I became aware of the words coming out of my mouth as I stood down counter, about ten feet from Pete.

"Do not fucking yell at me. I asked you twice for the ice cream and you've been standing there flapping your jaw. Now, make the fucking ice cream sundae and shut up!"

I stood, stunned, as a smile slowly took over my face. I started to laugh and then cry. Pete stopped what he was doing and made the sundae as if it were nothing. I served it to the customer, and as I walked back over to Pete's domain at the counter, he gave me a hug—and we both laughed.

From that moment on, while I no longer had a job waitressing at Tom's, I had a new freedom. I was free to ask for what I needed; though, it still took a lot of work and practice to become comfortable with communicating my needs. It was now clear: not only was it my job to ask for what I needed, but to ensure what I communicated was understood.

Pete didn't actually fire me; we both agreed that Tom's was not for me. He recommended me to a restaurant across the street owned by a family member, a casual bistro named Gargantua where the pace was a bit more leisurely. Gargantua was the beginning of my new independent life, where I forged relationships I still nurture today.

The Infinite Connection Between Food, Pleasure, and Hope

Consider how we've made the presentation of a broccoli casserole an expression of our condolences or a sweet potato pie our welcome to the neighborhood; culturally, we have made the connection between food, pleasure, and hope a palpable one. In my many reflections of food and hope over the years, I've begun to think of it as a respite. Hope is the rest we take on the road to having what we need or want. When we're tired, we stop and hope for things for a while. And when we're done hoping, we make plans to get them. Hope is a generator of possibility. Not sure what you want? Make a snack and hope on it.

And if food is the agent of hope, then money is it's warrior. Always, at the end of the line, we are taught that food or money is the answer (or will bring the answer) to just about anything. We use them to speak on our behalf, care for others, and pacify ourselves. This gives them a huge, undeliverable responsibility and creates a cycle of addiction.

In the cycle of human needs, we must first be full and safe, then we long to feel good about ourselves and belong to a community. If we've achieved that, we seek understanding, meaning, and balance in life. Finally, with all those things under our belt, we are free to achieve personal fulfilment and help others do the same. The resources we have can only influence these things, not offer them. So the question is: how can a slayer create a quantum shift in their cycle of needs?

My first summer in New York City, I was in between apartments. (A natural state of affairs for me, as I moved eight times in my first two years there.) I was nineteen and trusted people meant what they said. I'd made a friend, Frank, who lived a few floors down from the apartment I'd been staying in, and a couple floors up from the apartment I was going to move into (when it was ready in a month's time).

I'd had a peripheral, but good, platonic relationship with him for about six months, so when he offered me the opportunity to stay with him in his studio apartment for the remaining few weeks, I accepted.

"No worries," he said. "You take the bed. I'll take the floor."

"Are you sure?" I said in disbelief. "I don't want to inconvenience you, and I'm not going to sleep with you. Are you okay with that?"

"Oh, of course... Of course," he responded.

With that, I was comfortable, and I headed over with my suitcase. As I'm sure you've already figured out (this stuff writes itself), after two weeks of sleeping on the floor, he was certain he could leverage my appreciation by joining me in the bed. And, of course, that wasn't going to happen. As it went, our little arrangement ended with him throwing a fit and stealing money from my suitcase one night while I was at work. I left the next day. Believe it or not, that wasn't the most potent memory of the experience. Those are the facts of the story I laugh about today, and I have absolutely no regrets.

What is seared in my mind? Frank was an early bird like me, and every morning we would get up and sit at his little bistro table placed near the kitchenette of his 200 sq. ft. studio. He'd make tea and toasted pita. Serving it with honey and cream cheese—we'd eat, laugh, and talk about life as the sun rose on the day. I think those mornings were the most tranquil moments I had that entire first year in New York, and because of them, I now associate the feeling of renewal with pita, honey, and cream cheese.

Filling the Void

All of us, at some point, have a void to fill. The gap for me, that first year in NYC, was feeling safe and stable. So when it came to Frank—being around someone whose company I genuinely enjoyed, not having to leave the building I'd been living in for months, staying only a couple of blocks away from where I worked—all those elements were assets that far outweighed the inevitable impasse around sex.

I don't remember getting mad about the money he stole, either. I sincerely understood. I'm not condoning his immature, passive-aggressive behavior, but I had anticipated the eventual outcome and knew I'd be safe. I think he ended up giving the money back after all, sticking it in my suitcase where he'd found it. When I left, I split it with him for a rent payment.

Specifically, crossing a void is the conscious connecting of all our needs together. In the case with Frank, I was joining my need for safety, stability, clarity, and friendship without compromising my integrity. And, as with any integration, there are a few casualties—my friendship with Frank disappeared.

We learn to investigate the ethereal realms of idea and emotion, the information that propels us, by shifting our focus from what we're feeling or thinking to the bigger picture—the end result. When you gain perspective from your worry or query, you begin to see the space in between things as the intricate detailed information you must understand to resolve them.

For example: if you're bored, learning something new will bring to mind the energy causing the boredom; when you're lonely, finding things to do can make clear for you what you're missing; when you're sad, being of service to others can help you be mindful of what you're grieving.

Back to the question at hand: how can a slayer create a quantum shift in their cycle of needs? We start by believing it's possible. Once security and the basics are achieved, we focus our essentials on the mental, emotional, and spiritual bodies. The auric and chakra system are the energy fields that govern these frequencies of experience and are what we refer to when we talk about being spiritual. We are all spiritual—independent of our religious beliefs. You can use any form of ritual, meditation, or contemplation to begin cultivating your awareness of these other energetic dimensions. The first to address: your lowest common denominator.

Shifting Focus From The Lowest Common Denominator

Each of us have a lowest common denominator. Many ancient religions and rituals were created to instill in their followers the discipline and self-knowledge necessary for spiritual growth. If there is a deficit in managing 100 dollars, then that deficit will be amplified in managing 10,000 or 100,000 dollars.

It is the same for you spiritually. Let's say you are asking to be a millionaire or to lose 100 pounds but have an unspoken resentment attached to money or food. The pivotal information to accomplish your goal often lies hidden in your mental, emotional, and spiritual bodies. It is in the gap between what you want and what you are able to handle. In that gap, or space, is the information needed to obtain your desire. This is called the principle of the lowest common denominator (LCD).

In times of stress you will always resort back to the LCD of your thinking and feeling patterns. To create a quantum shift, the LCD is where you begin. It is important to know what your lowest common denominators are, and to understand yourself in a deeper, more conscious way.

Unconsciously, we use our judgment of others to become aware of ourselves. Consciously, we become aware of our LCD through the feelings and self-talk we generate about ourselves, they allow us to become clear on what we perceive as our vulnerabilities.

> **Write a few sentences to answer each of these questions:**
> - How much money do you need in your pocket to feel safe?
> - What was it like the first time you didn't have enough food or money?
> - Do other people control your finances or access to food?
> - Do you eat or spend emotionally?
> - How many meals a day do you need to feel healthy?
>
> Itemize these answers. Sit with them. How do they make you feel? What issues do they bring up for you? They may help to simplify your recognition of a complex emotional dynamic that underlies how you relate to yourself and the world—breaking down the most basic elements of your relationship to food and money. Once you have a deeper understanding of your feelings of safety, you'll have a better idea of where you need to focus your mind to make the needed changes.

What You Need to Change Your Karma: Soul Retrieval

Once you understand your comfort level (LCD), and the place you'll return in times of stress, you can, through compassion, begin to cultivate a new level of comfort. Spiritually speaking, when we experience a trauma, on any level, a portion of our energy stays in that space and time where the event or experience occurred. In addition, we leave pieces of our spirit with others when we are hurt and speak unfortunate words over them. It's called an energy construct. Throughout our lives and lifetimes, we leave little pieces of our soul in these other dimensions. Calling them back is a process called soul retrieval.

Retrieving these pieces of your spirit will allow you to claim peace and forgiveness and complete the karmic process of understanding that is the obligation of the spiritual pattern.

For years I struggled with my relationship to money. I've always been a great generator but felt more at peace with debt than with considerable reserves of cash. As I began to tackle the pattern, I realized the issue was not with money itself but with the banking system. Banks are beasts in and of themselves. I've always found their systematic, dry structure to be stifling. Nonetheless, I've no interest in hiding my meager fortunes in my Tempurpedic, so bank like a normal gal I must.

I've gone into debt multiple times, eventually paying it all in full—which I attribute it to my strong money luck. The other strong karma I carry is an integral need to be accountable to no one but myself, deliberately or by default. I don't like leaving messes for someone else to clean up.

A few years after relocating to Los Angeles from New York City, I met a man named Zach. I was living my pre-psychic career of working special events in the cosmetic industry—one of these was a temporary product launch at the Macy's Men's store in Beverly Hills. Zach, an employee, had flirted with me multiple times, and I found him intriguing, sexy, and slippery—all at the same time. He wasn't classically good-looking, but he was swarthy, charming, and had a seductive-swagger. I was definitely attracted.

Finally, at the store one day, he wore me down—charming me into giving him my phone number. Within minutes of him walking away, I heard a voice in my head telling me to turn and look. As I pivoted my body 180 degrees, my eyes focused in on a moment happening about fifty feet away from where I was standing. It was Zach. He was leaning over a counter, whispering to a new female employee as he slid her his business card. She blushed, giggled, and took it. I couldn't believe that my vision had zeroed in on that less-than-a-minute event. But on multiple levels, it would sum up who he was and our on-again, off-again five-year relationship. He was a liar, and I always knew it.

Shortly after going on our first date, I had a vision. It was me: as a white man in the 1800s, somewhere in Colorado, sitting on a horse directly beneath gallows with a noose around my neck. While another man on horseback slapped the horses flank—I watched as I dangled to my death. My reaction wasn't grief; it was pure vicious rage. No, I didn't date Zach because I was naive or because he was a good person. I spent time with him because I needed to know what that vision was about. Over the years I have had multiple emotions for Zach, but I understood he was a conduit for a richer mystery that needed to be uncovered: ultimately, I would discover it to be the foundation of my relationship to money and the karmic wound that underlay it.

It wasn't until years passed that I thought of Zach again. A memory flooded back to me that was somehow connected to him, but it's meaning wasn't obvious. I was in a historic Hollywood bank. I'd received a large check written from an account at the bank by a company who was paying me to provide psychics for a party they hosted every year. Cashing the check then and there, as opposed to depositing it in my own account, would allow me to pay everyone that night. The bank teller, with a blank face and no emotion at all, said: "I can't cash this check."

We went back and forth for almost fifteen minutes. It was not computing why they weren't cashing the check, it was written from an account at their bank. I don't remember the reason they gave. All I remember is standing there being taken over by the most powerful, dark, vacant, distant, unemotional rage. As the energy creeped in, I understood what a mass shooter feels: the power and overwhelming desire to annihilate. In that moment, I had no empathy for any of the bank employees; any humanity they had was removed from my vision in those few seconds. As I looked at them all, behind the bullet-proof glass, my eyes welled up with tears at the awareness of what I was feeling. I took my check and ran—not walked—ran from the bank. I sat in my truck, wailing for over an hour.

Piece by piece, vision by vision, my karmic history with money revealed itself. The appointed day of healing soon came. I was triggered by a short conversation with a delightful agent of the Internal Revenue Service. She was giving me some information, when the subtle echoes of anger washed over me. It wasn't her, the information, or the issue at hand. It was the subtle presence of my spiritual wound signaling to be revealed and healed. After the conversation with her, I sat back in my comfy chair and asked to see the story in its entirety.

In the early 1800s I was a young man going to find his freedom and new life in southwest Colorado from the Eastern Seaboard. Traveling by himself, and with the money from his late father's estate, he made his way. Stopping in a minimally populated western town, he found a room to rent and began to meet the locals. One, in particular, was the town's bank owner and con man (currently known in this life as Zach). Somehow or other, the young man was convinced to put all the cash he had into the bank for safe keeping. Understanding finally, after multiple attempts to withdraw his money from the bank, he'd been conned. As it turned out, the bank owner and the local law were in cahoots, which ultimately led to my dear young man's untimely death at the gallows.

While I'm certain there were many more details and others involved, I was satisfied and relieved. My grief was not for money or our formidable banking structure; it was for one murderous con man I had the unfortunate experience of meeting twice—back then, and now. I sat in total forgiveness, feeling complete nothingness for any of them: no anger, grief, or sadness; no love, desire, or longing; no absence or presence. It was almost as if it had never happened, any of it. I was complete, beyond ready to move on; I had been thoroughly transformed. My journey of over two decades ended with the only response that seemed fitting: hmm, okay.

Opening to Receive and Retain the New Pattern

Much as anger was connected to my relationship to money, grief and change correlated to my relationship to food. I binged so often those first few months in New York City that I gained fifty pounds. It took almost two years to ferret out all the emotional burdens that were contributing to my desire to eat more than I needed.

The process of releasing and transforming a karmic spiritual pattern is multifaceted and arduous, comprised of multiple experiences, people, and levels of understanding. It's like a big quilt, filled with details put together piece by piece and culminating in an expansive, masterful tapestry of your history. And like many quilt makers can attest to, an unfinished project gets folded up and put in a closet for a period of time while more fabric or threads are gathered. Once it's finished, though, you're free to do with it what you will.

One of the next steps is to begin to receive and integrate the new pattern: how you want to be and the changes you'd like to see in your life. You must call down in thought and form, from the furthest reaches of your soul, the antidote to the old pattern that has ailed you. For most, the way this happens is through grieving and the explicit and relentless desire for total change.

When we cry, focus, or experience all-encompassing emotion—it activates the body's life-force energy that moves through the endocrine system, energizing specific layers of your physical body and the subtle bodies (auric field) that govern them. This activation reveals the soul information they hold.

Contained in these layers of energy are the blueprints for the new patterns that will manifest in you and your life. It is in the storage of these karmic designs from which springs your destiny—a fate that contains multiple options to choose from—to create your new self. How it all breaks down and then rebuilds is completely up to you and your relationships. The plans do not create the opportunities, per se, but help you to receive and recognize the new options as they flow your way. It is your willingness to move against what has been habitual, taking deliberate steps towards the things you say you want, that moves you forward.

> **A few questions to answer:**
> - What are five things you get from money?
> - What's the first thing you'd do if you won the Lotto?
> - If you had to change your job or career, what would you most like to do?
> - What are five things you get from food?
> - What's the first thing you think of when preparing to cook and eat?
> - What would you most like to change about your eating dynamic?
>
> Answering these questions and contemplating their answers will allow you to explore the energy you have around your ideas, feelings, and habits regarding food and money. It is in this information you'll discover simple, yet impactful, realizations on how to make any changes you desire.

> As human beings, we cultivate a constant state of preparation—we are always working with what we have while we wait for what we want. Whether it be with grace and gratitude, or bitterness and frustration, we'll eventually get where we're going; the attitude determines the condition in which we arrive.

The Universe and Prosperity: Understanding Deficit Driven Choices

Does conjuring what you want require positive thinking? Well, to be accurate, you get what you focus on—any thought, positive or otherwise. A colleague of mine used to preface every prayer by asking for the highest and best, as if not saying it would automatically bring the lowest and worst. Being clear is a phase of the manifestation process—phrasing accurately your desires. When we go about the task of describing what we want or expressing our current condition, we often find we've not seen or accepted the circumstances as they are. It's impossible to build on something when you are unable to be honest about the starting point.

I've had many a discussion with a disgruntled client who sought to manifest a new job or circumstance, but then found themselves blindsided by an aspect of their life falling apart as they begin their prosperity work. They feel upset and betrayed, as if the Universe has been disloyal. The more they focus on having, the more things fall apart.

Simply put: as you focus on the object of your desire, all the reasons come to the fore as to why you don't yet have what you want. They arise in the space to be evaluated and renegotiated. This process can feel like things are falling apart, when they're actually falling away to create space for the object of your focus to be brought into the picture.

Your ability to manifest a life you want is based on energy flow: how easily you receive and how quickly you are able to let go of what doesn't serve you. Allowing conscious ebb and flow of energy—in relationship to the things you want—is a skill that is cultivated over time. For example, if the job you have doesn't bring the kind of money you want, makes you unhappy, or doesn't make you feel good about yourself for doing it, you'd think that letting it go would be easy. In fact, there is a lot more to letting go than just letting go.

The presence of grief, as we've mentioned several times, indicates where we have attachment based on our beliefs and ideals—like losing weight because you think you'll be prettier or folks will like you more. Consciously allowing the flow of energy in your life requires you to be receptive: ready, willing, and able to receive and manage what you want. As human beings, we cultivate a constant state of preparation—we are always working with what we have while we wait for what we want. Whether it be with grace and gratitude, or bitterness and frustration, we'll eventually get where we're going; the attitude determines the condition in which we arrive.

Start Where You Are

Things may seem like they get worse before they get better, but in truth, possibly you didn't see how bad they were when you started. Self-honesty is the first step of manifesting what you want. For example, if you want money, do well with the money you have. Are your goals in alignment with what you have? Do you spend within your means? Are you respectful of your money? Do you want money because you feel you lack other things? Taking a little inventory on the motivation for the object of your inquiry will go a long way in helping you get it.

You Can't Get What You Want, if You Don't Know What You Want

After you've studied your motivation, you'll begin to understand why you are in your position, and you can create a strategy to change it. This part is going to take a little imagination, thinking outside your normal box about the things you wish for. First of all, write out your top five desires about health and wealth. Now, think of five people you've heard of who have achieved these things.

If you have a money goal, choose the next logical level of acquisition for yourself and focus on people you know or people in the public eye that have the amount you want to create for yourself. Do your research—learn as much as you can about the habits of these people. Your aim is to learn how to have what you're asking for—not just get it, but have it. Let the Universe create the design of how you receive your objective. Keep in mind: anything is possible in its logical progression, and what is reasonable for you could very well be a miracle.

Manage What You Have

Notice the emphasis is not on how to manifest your target, but how you will experience having it. When you focus on how to get something, you become process oriented, which is really important if you want to teach someone else or be able to communicate how you got it. If that's not your intent—focus on managing well what you have.

If you want to feel healthier in your life, focus on doing things in moderation. Eating small portions, two-minute-interval exercises, and limit your time in places or with people who compound your stress. If money is your object, pay your bills on time, put money in your savings, and only spend on things you really want—no wasteful spending. It is the natural alignment of the Universe to amplify what you are already doing.

The Universe Responds to Action

The physical world is the last stop on the manifestation train. It's where ideas are realized, broken down, or reborn. Because the physical world is slower moving than any other creative level, an idea, in order to become manifest, must be in alignment with other things in your physical life.

For instance, if all you think about is wanting more money, what you'll wind up feeling is frustration at work, and what you'll wind up doing is living so far beyond your means that you'll worry about paying the bills every month. The Universe receives this as: *I'd prefer to have barely enough to get by, thank you.*

This translates in your life as attracting people and situations in crisis, being caught unawares, or constantly being asked to spend time doing things you don't like. The Universe multiplies what you do, not what you say.

Your Thoughts Promote Your Choices

Now, this is where your thoughts become important, they lead to every choice you make. Your karmic patterns contain images and feelings that lead to your thinking. At every level in between we have the opportunity to nurture, change, or erase what's already there. So, as you become mindful of thoughts and feelings without letting them dictate your choices, you'll get clear results. Relaxation is the optimal state to create from, so patience and self-acceptance are your most valued assets when it comes to figuring out what you want, getting it, and living with it.

Angelic Teachers of Manifestation

Every stage of manifestation can be fun when you embrace it. Getting comfortable with asking for help and working in the spirit of collaboration with your human companions or your spirit guides, and capitalizing on their support, will strengthen all you do. I love working with the angels and the many spiritual teachers of this process.

- Galgaliel: the angel of vibration
- Jamaerah: the angel of manifestation
- Amitiel: the angel of truth
- Metatron: the angel of thought

They are waiting to assist you when it comes to manifestation, if you'll ask. If ever there was a time in life to be brave, bold, and think outside the box, it's when you are creating a new life for yourself.

Living With Surplus: Having Too Much Equals Waste?

Unconscious bias is the way we use judgment as a guidepost to reveal our deeper truths. Let me tell you about one of my own biases. But I'll start with the simple portion of the discussion. I am bigoted toward fat—not other people's fat, just mine. For me, on a conscious level, having a lot of fat is synonymous with being unwell (that's just always how I've felt). But subconsciously, something else was going on.

Have you ever considered what makes you a bigot? No judgment here. We are all partial and intolerant about something at any given time—but when you strain it down to the core ingredients of your own bias, what you have left are the seeds of your own self-loathing. Whatever we despise in ourselves, at times, we reject in others. That's the simple portion of the discussion.

The complicated part is acknowledging and defining the multiple layers of long-held beliefs, ancestral traditions, cultural misunderstandings, experiential events, personal agendas, and mounds of fear that make up your karmic patterning.

One day I'd gone for lunch with a longtime friend and client. I was acutely aware of the amount of food I was serving myself from the afternoon Tibetan buffet, and the building anticipation of the most amazing freshly baked naan bread they served just after you sat down with your plates.

This stuff evoked the most profound pleasure for me. The sight and smell of it's soft, tender, lightly browned surface with the most delicate air bubbles—promoting blissful childhood memories of eating Navajo fry bread with honey—set off endorphins of joy that could easily bring a tear to my eye.

However, mindful of not being particularly hungry, I imbibed in a bit of the yellow lentil soup, ate a few bites of the chicken curry and enjoyed two halves of the beautiful naan. Already feeling full, I focused on the jovial conversation at hand.

Then, on the car ride home, all the emotion I'd been carrying got real. You see, for several days I'd been engulfed in a reality of being old and fat. *Fat and old*, had been reverberating in my mind repeatedly. Because my health and genuine feelings of youthfulness had always been a sign of success to me, the thoughts filled me with intense anger and sadness—propelling the outburst: "I am old and fat!"

To which my friend responded in horror, "Oh no, Tracee. Don't put that out there."

He looked at me and winced, slouching away from me towards the car door as he said it. For a brief moment I saw myself in his deep rejection of my words. As if saying it out loud is what causes it.

"Oh, it's already out there," I said.

Over the years I've done battle with fat. The first phase of my opposition were the many ways my consciousness sought to bring my attention to the subtle body dysmorphia that lay dormant, just waiting to be revealed. It would come out when a boy I liked suggested that my lean and muscular thighs were fat, or I'd be prettier if I were five pounds thinner. Five pounds? Today, I belly laugh like a villain at five pounds.

It took me years to recognize that overcoming weight was just the first skirmish in the war. I had to keep going back, deeper into my history each time, to find the winning strategy. The problem wasn't the fat, the issue was the unconscious notion I held deep within—to be thin equaled death.

When I was a child, I'd say under ten, a girl from the neighborhood and I would hoard food. She and I would steal food stuffs from our respective kitchens, anything from packets of Saltines and butter to leftovers. We would hide our cache of nourishment in the evergreen shrubs outside my bedroom window and meet periodically to indulge in our extra meals. I never ate too much but couldn't stand the feeling of being hungry. I never questioned why I was doing it, and surprisingly, I never got sick from it. Sometimes our collections would be out there for a few days.

Next stop on my train ride back through time is my miracle birth. I was born at seven months during the sixties. Weighing in at 2.2 pounds, I was promptly placed into an incubator where people could look but not touch. I do not have any direct recollection about my time in the incubator, but I know that touch and affection was a struggle for me for many years—either getting too much or not enough. It seems fat makes a very nice incubator.

All of these unconscious layers, along with very little parental input growing up, drew to me others who were in conflict with my independence and promoted in me a highly critical self-view. I've always known that my relationship with food had connections that preceded the habits I learned in my upbringing. It took years of working with different healthy lifestyles, much contemplation, and the multiple soul-retrievals I endured for me to bring into balance what took centuries to create. The final step was the revelation of my father's dear Uncle Dornblaser. I needed to tell his story, grieve his loss, and make peace with feeling hungry.

Love, Not Shame, Your Fat

As I've just touched on, I have struggled with my own relationship to fat—and the many layers of spiritual and emotional need—leading me to carry more of it than my body required. I'm not judgmental about other people's relationship to fat—whether it be a circumstance, a proclivity, or an unaddressed response to one's inner or outer world—it is a person's health that I give the most value. However, each individual has their own karmic pattern that will bring to them their greatest knowledge regarding balance and self-esteem on any level. This will be their highest priority and most certainly guide their relationship to weight.

When we carry a lot of fat in our bodies, it isn't about vanity or the lack of it, it's about the existence of safety on many levels—either currently or karmically. Biologically, our body is intrinsically trained to hold on to the fat we eat instead of using it for current energy needs. The cells of the body communicate to one another when fat is being processed, essentially, deciding whether to use the fat for energy or send it to a fat store. Your body can harbor fat in many places, not just the belly, arms, or hips which are common for both men and women; but the organs and other tissues as well.

The storing of fat in your body is to keep you safe and alive should you ever have to go without a meal for a day, or even a season—as was common in different times, when food was not so readily available. Your body can also hold the spiritual memory of starvation and illness from past lives, that trigger the biological need to hold on to fat so as to never have the unwanted experience again. These fat cells, in turn, can carry the current life memory of any form of habit, discord, or traumatic event.

We have a tendency to hold on to extra fat as a physical barrier to our emotional traumas or sensitivities. I know many abused men and women (including myself) who've gained a substantial amount of weight in response to a trauma and the grief that comes after. I gained about sixty pounds within a year of addressing my own grief around the loss of my personal power after being raped. So, when in the process of assessing your own weight and health, be conscientious of why you carry the weight you do and the energy that lies beneath it all.

The Slayer's Altar and Ritual: Living Wealthy

Collaboration is key to a new start.

Wealth isn't just about having money, it's about expansion in all aspects of your life. It includes feeling confident in accessing, managing, and utilizing all of your resources. Each component of this matrix is vital to sustaining balance. If you don't have confidence, you may not react in a timely fashion nor trust your instinct when opportunities arise. If you are unable to manage what you have, being overwhelmed will also limit your prospects. If you lack trust, you diminish your options for collaboration with others.

Living a healthy and wealthy life will always include working with others. No matter what resource or goal is the focus of the Slayer's Ritual for you, the intent is to recognize all the ways you will collaborate with yourself, others, and your universe to achieve your aims.

This ritual is intended for you to reveal the deeper story you may have about your relationship to food and money, and the way you integrate your network and resources. Take a few moments to gather the necessary items, and be prepared to spend the time to follow through on the process.

The Altar

What You Need:
- Seven-day red jar candle
- Tobacco, corn, or cornmeal
- Paper and pen (not your digital device)

How to Proceed:
Clean and clear a space in the western direction of a room in your home, ideally the kitchen. Put some corn, cornmeal, or tobacco in a small bowl as an offering of gratitude for all you will receive from your Creator.

Sit in the space where you are creating your altar and take four deep breaths, breathing in through the nose and exhaling through the mouth. Close your eyes and imagine a light turning on in your head, throat, heart, stomach, lower abdomen, and the perineum (this is the space below the pelvic diaphragm and between the legs). Now, sit quietly.

Ask yourself: on what main topic would you like to focus the energy of this altar regarding your dynamic with food and money? Write down whatever comes to mind. If you're looking to manifest something specific or are looking for a particular outcome, write it down now.

Create clarity by using as few words as possible to express your thoughts. Also, gather any notes you've taken while reading Part One.

Now, after organizing your intent for this altar, you're going to gather together a few objects that represent the answers to the following questions. Where they come from is not important; the ingenuity you use to get them is the point. They can be from nature, bought, borrowed, or something you already own.

- What is your first adult memory about money?
- Who handled the money in your childhood?
- What represents your mother's feelings around money?
- What represents your father's thoughts about food?
- What is your first childhood memory with food?
- How do you want to feel about yourself that you don't already?
- If you had limitless resources, what is the first thing you'd do?

Take each of the objects that represent your answers and place them on the altar, or in the altar area. Fold your papers full of notes and place it underneath the candle. For the next seven days light the candle and allow it to burn a few hours every night until it's down to the socket. Each morning, take a few notes of any dreams you had or any thoughts and feelings that have come to the surface. At the end of the ritual, if you have a fireplace or firepit, burn all your notes.

This ritual will bring together clarity on your spiritual patterning regarding food and money, and the decisions that have followed them. In addition to this new self-awareness, you will begin to understand the elements of your life and self that you'd like to change. You'll have a new foundation of thinking that will set you up for success.

PART TWO

AFFINITY

Your Karmic Relationship to Romantic Love and Your Ancestors

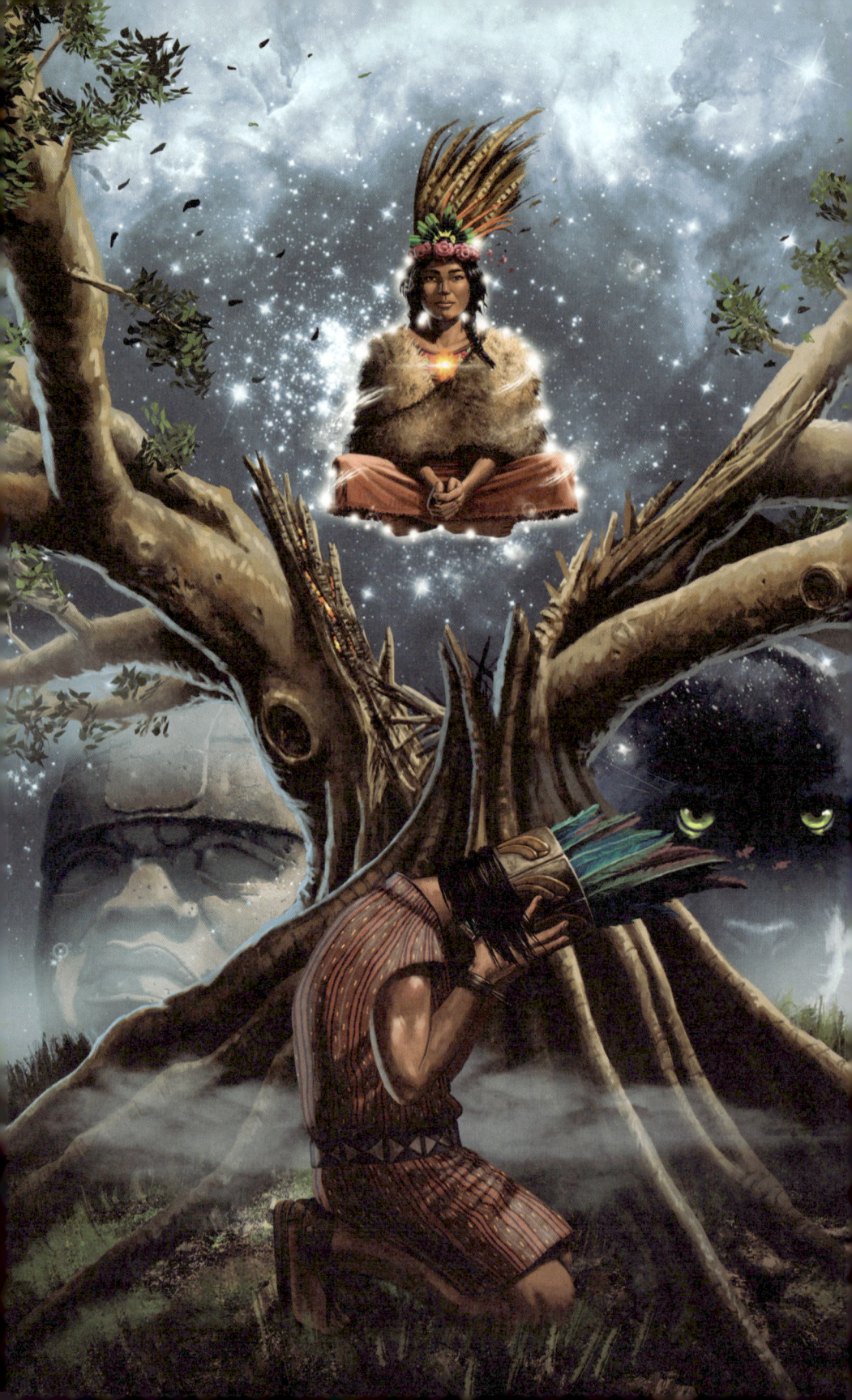

Betrayal is Karma's Middle Name—New Directions Come in All Forms

The Slayer's Weapons:

Independence, Trust, Joy, Fidelity, Truth, Tradition, Culture, Betrayal, Boundaries, Self-Expression

The Karmic Story:
The Once and Disappointing King

No one really knows what happened to the village of Zac Zac U Ut Tun. It is a secret still held in the ground, yet to be discovered. It is the story of King Tzon Halal and his deep love for Xulab, his thirteen-year-old daughter—and the pivotal choices that changed the Xi people forever. But more than that, it is the story of a father's abiding faith amongst the confusion of a changing and turbulent time.

The rains had been pouring for many days, now. The caves had become full, and for a third year in a row, the maize in the fields below had been rendered useless because the plants had become too saturated during their early growth. Once again, King Tzon Halal sat at the highest point on the mountain waiting for instruction, a message from the Jaguar God. But still, nothing.

The little village had been a safe haven for many as they came from all over seeking asylum from their warring tribes. Tzon Halal had been gifted with the honor of leadership from the others that had moved with him to the plateau where sat the mountain caves. Not a king by blood but by wisdom—he was a young, vital man who was believed to be a Nahuale' (a shaman with the ability to shapeshift into a jaguar).

Although he carried insight and discernment beyond his years, it was his affinity with the Jaguar that gave him his power with the people. His connection to the stars and ancestors gave him his confidence. So much so, he planned to name his daughter Xulab (meaning "star"), as she was a star yet to be born.

It was a tragedy when Xulab's mother died in childbirth and left Xulab and her father to fulfill the promise of new life that she'd made to the community. Xulab and Tzon grew to be as close as any two people could, with a mutual respect and an unbreakable spiritual bond. Tzon adored and nurtured his daughter, knowing that one day she would take his place as the leader of their people.

Xulab was born with the ability to predict the most valuable elements of growing maize: the richest soil, the moon cycles that nurtured planting seeds and harvesting crops, and most of all—the weather. Xulab was connected with the gulf ecosystem as though it had become the mother she never had.

She foretold every major storm that came through the area since before she could walk. When Xulab was a baby, she could feel the psychic pressure of a large storm weeks in advance. She would cry in a particular rhythm that the adults around her eventually understood; inevitably, communicating with words which allowed for the precise and proper planting of every crop.

For many years, Zac Zac U Ut Tun enjoyed much prosperity. Food aplenty and pleasant relations with all the surrounding villages and other tribes. The people were able to live in balance with Earth, their mother, and the stars, their father—but most of all, with the Jaguar: their leader, who was the god of the underworld. No one was prepared for the tragedies that befell the bourgeoning settlement, one after another, and the cords of integrity and tradition that would begin to unravel in all of them.

In general, King Tzon Halal had no detractors. However, with the consistent challenges, multiple storms, and changing weather, the people were beginning to look for someone to blame. The food resources became scarce. The local water hole was poisoned with some sort of bloom due to the abnormally hot weather for the region. And still, there was no sign of the Jaguar. Everyone, including the king, was beginning to feel abandoned.

Womanhood was beckoning for Xulab, now in her thirteenth year of life. She awoke from a dream of her mother one night, and it was troubling her. In the dream, her mother was crying and reaching down to her from the stars with blood on her hands. Xulab couldn't shake the feeling of deep anxiety it left in her, but even so, she took it as a sign of the arrival of her first blood and left it at that.

Meanwhile, once again, Tzon Halal found himself praying on the mountain. It was tradition during a time like this that a sacrifice of blood would be made to elevate the human into their higher consciousness to communicate with the gods. The people had been requesting it. However, normally it was to come in the form of a bloodletting from the tongue of the queen—but there was no queen. Finally, the Jaguar spoke.

The king came down from the mountain with a message for the people. The Jaguar requested Xulab's first blood be given to the Great Mother when the moon turned red.

It was to be a celebration, and the preparations began immediately. Sacred Anh' (flowers and plants) were collected for her adornments, as many as could be found that hadn't been dampened or washed away. The hallowed bed where she would reside for seven days was laid upon a mountain ridge, under an old rubber tree for shelter. There she would allow her dynasty to breathe life into the Earth for all the people.

Part Two - Affinity

Although the harvests had been thin this season, the people of Zac Zac U Ut Tun were hopeful, because there was much for which they could be grateful. The people of the community made a beautiful presentation of foods and created the sacred circle to be joined by everyone. Still, Xulab's anxiety was waxing with the moon, and it was almost unbearable. She prayed for the strength to hold herself together for the less than twelve hours until the eclipse, but the psychic pressure was mounting, and she knew there was a storm on its way.

The villagers danced and prayed as the full moon became red, but there was no joy for Xulab. She sat by herself under the tree, knowing the storm on its way was a power that hadn't been seen in lifetimes—surely not remembered by anyone in Zac Zac U Ut Tun. On her mind again was her mother, reaching for her through the stars. It made her panic. Within hours the pelting rains had become relentless, and the lightning and thunder were terrifying for Xulab.

In the village, Tzon Halal was beside himself with worry; he could feel her terror. However, it was a tradition of this particular rite of passage that she must commune with nature on her own, and even Xulab had encouraged her father to release his concern. Surely, she would be fine. He had faith that the Jaguar would take care of his daughter.

The winds were now blowing with such an extreme force that the rubber tree's canopy surrendered to their authority, almost touching the ground. Xulab, wrapped in a blanket, now clung to the tree trunk.

The night pressed on, but there was no sleep for anyone. The tide was at its peak and the water poured into the village. Everyone grabbed what they could and made their way up the mountain following Tzon Halal. A massive lightning strike and the crack of a breaking tree was heard. A deafening slap of thunder that echoed through the gulch came soon after. Tzon Halal was less than one hundred yards from the ridge when he began to run.

"Xulab!" he cried. "Xulab!"

As he made it past the final rock formation, he could barely see through the rain, but he could make out the giant rubber tree torn in two. Lying at the base was his precious daughter Xulab. The lightning strike left its mark directly in the center of her chest as it hit her first before splitting the massive tree in half. Tzon Halal fell to his knees, cradling Xulab in his arms. He wept uncontrollably as the others began to make it up the ridge.

The storm raged on, and it would take another four days to subside. The waters overtook much of the land, and the settlement was completely flooded.

No one knows who the gods ordained lucky enough to survive from the village. Only Xulab, her mother, and the rich layers of rock and earth that hold the secrets of the once thriving community of Zac Zac U Ut Tun know for sure. As for Tzon Halal, he'd already sacrificed his greatest treasure. He joined the Jaguar in the land of the ancestors with his wife and beautiful Star.

The Impact of Our Ancestral Relationships

Always in my life, a story that needed to be told would reveal itself in pieces and layers—over time. For years, jaguars have been a part of my story. They've come to me in dreams over and over, the grandmothers and grandfathers of our galactic ancestry (as the Olmec people considered them); however, it wasn't until the emerging of this story that they began to speak to me.

One night in a dream, I was living in an adobe house with high vigo (log beam) ceilings and all white interior walls. It was a unique multi-leveled design that was reminiscent of the Pueblos of New Mexico, the state where I grew up. I appeared to be entertaining a group of friends. Some were in the dining room and some in the living space near the fire. Some were sitting on large white adobe banquettes that lined the edges of the rooms and encroached upwards on the walls three feet at a time to different levels, like large stairs. All the areas in the house were visible from these steps.

The front door opened, and in walked a massive black jaguar. You could see his muscles ripple underneath his sleek black-spotted coat as he walked through the door. I ran to him like he was my long lost father. I welcomed him, and in he trotted. With only a few leaps, he was across the room and sat on the highest banquette of the living space. He surveyed the room, and as he jumped from place to place, the guests of the party were a little unnerved but joyful to see him.

When he made his way back to where I was sitting, he jumped up beside me and licked the side of my face, sticking his long prickly tongue directly in my ear, all the way to my brain. It didn't seem weird at all. He needed to tell me something. The giant cat made his way around the room, hopping from one ledge to another for a few more rounds, finally circling back to me. He butted his forehead against mine, once again licking my face. Turning around, he bounded out the door.

Although the jaguar's message was not yet clear, around the same time frame I reconnected with a man I grew up with. I did not know him well—his cousin Daniel was a beloved childhood friend of mine. Daniel and I had known each other since we were three, but he'd met with an early and untimely death. A day or two before I'd been told of his death, he'd come to me in spirit. Daniel and I shared a deep karmic love, and in the dream-time vision he danced with me, holding me tight—there was no need for words.

A few days later my mother called me in Los Angeles to let me know that Daniel was gone. I understood then, the dream had been to let me know he was leaving, Since his death, he's joined me many times in dreams and psychic visions. And again, in this most recent jaguar dream, he was making his presence known for the sake of his cousin Miguel.

Daniel had been pushing me (psychically) to reach out to Miguel on more than one occasion, but we hadn't spoken in years. He thought Miguel hadn't dealt with his death. It was awkward, to say the least, because I was being requested to intervene in something that wasn't my business. So I prefaced my conversation with Miguel in a text, saying I'd like to have a conversation with him about Daniel. He accepted.

Once Miguel and I got past the difficult first five minutes of conversation, we stayed on the phone half the night. I could feel Daniel's presence the entire time. About an hour into the conversation, I experienced a powerful energy download. It felt like a lightning bolt to the center of my chest. It didn't hurt, but consequently, I didn't sleep for almost seventy-two hours. I was teaching a workshop at a resort in the desert at the time, and I was grateful to be working so that I could stay busy while processing such a powerful energy exchange. The experience was full of surprises; not the least of which, Miguel had avoided any real conversation about his cousin, and his avoidance spoke louder than words. The energy shift I experienced is called a kundalini (life-force) activation. It triggers the soul's sacred information to become active and, eventually, conscious.

My need to connect with Miguel was still a mystery for a few more months. The following few conversations we had became more and more awkward, but I was still experiencing the intense energy connection with him whether or not we spoke. One day, in a text chat, Miguel sent me an old photo of himself and his two young daughters—my heart exploded with emotion and grief. In that photo, Miguel looked exactly like my father before he'd gotten sick, and his daughters were about the age I was when I lost him.

He died of cancer when I was eleven years old, and I'd forgotten what he looked like healthy—my strongest memory was from the last week of his life and his eighty-pound form. Helping Miguel move toward healing his separation from Daniel was helping me with the healing of my own relationship to my father. My karmic story was unraveling…

The Slayer's Path: Leave No Stone Unturned

Most of us when contemplating karmic relationships think about the romantic, love-based, or familial variety. But when it comes to deeply personal relationships, there are often multiple layers that create each one. Understanding them requires you to look at all the factors that created them, those aspects that make sense and also the ones that don't. This type of spiritual relationship sits firmly in the soulmate category, and will be fully unearthed in the pages to come.

What Are the Initial Tell-Tale Signs of a Soulmate?

- Experiencing love at first sight
- An intense calm or humor
- Extreme sexual connection
- Feeling like you've known someone forever
- Having a past-life flashback or extraordinary sense of familiarity when meeting for the first time
- Telepathic communication
- An experience of fear, loathing, or premonition immediately or early on

All those intense feelings that two people experience in the first couple of meetings are created from the past-life connections or the intertwining energetic patterns—the spiritual lock and key—that is found in all soulmate relationships.

Are soulmates good or bad? They can be both. We engage in soulmate entanglements for our development on every level. These relationships often represent a dynamic or situation that needs resolving. Ultimately, when the relationship is based on a past-life experience, everyone participating in the connection must have a complete understanding of each other's position to be released from the pattern.

It might appear at times that your experience with a soulmate is destined, and certainly, it can be true. However, we all have soul groups: thousands of souls with whom we incarnate in multiple life experiences over time. Often, family members have lived multiple lives together and have traversed a wide array of relationship dynamics: marriage, friendship, rival, parent, enemy, lover, or foe. That's why a slayer must leave no stone unturned when seeking to resolve or nurture a spiritual relationship.

What is a Soulmate?

The common perception of a soulmate is the person who is the love of your life, and the belief that there is only one. The truth is we have many soulmates in a lifetime. They are people with whom we have previous life experience and spiritual connection. Reconnecting with them is a sensation unlike any other. Sometimes it's an instant emotional reaction to someone upon meeting them, and for others, it's a subtle knowing or familiarity with a person you've not met before.

A soulmate relationship isn't always a loving, happy-go-lucky, happily-ever-after scenario for everyone. In fact, consistently, the connection often brings two people back together to heal a dynamic or event left unresolved. Not necessarily incomplete between the two specific souls coming together, but more often than not, it is the attraction of two people with life patterns that intersect and need to be healed.

We attract in our spiritual partners what we need when we're ready to transform or develop the spiritual patterns we have in common. *Every lock has a key* is the principal at work here, and during your lifetime you'll have many relationships with those who hold pivotal information for you or you for them.

Everyone has a soul group. They are those with whom we have connection and affinity. They may appear in our lives just in time to give us support, teach us a lesson, or love us unconditionally. They are the souls with whom we share eternity. The most important thing to consider as you contemplate your soulmates: it takes cultivated unconditional love to be a soulmate. These spiritual beings love you so much they come back to play a role (good or bad) in your life, as you do for others. No matter the timbre of the relationship, a soulmate deserves respect and honor. Below is a list of the many types of soulmate relationships.

Lovers

Lovers are the people with whom we have sexual relationships. They come into our lives to give us connection and encouragement for a while. We attract lovers that give us emotional nourishment even if we inevitably outgrow the source. The attraction we have with a karmic lover can be intense; usually, it is evidence of the healing on its way to us through this powerful soulmate relationship.

I had a lover I really liked and to whom I had an intense attraction. I spent time with him periodically over three or four months until one night, while we were together, I had a flashback of the rape I'd experienced a few years before. Of course, I plummeted into a deep grief response. As I did, he held me and reminded me of the strength, value, and love I carried inside me.

Unfortunately, it became evident that he wasn't a very good person—he lied about another relationship he was in. I found out when the pregnant woman confronted him at a local bar where we were having a drink—he was cruel and disrespectful to her. But, although we didn't remain lovers or friends, I was always grateful for his compassion when I needed it.

Beloveds

Beloveds are the husbands, wives, and long-term partners we choose and the families we are born to. These soulmate relationships can be our biggest teachers. Everybody contends with expectations in a relationship, but it is a unique experience to transcend or transform the unconscious expectations of a karmic beloved that are revealed from coming together with another based on the spiritual energy from a previous life or a current relational dynamic. This relationship may take a lifetime to experience, transform, and express itself fully.

It is rare for two people to reincarnate into a lifetime together and engage in the same type of relationship they may have experienced before. The intense connection and deep-seated love we share with our beloveds are based in the requirement of a long-term relationship to reveal the teaching or healing over time.

The goal of all of these soulmate connections is to cultivate love on every level: unconditional love; love with boundaries; and, ultimately, unshakable love of ourselves and the Creator. They are the faith builders that give us our life's blood. Next time you cross paths with a soulmate, fortify yourself with love, kindness, and (most of all) forgiveness; jump in with confidence, knowing the greatest outcome is illumination.

Are All Relationships Karmic?

All of our relationships are based on spiritual patterns and how we nurture, deny, or transform them. No matter if they are ancestral, familial, or romantic—the conditioning that occurs from our responses, and the multiple returns from our environment, are the building blocks of our world view as we develop. While not every relationship is dramatic or deeply intense in nature, we all engage in our associations based on what we know about ourselves consciously or unconsciously.

We make choices and glean information from our triggers and desires— with all the emotions that come with them. Because we relate to all relationships in the way we do, for the same underlying reasons, the type of relationship doesn't matter. Throughout the following pages I'll use the word partner to signify all manner of relationships: ancestral, familial, romantic or casual. They are all spiritual partners in the matrix of life.

The Spiritual Lock and Key

Everyone has an unconscious lock and key. It is the part of their spirit that expresses itself through what it attracts or provokes in others. One person energetically provokes another to express themselves in a particular way and vice-versa.

Here are a few examples of what that looks like:

- You desire to be treated with respect, but you deeply fear hostility and continue to attract it.

- You dislike a certain experience like having your hair pulled, yet your partner does it continually.

- Maybe you find cursing abhorrent; yet, no matter how many times you express your displeasure, others continue to use foul language around you.

These are the small subtle ways we connect the spiritual fibers of our relationships. They may be misconstrued or experienced as negativity, but these apparently meaningless irritations and idiosyncrasies that occur continually, are all indications of the underlying, unspoken, spiritual trauma that reverberates from our energy. Inherent in those same vibrations is the way to reveal and resolve that pain or discomfort.

What we may not be taking into consideration when we experience or witness an extreme emotional response to something, is the unspoken information that is being triggered. A person who has experienced abuse in their lifetime, or any form of racism or bigotry, may be set-off by any appearance of disrespect. The person who doesn't like their hair pulled may have had a concussion from falling forehead first out of a tree. A person who doesn't like cursing may be an ultra-sensitive and feel the impact of the harsh language viscerally, or may have had an alcoholic parent who used gruff language. No matter how you slice it, unprocessed pain from any time in our conscious or spiritual life remains intact and finds ways of being brought to the surface for healing.

> **If you find yourself with a specific partner who triggers you continually, contemplate these things:**
> - Consider that the discord in your relationship may not be caused by your partner or a product of the relationship at all.
> - Ask yourself what feeling is provoked when you are triggered by your partner.
> - Take some time away from them to reflect on those feelings and get to the origin of the emotions.
> - Let your partner know clearly that you understand that they are not the cause of your pain or discomfort, but what they are doing is making the wound you carry obvious to you.
> - Make an agreement with yourself and the specific emotional wound in question that you are ready to receive healing on all levels.

In our culture, we love drama. We support it in many ways—daily. So if you find yourself with a little extra, know this: the quicker you embrace it and get to the core of its message, the more peace you will have for yourself and in your relationships.

Familial Relationship Patterns

We choose the energetic building blocks of our spiritual destiny prior to our incarnation on this planet. We either sit with a spiritual council, picking and choosing the important details of our destiny, or our soul's vibrational content attracts to us the nearest willing participant in the spiritual blueprint of our life-design. In both cases, this includes the souls we choose as biological family. However, it's not as clear cut as choosing Elvis to be your dad.

Our biological family are those souls with whom we must process intense deeply rooted spiritual dynamics by carrying the same DNA imprint. It doesn't matter if we live with or without them for a period of time, or never know them at all. These souls and our connection to them, anchor the patterns that keep us joined in the spiritual realms until any conflicts can be resolved.

Parental Relationships

We have spiritual agreements with others from our soul group (people with resonating goals and ideals with whom we'd like to work through some of our spiritual patterning). The souls we choose as parents will be the most formative, consistent allies in this process, regardless of whether those relationships cause beauty or strife. Essentially, we choose our parents because their spiritual habits and traits will allow for our deepest growth within the human experience.

My birth story has had a tremendous impact on my perception of life—it was a fundamental building block of my perspective. I was born prematurely in the '60s, at seven months—just surviving was a miracle at the time. My mother and father were the perfect parents for me. Now, by no means am I saying they were perfect, but they were exactly who I needed to give me space to learn to nurture myself and become accountable for who I am.

My father was in entertainment. He died around my eleventh birthday, but before that, he wasn't very emotionally present in my day-to-day life.

My mother was a great homemaker. She denied the expression of emotional pain like a star athlete. But it was no wonder: mental illness ran in both sides of the family. The expression of emotion or pain was looked on as weakness. Spiritual sensitivity and intuitive ability also came from both my ancestral lines.

It was only as an adult I was able to process the grief of feeling emotionally neglected, which I held on to for all of those years. I eventually came to understand that what I perceived as emotional abandonment was the opportunity to release myself from the dynamic of victimization I had carried for multiple incarnations. I was able to recognize the spiritual determination it took to be born premature and without any real physical touch at such an influential time.

As I came to understand my extreme empathy and spiritual sensitivity, it became clear how I was impacted by the energy of others, to the point of illness at times. It then made sense to have parents who were physically present in such a strong way but not emotionally engaging. I needed to figure out who I was without the opinions or input of others. Ultimately, they positioned me to be fully accountable for myself on every level.

Of course, there are many more details to my story. But essentially, what I'm trying to say is that each of us can be reduced to the few spiritual patterns that attract, create, and support everything we do and drive our perceptions and decisions.

Karma of the Same Sex Parent

Our same sex parent (or the gender with whom you most deeply align) is the most influential. We have a tendency to energetically connect to the parent with matching hormones in our formative years. In addition, one of the things we are seeing with many gender fluid people, is an expansion and refinement to how they express their physiological breakdown and the patterns that are created from a gender specific hormonal cocktail. In general, these humans experience hormones the same way as folks with a traditional gender relationship, but their spiritual imprints hold completely different traditions and meanings for them.

It is the imprints of those specific traditions and meanings that we tend to emulate in our formative years and then attract or pursue in others as adults. These imprints create an affinity or conflict with our same sex parent and clear the way for karmic healing.

Karma of the Opposite Sex Parent

Many times in my life my father has sought to connect with me spiritually, but it wasn't until just a decade ago that I could really be open. Although I felt his subtle presence for years, I had very little physical memory of him. I also carried an enormous amount of grief for him. Both of these obscured my conscious connection to him.

One day, a decade ago, I was living in Los Angeles and sitting in a coffee shop waiting on a man I was dating. He was late, and as I looked down at my phone to check the time, I saw my father piercing through the veil and sitting on the chair across from me. He looked at me, gave me two thumbs up and a corny smile, and then disappeared. I burst into laughter. You see, my dad was quite a funny man and was known for his practical jokes and sarcasm, but I knew exactly what he meant. It was his acerbic disapproval of my coffee-date (who, incidentally, never showed). Dad was mockingly saying, "Good job!"

It is our relationship with the opposite gendered parent that delineates a whole host of our behaviors and feelings regarding how we relate to others, and our self-esteem and confidence to do so. Is the relationship we have with them conflicted or supportive? Are we embraced or rejected? Do we have many things in common or are we opposites? Do we communicate well or not at all? All of these factors, in addition to their presence, and time spent with us, will create an impact long into adulthood.

The opposite sex parent will greatly influence our relationships with our partners of the opposite sex, as we set up spiritual dynamics with them early in childhood. This can carry on into other significant adult relationships, especially romantic ones.

Being an empath, navigating romantic relationships has been a powerful, yet frustrating experience. I easily connect with people, whether in a sexual relationship or not, and know things about them from just being in their presence. It may come as a shock, but the boyfriends I've had haven't really liked that. It took me several years to master the information and my ability to hold the secrets of the people I most cared about.

It was natural for me to be immediately comfortable, confident, and openhearted in getting to know the object of my affection at a rate that didn't offer the same opportunity to my partner. I didn't need to be in their presence to feel their presence. Therefore, intimacy couldn't happen in a way that was comfortable for both of us. I didn't comprehend how to unlearn the information that would come to me when we were beginning to get to know one another.

As I spoke of earlier, there was a multilayered message of love linked together for me from the ancestors. It began with the original link from the jaguar—to my friend in spirit Daniel—to his cousin Miguel—to my father—and finally to the dream that portrayed the story of Tzon Halal and his beloved daughter, Xulab, locked in trauma for an eternity. I finally understood my comfort embracing a spiritual-telepathic relationship dynamic with people. After all, I had spent my entire childhood in a psychic relationship with my father and years later, after the grief for him had passed, the spiritual relationship dynamic had not. Now, I was being given the opportunity to break the cycle for all of us, by finding and embracing forgiveness.

Parent-Child Relationship Questionnaire

Take a few moments to contemplate these questions for yourself. It doesn't matter if your parents are living or deceased, you no longer have a relationship with them, you've never known them, or maybe you come from a blended family with multiple parents and step-parents. All of these circumstances are potent factors in how you relate with your lovers, so dig in.

1. What is your first childhood memory with your same sex parent? Why do you think it's valuable?

2. What is your first childhood memory with your opposite sex parent? Why do you think it's valuable?

3. What is your happiest memory with each parent? Why do you think it's valuable?

4. What is your worst memory with each parent? How do you think this impacts your romantic relationships?

5. What characteristics do you have in common with each parent? How do you think this impacts your romantic relationships?

6. In what ways do you differ from each parent? What would you like your parents to know about you?

Ancestral Karma

Ancestral karma is the culmination of ancestral family traits, behavior, and choices that do not get reconciled within the lives they were created. It consists of energy patterns passed down in DNA—or the familial traditions that move from generation to generation in a family line. It can show up as hereditary illness or shared proclivities, but also a soul can incarnate into the family line to help break the cycle of those hereditary dynamics.

Keep in mind that you have a biological family and a soul family. Your spiritual family consists of those souls with whom you have shared past-life experiences, or that you have many things in common, such as ideology, interests, and beliefs; you vibrate at a similar resonance or are from the same oversoul (a collective soul group in another dimension).

Many spiritualists have experienced sitting with a council of their spirit guides in another dimension, prior to incarnation on Earth, to decide where and with whom they would like to incarnate for the best learning advantage.

It is unimportant whether you believe your choices come from such an angelic encounter; or more simply—your vibrational resonance determines your attractions in life. Essentially, they are the same no matter where you conceptualize the beginning of the process. The biological family dynamic is vital to your spiritual education as is your soul family.

Family Dynamic Helps Prepare You for Life: Charles' Story

I worked with a manager, Charles, when I first arrived in Los Angeles. We met on the set of an infomercial that had the funniest crew I'd ever worked with. Charles had the best sense of humor, and we had a connection that revealed our similar spiritual imprints—and thus began our professional relationship.

A few years later we were developing a talk show about communication when he told me about his mother and family dynamic. He was born in the deep south in the early 1930s to a single mom, and he was the second youngest of his twenty-two siblings. We were all sharing childhood stories, and he blurted out:

"When my mother needed a break, she'd check herself in for a 72-hour hold at the local asylum."

To which we all laughed, including Charles. I sat for a moment and digested what he said.

"Are you serious? You seem serious."

"I do not tell a lie," he responded.

He began to speak about how much he owed his mother, and in retrospect, what an impossible job she had managing all twenty-two of his siblings (part of the family dynamic was that all the older children embraced responsibility for caring for the younger ones). Charles' mother was in her late forties when he was born in approximately 1935. We decided that he was made from the stuff of miracles and magic—a king in his own right.

Charles was around my mother's age, and I was deeply touched by our familial connection to mental illness and the refusal to accept any sort of stigma about it. He was very courageous in his forthright attitude. I figured if he could do that in his generation, I could certainly do it in mine. I learned that if I wanted to be of service to others, I was going to have to do the hard work of self-realization and healing—setting aside any fear, shame, or anger that I felt, as it really was time to leave it behind.

Charles' birthright created in him independence, confidence, compassion, people skills, negotiation skills, humor, determination, success, and longevity. All the elements he needed for his career in the entertainment industry and in his life—all he gave to others, including me. Even though Charles and I weren't related, he will always be an integral part of my spiritual family.

Ancestral Curse

An ancestral curse is a form of energy sent to teach a lesson. Either directly or indirectly, it is the presence of a pattern created from cultural habits or focused intent. No matter how it got started or why, we call this form an energetic construct. A family curse is an intended boundary to be realized by current and future generations. Let's say your uncle gets cursed by someone he wronged, and during the course of his life he doesn't make any changes to himself, or get the intended message. The curse will stay with his soul—or be transferred down to subsequent generations of his family who exhibit similar dynamics—until it can be reconciled. However, it can't affect anyone who doesn't have some form of resonance to it. It's called *agreement*.

In times of oppression, people use the energy they have in a way that is not discernible by everyone (usually the oppressors). Curses can be put upon specific families, groups, people, and concepts, and are revealed in the health, prosperity, and beliefs of those afflicted. However, those afflicted must agree to the curse. An agreement comes in the form of grief, guilt, anger, or a similar response to the nature of the energetic construct while having no conscious awareness of its presence.

Many years ago, I was called to a client's home to do a house clearing. She had just moved in with her fairly new boyfriend who lived way outside the city limits—on many levels. He was a low-level drug dealer, in addition to creating his own rooster farm—cultivating birds for professional cockfighting. My client Molly hadn't had a decent night's sleep since she moved in, and she was sure someone had put a curse on her.

The energy of the home was intense for many reasons, such as the dynamic of their relationship and the events that occurred on the property. But more than any of that, the energy in a back bedroom was so dense with darkness it was palpable. It hit me in the gut as I entered the room. There were boxes piled from floor to ceiling and no room to walk around. I turned and left, closing the door behind me—which suited me just fine.

After the initial assessment of the house and property, I set up the necessary crystal grid to begin the clearing of discordant energies, I went to the kitchen where my client was washing dishes. As we were speaking of the heaviness in the back room (the door was visible from where we stood), a swoosh of dark energy came barreling out of the room at us. We both ducked. Standing at the kitchen sink, our jaws dropped. We began to laugh; it was surreal. I saw the face of a woman wearing a conical hat. Yes, it was quite literally a witch on her broom! She moved so quickly, it created a black swoosh.

My client saw the face of her boyfriend's aunt, who was a known bruja in her community. We shifted the energy in the place and forced the bruja's energy out, by sending it back to her. Molly wasn't quite sure why her boyfriend's aunt didn't like her, but she was clear she had no interest in being bullied on any level anymore. I told Molly that the aunt believed she was a gold-digger and was seeking to protect her nephew.

My client laughed and said, "Well, I do like money—but I make my own."

After the clearing, Molly was able to sleep and had no more spiritual issues with her lover's family.

So, what is the magic of a curse? It is the moment a person understands the lesson the energy is meant to teach or inspire (in any incarnation). The afflicted person detaches from the energy. The construct that remains can be removed by a third party when the energy is no longer relevant. It's like a ghost that is fed by the behavior or dynamic at play. If there is no energy to feed the curse, it can dissipate over time and become listless and weak. But ultimately, it must be transformed or given back to the one who put it in place—in this case, the boyfriend's aunt.

The Ancestral Spiritual Patterns that Direct Disease and Congenital Defects

The presence of a long-held pattern of thinking and behavior that creates an imbalance for the physical body can manifest itself as disease. There has been much research in the past decade confirming that energy and emotion create an impact on how the physical body works. Each of our cells respond to all the elements of the climate that nurtures them.

If the climate is harsh and destructive, cells will adjust to this energy based on the person's willpower, physical ability to respond, or activated karmic patterns. Your karma can support getting or avoiding disease, or the strength with which you respond to it. In my family, cancer has been present in this and previous generations. I've made it a life mission not to have cancer, and to eradicate it on any level. I make efforts to grieve often, and address the things that give me pause, resistance, or conflict by discovering my honest feelings about them and then communicating those feelings if necessary. So far, I've been successful.

The object to healing is finding the source of discord and disinviting it. Cancer can be passed down from generation to generation, whether it is sourced from DNA—or the matter of spirit looking for expression or transformation. In my family, cancer was a note from both lineages on self-acceptance.

Cancer Never Wins: My Mother's Story

The spirit of my mother's cancer took a visit upon me one day, as it passed by in a maroon colored sedan...

Let me say first that my mother's self-worth—the view that who she was and what she needed didn't matter—was forged early in life. It was formed, in part, by a mother whose practical mind and low expectations for a woman's possibilities were a struggle for a creative young woman in the 1940s, in addition to a restrictive cultural view. My grandfather's contribution was the rampant rage, self-loathing, and self-centeredness that I believe invaded his life early on as well. It had been living in him since before my mother's birth. Certainly, that wasn't all he contributed; he was a good man at heart. But he was deeply troubled on many levels from the multiple traumas he'd experienced in his own life, and he had no way of managing all the pain.

The maroon colored vehicle was the curse of a broken promise to a little nine-year-old girl. As the story goes, my mother's father had committed to taking her to the movies early one Saturday afternoon. Even so, he started a project to transform his old vehicle with a new coat of maroon paint. Every time she reminded him of the promise, he became more focused—yet less productive—in his mission. Finally, he retired from it—only because the sun had gone down—not mentioning the movie again. My mother was so deeply disappointed and left with a feeling of unworthiness, the maroon colored paint became her trigger for remembering her father's rage.

Entertainment resources were limited in this small farming community and nothing was close by. This was probably the impetus for my mother's interest in singing, fashion, and—ultimately—bigger city living. Consequently, her talents, her need for self-expression, and all of her father's broken promises pushed her out of the house and into a full time job at the age of sixteen. Her father's mental illness and consistent violent rages became too much to tolerate; she left and never looked back. No doubt carrying, packed deep in her luggage, a belief that men should be feared, that her needs were only important to her, and that whatever she was to accomplish, she'd have to do on her own. Notions she sustained for the rest of her life.

Of course, there was love, loyalty, and certainly compassion to the degree there could be. But somewhere, somehow, something went wrong, and there was plenty of anger, sadness and pity to go around. At the end of the day, when you take away someone's choice—whether it's through not giving them one or their lack of fitness in making one—it leaves a deep well of pain and powerlessness for the entire family.

It wasn't until many years later I learned what a painful trigger seeing a maroon vehicle had been for my mother. It affected her with subtle anxiety every time she saw one, even to her last days.

Internal rage was one of the few things my mother and I had in common. So much so, only once did she and I ever flirt with doing battle. I don't remember exactly what we were arguing about but I'm sure it was fueled by our deep emotional divide—my extreme empathy and emotionalism, and her belief that showing emotion was weakness. In addition, I was sixteen and wise beyond my years. Or, maybe, I was just sixteen.

Either way, my mother got angry at my sarcastic retort to something she said and responded quickly with a hard whack on my upper arm. Unleashing the rage that flowed from the center of the earth up through my feet, without even a consideration, I smacked her back. Our eyes met—frozen in time—in a way I'd only seen between two lions in the wild on National Geographic. For the first time, I met my mother spirit-to-spirit; I saw directly what I'd always known was there. Then the moment passed, and that was the end of that.

Until a sunny afternoon, thirty years later, in Beverly Hills, California. Mother was in town, I was driving her up towards West Hollywood when a man in a maroon Miata sped by, darting in front of me, forcing me to stop short.

In frustration, I honked and called him a name in my normal car tone. My mother's reaction, however, shocked me. She once again whacked my hand as hard as she could, but this time I saw the deep and abiding fear in her eyes, and I felt only compassion. I looked at her, and calming my voice, I asked her what was wrong. She said she was sure the guy would attack us. I laughed and told her not to worry: "I can take that motherfucker, easy." Whether it was from relief—or my freedom to use a well-pointed curse word—she laughed, and the crisis was averted.

Flash forward several years, my mother was diagnosed with lung cancer which spread to the brain and lead to her death nine months later. As I spoke about in volume two of this series, I'd been alerted to my mother's pending illness in several ways in the two years preceding her diagnosis—including a tipsy chat with her over margaritas one night. She told me I would need to take care of her. I passed it off as a *when I get old* conversation. But two years later, when the diagnosis came, I understood the following days would be her last.

One night near the end, mom was watching television from the hospital bed we'd moved into the den. I sat with her, reading a book, when her drunk husband entered the room. Coming up behind the chair I was sitting in, he began to yell and scream at me, attempting to further a conflict I'd successfully quashed fifteen minutes before. He had been yelling at me to get off of the phone. In his inebriation, it hadn't occurred to him I was on a professional call.

None of his behavior was rational—and no doubt it was grief driven—but regardless, I wasn't participating. So, when he came in yelling at me, I turned to look at him with the force of an army and said, "You will not continue to speak to me this way."

My tone was calm, but my vigor was unwavering. He stopped, looked at me, waived his hands in the air, and said, "Oh, balls!"

He walked out of the room, not to be heard from again for the rest of the night.

I have to admit, his response made me laugh. Because, who says that? But, as I looked over at my mother, she had this look of fear, then laughter, and then gratitude. It was in those moments, I finally understood that no one had ever championed her. Twenty years with an alcoholic had taken its toll, and now she was done. She had lived with those angry outbursts, triggered repeatedly, which had caused her emotional retreat from the relationship and sealed her fate.

I'd had no idea how much she was suffering. Mom was prone to keeping her feelings to herself, but that night, she looked satisfied. Someone had put the bully in his place, and I was happy to have been the one to do it.

While my mother and I were kindred spirits when it came to appreciating solitude, we were opposites regarding addressing the pain in our lives openly and deliberately. My mother was made of strong stock. She never told me what to do (except to clean my room). She valued me as a person and respected my unique outlook by never judging or making fun of me (a trait our family was famous for). Those last nine months together, I was able to offer her some peace by showing her faith—experiencing with her our telepathy. I introduced her to the multi-dimensional world; one that she'd been afraid did not exist.

Our family patterns—whether they be putting off honest communication and living in fear or looking at emotion as weakness—must be transformed and transmuted to a new life force that can change how our body responds. This won't necessarily dictate the absence of illness, as it is one of our most powerful teachers, but we must learn to be empowered in it.

Regardless of the body's survival, it is the peaceful spirit that can move on. My mother, on some level, was ready to transition, and cancer was the way to take all of us through the process of getting on board. I am certain of that. It's why she gave me advance warning. During the last few days of her transition, she was delighted. Her body was in bed and at peace, and her spirit danced about the house like never before—joyful, loving, and free.

Karmic Romance

A karmic romance is a non-platonic experience we have with a partner that is based in our unconscious spiritual patterns. Often they are marked by an intense sexual and emotional attraction and can run hot and burn out fast. These relationships are strong teachers about attachment and connection. For those with whom we share a sexual intimacy, we also share pieces of our spirit.

We can receive much subliminal information through the intimate sexual dynamic, which often occurs prematurely, prior to actually knowing much about the person and their current life conditions and circumstances. Once we've gotten to know our romantic partner a little better in the physical world, we may find that we have no compatibility, matching values, or we just don't like the people we find them to be.

Whatever the case, there is always purpose in such relationships. In the beginning portion of the relationship, we are apt to learn what we most love in ourselves by seeing that mirrored in some way in our partner; conversely, towards the end of the relationship, we become witness to what we most dislike about ourselves. Often, these karmic encounters will bring out and support the worst in us, either in triggering previous loss and grief, or behaviors we have a difficult time curbing or mastering. Sometimes, they provoke us to treat our partner or ourselves with disrespect.

Of course, not all karmic romances are star-crossed or steeped in loss. However, the relationship must move through its power-struggles (which is usually the purpose), transforming into a relationship that is balanced, communicative, and serves the needs of both parties—hopefully with love to spare. Rest assured that the karmic love-rush will give way to a deeper—and at times—more mundane bond. This is the point at which many people give up on the relationship because they interpret the shift in intensity to mean an absence of feeling or love.

"WE CANNOT DIRECT THE WIND, BUT WE CAN ADJUST THE SAILS."[1]

– BERTHA CALLOWAY

Soulmates: Sheila's Story

I received a call from a client one day, asking for a session. I'd not spoken with Sheila in almost a decade. She claimed she'd found her Twin Flame (a soulmate with whom—and for whom—you connect on all levels and have an abiding unconditional love). She was anxious to bring him in for a past-life session. We set the appointment for the next day. She was so excited to introduce him to me. I do a lot of counseling with couples, but rarely do they call because things are going well—most of the time it is to work through a karmic pattern.

They arrived at the appointed time and quickly sat down. Sheila began to explain that they'd met three days before and it was love at first site. As it turned out, her new love didn't have a place to stay so he'd been living with her since they met. In spite of all the love they felt—they weren't getting along. Jack was twenty-five and Sheila was ten years his senior.

Like Sheila, though, he too was feeling intense emotion in the union. He usually experienced a lot of insecurity in relationships, but the confidence he experienced with Sheila even surprised him. However, notably, he was less attached to the idea that they would be together and was more along for the ride. Conversely, it was clear that Sheila had spent a lot of time in contemplation of what it would feel like to meet her beloved, and this experience matched all her expectations.

At this juncture, my goal was to encourage them to let go of their ideas of where the relationship would go and focus on what they were doing together now. We walked through a few questions, and once they were comfortable and the nervousness they'd walked in with had subsided, we began the past-life session.

As they opened their eyes from the past-life visualization, both Sheila and Jack had tears in their eyes. Both of them recalled a few different past lives together but the one that unearthed the most matching memory, was a life in which Sheila was Jack's mother. The life took place in the early 1900s in the United States, somewhere in Middle America. They lived on a homestead with the other members of their family; Jack was the youngest of eight siblings.

Sheila was being forced to contend with her past-life grief and devastation, in this meeting with Jack—today. In their life before, Sheila had been giving her three-year-old daughter (the spirit that was Jack currently) a bath, and she drowned in the bathtub while her mother looked away for only a moment.

Sheila, unconsciously, had so much guilt from that loss that upon meeting Jack in this life, all she wanted to do was take care of him, be with him, help him. And the only way all that love made sense to her was to be lifelong partners. After the session was complete, they both felt lighter. Sheila felt a calm that had eluded her for the past 72 hours.

She called me the following week to report that it was over between her and Jack. A few days after the session they decided to just be friends, and she hadn't spoken with him since—a common outcome to a karmic relationship. Two people in a karmic reunion come together to resolve an energetic conflict; once resolved, everyone can easily go their separate ways. No attachment and no guilt—only love.

Incompatibility In A Karmic Relationship

Incompatibility in a spiritual bond is often immediately overlooked at the beginning. You find it endearing when your partner holds views and values that don't align with your own. Of course opposites attract, but can they stay together?

I've always loved a good debate or a fun adventure, but there is a fine line between a person who is interesting, passionate, and will take a risk with care—and a person who needs to participate in high risk behavior.

What is the difference between *compatibility* and *karma*?

- **People who seek conflict:** A person who seeks conflict oftentimes sees the world through a personal lens. This means everything is happening to him/her. Life cannot be peaceful if it's happening to you. Inviting this person into your life requires a prerequisite of extraordinary communication and boundary skills. Choosing this person is *karmic*.

- **People who lack self-awareness:** Folks who are unaware of their deeper feelings or what drives their behavior often create conflict as a spiritual way to understand themselves. Not that they deliberately seek it, but that it is, in fact, the outcome of their lack of self-awareness. This phase of development isn't necessarily who you are, but where you are in the process. Of course, we all lack self-awareness regarding some aspects of ourselves—so a person's attitude to self-understanding and change is paramount to their relationship fitness. This is a *compatibility* issue.

- **Someone who takes your inventory:** This person is actually in the best place to have a breakthrough if they stay engaged in the process of understanding. If they're only interested in looking at what you're doing and how it makes them feel, there may be some challenges to this relationship. Choosing this relationship, in this condition, is *karmic*.

- **A person who focuses on money:** This person is seeking to create stability on some level in their life. People who are generous with money or give it easily, can sometimes be manipulated, if they're not careful. On the other hand, a person who is stingy or withholds money has experienced lack or has been taken advantage of in some way and is looking for safety through the control of their finances. Choosing this relationship is often *karmic*.

We are all human and imperfection is our specialty. It's our purpose in life to learn and grow while cultivating a stellar attitude. It is possible to mold harmony out of conflict, raise fear into joy, and transform confusion into clear cut boundaries and communication. Letting others be exactly who they are is a sign that you accept, love, and embrace yourself—that you will create lots of good karma.

The Warrior's Hidden Motto: Trust No One

The warrior's most valuable tool is trust: trusting oneself, others, and the Universe. However, trust can often come at a price—at least that's the message many will take from their karma. The truth is, when we begin to recognize the flow of information that the many spiritual patterns bring us, we begin to bear witness to the subtle occurrences that happen before a big event takes place.

Trust doesn't dictate that bad things don't happen; trust paves the way out of them if they do. Likewise, it's not your karma or your fault that something bad happens to you. If you have been victimized—it is the perpetrators' choice, and therefore, their fault. Things happen to us to stretch our hearts to bleed more compassion. Some hearts, in the face of tragedy, pendulum all the way to the other side and harden just a little more. This is all before they're once again brought back to their natural state of empathy and compassion—with the applied pressure of lifetimes of experience to guide them.

The most important thing about trust? If you will open up to it, it will show you the best possible path to get you where you need to go.

> Anger and blame are truth seekers, not healers. If you'll embrace your souls deepest desire to heal, your spirit will lead you through the pain to the freedom and forgiveness of an open heart.

Drama Equals Trauma

I hosted a healing group one time and a man I was dating attended. We were just getting to know one another—he wasn't a big believer of metaphysical philosophy, but deeply connected to spirit. Everyone was taking turns sharing their week when a woman, out of turn, started screaming and crying. We were all a little startled; I turned to her and asked what was happening. She continued crying while pointing at another woman across the room. I took a deep breath, encouraging her to calm down, and asked her if she could wait until it was her turn. (This technique was a part of the boundary setting that was often needed in the group.) She quieted.

Just as soon as the next person started, she began to cry and hyperventilate, holding her throat. My date turned to her and said, in a solid, firm-yet-calm voice:

"Hey, are you okay? Is this a 911 situation? Because I will call them for you."

She looked at him and became silent and the tears stopped, as if surprised that someone was concerned—then shared when it was her turn.

I was impressed with my date. He didn't diminish her in any way and showed concern, going directly to the core of *Are you safe?* —keeping to the parameters of the group which were: everyone gets to speak and deserves to speak uninterrupted. Unless, of course, there was a physical emergency.

Oftentimes, the folks who seem addicted to drama or a negative perspective are just having a completely different experience than others in the situation—no less important or valuable, but definitely different. This is very common in a karmic relationship.

I'd like to relieve you of the term *drama* or the idea of being *too negative* when it comes to interrelationship dynamics. It quickly diminishes the concern at hand, and when you seek to lessen the impact of something for which you do not have all of the information, it disables you from getting that information accurately.

Instead of *drama* or *negativity*, let's use the word trauma. Any sort of drama a person expresses is sourced from some level of trauma: past or present. People like to resort to terms like *crazy*, *messy*, or *dramatic* because it's easy. It's common in relationships to project pain onto a partner when they are not the cause.

Actually, when this happens, you can take it as a compliment. Seriously, if someone is projecting their pain onto your relationship with them, they are doing it for one of two reasons.

First, they feel safe with you. People who have lived through tumultuous experiences or abuse of some sort have difficulty expressing it, unless and until they feel safe.

Don't get me wrong, I'm not saying, "Hey, it's okay they treat you like a jerk; they feel safe. Take one for the team, bro."

What I am saying is their experience of safety and trust in you allows them to dig a little deeper into the landmine wounds of their soul—consciously or unconsciously. This, in the land of human transformation, is a glorious momentous occasion and opportunity for healing.

The second reason: when people first come together they meet spirit to spirit. For many couples this spiritual introduction is unconscious and can be karmic in nature. It is the presence of *reaction* and the illusion of *drama* that let you know there is a deeper meeting of the spirit. I call it the 50/50 Rule.

THE 50/50 RULE

"THE OPERATING RULE OF THUMB AS THE BURGEONING INDEPENDENCE GROWS INSIDE OF YOU, AND ULTIMATELY IN YOUR RELATIONSHIPS, IS CALLED THE 50/50 RULE. IT'S THE UNDERSTANDING THAT EVERYTHING THAT YOU ENCOUNTER ON EVERY LEVEL—FROM THOUGHTS, FEELINGS, EXPERIENCES, AND EVENTS—IS SOMEHOW CONNECTED TO YOU, AND YOU CONTRIBUTE HALF OF THEIR PURPOSE. THE IDEA IS THAT YOU NEED THE WAY THINGS ARE HAPPENING IN YOUR LIFE AT ANY GIVEN TIME, AS DO THE PEOPLE WITH WHOM YOU PARTICIPATE. THE INTENSITY WITH WHICH YOU SPEAK TO SOMEONE IS A DIRECT RESULT OF THEIR DENSITY AND VICE VERSA."[2]

– HEAL YOUR SOUL HISTORY:
ACTIVATE THE TRUE POWER OF YOUR SHADOW

The Slayer's Dilemma: Blame

Personal accountability is sexy. Nobody likes to have the finger pointed at them, especially when every person who has contributed to a situation has accountability towards its outcome. This is a spiritual perspective, and very valuable to embrace, especially nowadays, when suing over ridiculous matters is so popular and prevalent. People aren't looking for accountability; more often than not, they're looking for a payday or to soothe their own trauma or guilt in some way. By all means, I know there are careless people and corporations who— if no one takes them to account—won't be held accountable. It's possible that being personally accountable comes with holding others responsible as well.

When Blame Raises It's Ugly Head

However, in karmic relationships, the one playing the blame game will never really find happiness as they will never fully experience their own power. They are giving it away, with the blame, to someone else. When understanding blame from a broader perspective, it's imperative to contemplate how, as a society, people's actions are guided by factors such as non-existent boundaries, convenience, expense and money, and fear. Following, are some options for you to consider when the beast of blame rears its ugly head.

Look at the Big Picture

When it comes to putting the blame on only one person in a situation, the facts of the matter just never prove true. Every physical world event has a series of choices that were made by a series of people that contributed to creating it. Those choices were influenced by many people and experiences. Focusing the blame on one person is only a deterrent to the resolution or completion you're seeking by pointing your finger in the first place.

Look a Little Deeper

Every physical world event has a genealogy—a family history. Every choice is made or influenced by a series of people. Take an event that's important to you. Sit down and write out all of the people that touched or influenced the deciding factors resulting in that event. Begin with the incident itself and its decision makers, and then go back further in time chronicling everything from why the people involved may have done what they did to the influences on their life. More healing and resolution will come from understanding this history than blame can ever manifest.

Be True to Yourself

Anger and blame always go hand in hand. While they're present, the truth will often be obscured. For instance, people tend to blame the last person to make a choice in a situation, believing they are the cause of the event—an unfortunate position indeed.

While having an object on which to focus your anger is often satisfying for a little while, the satisfaction doesn't last and reveals the inevitable sorrow underneath. Grief, and the expression of that sorrow, is the hero in this story. Accept the loss (or the change) the event created, and grieve it's passing. Allowing yourself the process of mourning—consciously changing how you conduct your life in a manner the event has dictated—is the only way.

What Bitterness Brings

I worked with a woman once who caught her husband cheating. She was rightfully angry, but to her own detriment, she was stuck in the bitterness and resentment of the betrayal. I did my best to encourage her to understand that her resentment towards her husband only hurt herself. He'd moved on, and it was this that was the most painful for her. She'd been using her resentment to stay connected to him.

After we spoke, she cried out of sadness—instead of self-pity and anger—for the first time. Her grief cleared the way for her to accept that the man she'd married didn't (and couldn't) love her in the way she wanted. From that point on, the divorce went smoothly, and she's now in a relationship that brings her enormous joy.

Having gone through the process, she has the opportunity for freedom from anger, bitterness, and resentment. Most importantly, she has freedom from attachment to the people, places, and things that brought her suffering—allowing love and forgiveness to easily take their place.

Anger is the Truth Seeker

I want to be clear that there is a righteous place for anger to exist and a real purpose for it. Anger is the energy that brings your awareness to things you may not have perceived previously—about yourself and others—and is the precursor for grief. Grief can't come if there is no real knowledge of the truth about what has been lost, and that won't happen fully without genuine emotional process.

You aren't served by pointing your anger at another. It's easy for the target of your rage to tune you out, and then your attempt to jolt them into awareness or accountability is not successful. Know that silence spawns the real truth. Being tranquil creates a space for the other person to become present to the error of their ways—if it's possible for them to do so. Anger and blame are truth seekers, not healers. If you'll embrace your soul's deepest desire to heal, your spirit will lead you through pain to the freedom and forgiveness that serene communication can bring.

How Karma is Revealed in a Partnership

Look, everybody has issues. So when it comes down to unwanted habits in a karmic partnership, there are two categories. The first category is the *danger zone*: a person who is dangerous to themselves or others, or just too selfish to really consider another's well-being. The second category is the *incompatibility zone*: a person who is seeking conflict with one who seeks self-awareness and harmony.

A person's past will tell you a lot about their future. Of course people can change and they certainly don't have to live as a hostage to their previous life experiences, but oftentimes they do. Making changes within yourself takes an enormous amount of work, time, and energy.

Many people don't have access to the information or assistance they need to find positive coping strategies. Some ways of coping are negotiable, and others are deal breakers. If you or your partner have been abused, betrayed, or unloved in any way, it can make a new love difficult. However, with the right support, you can negotiate your way through.

The way a person has related to their life experiences and been supported in coping gives indications of how they are likely to engage in a relationship with you. The alternative to change is to accept people as you are receiving them in the moment.

Isn't that a gem? To accept someone as they are?

You must be willing to recognize the subtle communications we all make as we meet and get acquainted. Danger Zone dynamics, in this context, have the potential to be literally life threatening. Incompatibility habits are the anti-namaste experience: the God in me does not see the God in you.

Addiction

In the beginning of a relationship, an addict will always tell you who they are, either directly or indirectly. Remember that, always. It is imperative that you listen to your gut instinct—your subtle good or bad feelings that get your attention when someone is saying or doing something that reveals information about them or the situation that will be important for you to have. A sociopath I dated told me on the very first date exactly who he was. My intuition showed me the moment over and over again in my mind, but being enamored as I was, I put the subtle presence of his habit aside for later review.

Abuse Patterns

Someone who has opinions about you or your behavior as early as the first date, or who needs to know what you are doing and who you are doing it with—within the first month—can be an indication of someone with control issues.

As you become sexually active, take heed of a partner who won't use birth control or condoms. Sexual coercion and intimate partner abuse are more common every day. When a lover wants to get pregnant immediately or wants you to get pregnant immediately, it is a sign of control that can easily be misconstrued as love.

Other potential abuse revealers are statements like "That guy cut me off on the road so I followed him for five miles," or "They made me so mad I popped them in the mouth." Any indication of violence without the concern for the impact on others, having no remorse, or the presence of complete entitlement are views that you might not be interested in for your new significant other.

Low Self-Esteem

Stories of self-sabotage by a partner who starts a conversation with "My last DUI...," or "Nobody likes me," or finally, any indication of self-harm are signposts to needed help beyond which you can give in a romantic or familial relationship. However, it's common for these folks to hold you emotionally hostage and to keep you engaged in the relationship.

What they've done to others, they will do to you. People who cheat on their lovers do it because of their own fears and insecurities in a relationship. If they are unable to talk about sexual or intimate emotional needs, it may be easier for them to cheat than to speak to you about what they want. The biggest red flag in this arena is someone who will justify their cheating or blame it on you or their previous partner.

Being a Caretaker

This is the most frequently engaged type of karmic relationship. It draws on a person's desire to nurture but usually ends up enabling one or both of its participants in not being accountable for the circumstances in their life.

I saw an elderly lady on the street the other day pushing a cart; I'll call her Betty. On the cart, Betty had at least fifty plastic grocery bags filled with stuff. They were tied together, then tied to the cart. Betty had taken great care not to over pack any bag so that it could sustain the weight it carried. I was really quite impressed with her strategy and organization. I thought to myself, *that really is how we all are*—carrying our baggage from relationship to relationship. Some with more bags, some with less. Some bags filled to the gills and others with plenty of room for more.

Now, all those bags could have been filled with the cash from her 401k, but I suspect they were filled with things that had personal value to her. In time, they would be discarded when they were no longer useful or when space was needed to carry new things. It's the same way in karmic partnerships: romantic or platonic.

We all come with baggage, and frankly, if one partner has more bags than the other, it makes finding common ground difficult. This is the concern of a connection based in caretaking. Can you help your partner with their inventory? If you or your partner barely made it out of a previous relationship with your sanity or worse, you'll want to take time and be clear about entering into this dynamic.

Sexual Proclivities Outside Your Value System

I have counseled numerous people who were requested by a date, or a short or long-term partner, to engage in sexual behaviors for which they had no interest: threesomes, bondage and discipline, sadomasochism, and multiple sex-partners. All of whom reluctantly participated because their relationship was threatened if they didn't. Indulging in your sexuality any way you please is perfect when you have a conscious, willing partner that has the same desires. If you want an open relationship, negotiate it up front. I find that creating an open relationship down the line is usually an indication that the relationship may be over.

How to Manage a Karmic Relationship

In order for someone to heal they must first acknowledge that there is something to be healed (or brought into balance). A person can't fix what they won't face. The next step is forgiveness. If your partner can't forgive their previous relationships, they won't completely trust you. So, the first order of business is to recognize what the problems were and find their origins. This is something you must do for yourself.

Remember, it's not over till it's over. If you or your ex-partner still suffer or have strong feelings around your previous relationship, consider that if you enter a new relationship, you're inviting somebody in as a third party—specifically when it comes to the energy and emotion of the new union. Jealousy won't help, it just alerts you to the situation—the presence of that third energetic connection. As a third party, it's important to understand both sides of the dynamic at work. If you don't know how it was put together, you can't take it apart.

Your goal is to steer clear of participating in the same way as you have in other situations, and that takes practice. In a relationship like this, it's important to be willing and able to encourage your partner to talk about what happened and to listen to one another. Hear what is—and is not—being said. Most of all: don't take sides, consider both sides. Put yourself in both positions and consider what you would do and did do in similar circumstances; that way, you have a clearer understanding of the mechanics. This is something that lovers have difficulty with when they're juggling their own pain.

Make no mistake about it—frustration, anger, control and trust issues, all stem from unresolved hurt and trauma. Most of the time, especially in a new relationship, it's not what you've done that causes a conflict, it's what your partner fears you will do based on their experience with others. Your new partner may overreact one night when you say you're going out with your friends. A common response is to get pissed-off, leave, and deal with the fallout later.

I don't recommend it. It's much more efficient to address it directly by asking questions. For example, your lover doesn't want you to go out for fear you'll meet someone else your attracted to—and yes, you might. The issue isn't who you will meet, it's what you will do when you meet them. If you are not yet monogamous with your friend and want to be, you've got to address that. If you are monogamous, they've got to find a way to trust you, and you've got to be trustworthy. It's necessary to take a risk and be honest, even if it means you and your partner go in different directions.

In our karmic connections, there are bags we see and ones we don't. I wish everyone was as obvious as Betty, but they're not. Asking someone who is still reeling from the conflict of another relationship to be patient is a triumphant thought, but not necessarily realistic. So, if you're the one with the objectivity, then you are the one that holds the responsibility to communicate, set firm boundaries, and love unconditionally.

New relationships are full of disagreements about small things, their existence eludes to more important needs underneath. You can communicate in a neutral firm tone how you feel, or you can fight. It comes down to your ability to hear with empathy and compassion and be clear on your limits. It's imperative to be able to set a boundary with sincere emotion and then back it up with an action.

It's easy to get angry at not being valued or respected, but getting angry never helps. It just allows your partner to make you and your anger the problem. Nine times out of ten, the person just didn't give their missteps much thought. You are now giving them the opportunity to reflect and consider you differently.

Being able to see another's problems objectively is always easier than seeing your own. You can't help someone else if you haven't been able to help yourself. If I had a dime for every client who sat disgruntled on my couch going through a break-up, angry they just spent years of their life preparing their beloved to be the love of someone else's life. That feeling is tough medicine to swallow. If that's you—you're in no position to help anyone else. Not even for love.

Love means being ready, willing, and able to see your deepest inner pain or joy, and to embrace it head on. Sometimes helping another means letting them witness your vulnerability, your trust, your joy, and your pain—showing them how it is, instead of telling them how it should be. Most of all, show up and be fully present—or be honest when you are unable. Love while you can and be truthful when you can't.

> "To be deeply loved by someone gives you strength, but to love someone deeply gives you courage."[3]
>
> – Esther Huertas

The Slayer's Motto: I Carry on the Traditions that Make Sense

The family traditions, relationship habits, and personal behaviors that guide our lives were all created at some point for our safety, survival, or a belief that was held for our well-being—whether or not they were born of an absolute truth, or just something we believed suited us for a period of time. As we grow and expand our understanding of our world, our power in it, and our humanity, these same traditions become outdated, and our circumstances change.

Having said that, it's common for your community, friends, or family to consider you disloyal at the prospect of changing those same traditions, habits, and behaviors. Peer pressure is one of the main reasons people don't change, but change you must. It is an inherent part of life.

Dating Outside of Your Spiritual Patterns

Boundaries are the key to any good relationship. How graceful and articulate a person is in setting and respecting them, is a valuable skill set. One of the things I hear often from people is the consciousness of time. How they spend it, feel a lack of it, or don't want to waste it. I read in a guy's dating profile: "I don't play games. So, one strike and you're out!"

While time is important, it's essential to leave a potential lover feeling optimistic about getting to know you. After all, if you've chosen a date, hopefully you'll be able to let go of time—at least for the time the event warrants.

However, before we move to the end of the rendezvous, let's take a quick look at how it started. Nine times out of ten, if you've been deliberate in choosing your date, there shouldn't be any big surprises. Did you pay attention to your inner voice while communicating? Did you feel comfortable in sharing information, and did your potential match easily share with you? Last, and most importantly, did you get their last name?

Yes, you heard right. I know it sounds simple, but you'd be surprised how many people are willing to meet someone they've met online—only knowing their first name. Look, any good employer is going to check your social media before they invite you to an interview, and dating is the same way. It's an interview: for a friend, lover, or partner. It allows you to get to know the deeper layers of a person, especially when you have a tendency to choose karmic relationships. The way to work yourself out of the pattern is get as much information about the person from multiple sources, and let them know you're doing it. A background check isn't out of the question.

Every date is unique: coffee date, lunch date, athletic date, happy hour date or dinner date. Each of them have an implied time frame. For example, you'd expect to spend 30–45 minutes having coffee. If you've done your homework—trusted your gut and done a little background check—and still decided to meet someone, honor that by showing up and getting to know the person a bit, even if there isn't any immediate gratification. Respect that they've taken time out of their day to spend with you, as well. In the following paragraphs I offer some ways to act outside your spiritual patterns in different dating situations.

You're having a great time: You're having a magical time on your first coffee date—but don't be afraid to end the date when you're having a great time. Remember the first few dates are setting up the energy and the flow of the relationship. If you spend a lot of time at the beginning because it's a blast, but won't be able to sustain that same time expenditure in a few months, set the boundary now and leave them wanting more. Let them know what a great time you had and that you look forward to seeing them again.

Friends are good to have: Let's say you show up for your date and there doesn't seem to be the spark you had in your phone or online communications. The person is circling the friend zone. That's okay. It could be a temporal stressor and they may not want to give you the details, or they could be nervous and shy. It's completely appropriate to ask how they're doing and mean it. If honest conversation doesn't bring out that mojo you were hoping for, and they're still in the friend zone at the end of the date, consider this: it could take multiple dates to get the comfort level both people need to become intimate on any level. Be honest and suggest having a friendship before going further.

If you're bored, you're boring: You show up for your happy-hour date and within 15 minutes you are bored out of your mind. The truth is, while your date may be quiet or uninteresting, you really just don't feel like doing the work to make the date interesting. Possibly, you have a lot on your mind and are finding it difficult to focus. Again, it's a great opportunity to ask yourself why? No date or experience with another human is ever a waste. Make sure you get all the learning you can from your experience.

Engage with compassion: You arrive and your match is late. When they finally arrive, they are completely nervous, and it's making you uncomfortable—and they look nothing like their photo. This is the bummer trifecta. My advice is: stay. Take stock of why you're uncomfortable and have some compassion for your new acquaintance. Most often we have attractions towards others because they mirror us in some way. If you were attracted during your communications, there is a reason. It's a natural response to point out the things you don't like about someone—because they're most certainly the things you don't like about yourself. If you go in knowing this, not only can you grow as a person and glean some valuable information about yourself, but letting go of your judgment may just clear the way to having a good time.

Every reason to leave: The only reasons you should arrive at a date and promptly leave: if your date has obviously lied to you, is acting erratically, or you feel in danger. In that case, worrying about their feelings isn't relevant. You can feel free to say, "I'm sorry, I just can't spend this time with you today." Then leave out the back door if you have to. I do have to say I've only had to escape a date once. I mean, even the guy who lied and said he was 40 when he was 60—and pounded four beers in thirty minutes—was enjoyable and interesting for 45 minutes. When he asked if I'd see him again, I smiled and said, "No." We both chuckled, and parted ways.

Of course, you've heard you should never burn a bridge as you may need to cross it one day. I was instant messaging with a guy one time—it was a holiday—and about the third sentence in our first communication he asked me what I'd done that day. I responded that my cat was sick, and I'd spent the day caring for him. His response floored me.

"I'm allergic. This relationship is so over."

Don't get me wrong, I get where he was coming from. The truth is, not every person we meet will be a friend or a lover. But we need all kinds of relationships: colleagues, clients, connections. Most importantly, treating others with goodness supports us on every level.

Learning to engage with others beyond your fears, beyond negative or positive expectations, and beyond unwanted habits is necessary. It becomes a new opportunity in getting to know yourself, testing yourself, reinventing yourself, and being yourself with an audience—and, just maybe, learning how to be compassionate towards others. Embracing these fortuities paves the path to making new friends and relations in ways that we didn't have before technology. Being willing to take people as they are, and give them value, can only bring the same back to you.

Helping Friends with Karmic Relationships

Relationships and personalities are a balance no matter which direction you're coming from. You've probably learned this by now: life isn't fair but it will be even. Not everyone will like you, but some will adore you beyond words. There truly is a reason for everything. When and if you don't like someone, somewhere in your spirit you have a deeper connection to whatever it is you don't like.

So when it comes to tolerating or making friends with your friend's partner—it's a balance, like any other relationship. It's not uncommon to feel jealous or protective when your friend has a new alliance. But be wary. Your feelings are your responsibility, as is your intuition and your actions. Your friend's choices are theirs alone.

If your friend's mate makes you feel uncomfortable, it's important to ask yourself why. Do they trigger you about an issue that you have? Are you recognizing abusive or selfish tendencies? Maybe you know they are cheating or they've approached you in some way. Whatever the case, saying something is a commitment and can cost you the relationship.

If you find, with further reflection, that your discomfort is generated from an issue that you have, this may not be time or place to work it out. However, what if you find that the person in question is indeed questionable? Then it may be important enough to risk your relationship.

Remember that your friend is fulfilling their destiny by making their own choices, and it may or may not be appropriate to intervene. Or, more accurately, you may not be able to intervene, as it's your friends spiritual pattern in play and seeking to interrupt it may only alienate them. Consider asking them what they would do if they knew a friend was being cheated on? And, would they want to know?

There is a difference between a person who hasn't yet learned how to do things in a positive way and a person who has criminal tendencies. Many criminals lack empathy and don't care about the impact he/she has on other people. If you feel their mate doesn't have their best interest in mind, tell them you care for them and the things you see their lover doing you feel are hurting them. List each one as you see it. If you believe your friend is in danger, say something. A growing and expanding human being, caught up in a karmic dynamic, may not believe or consider that they have a choice in the way they achieve their goals.

If, for some reason, you don't see a future for your friend and their new mate, whether to say something is always a tough choice. Remember this: it's none of your business, unless you perceive them to be in imminent danger. What's important for you and what's valuable to your friend may be completely different. Your friend has chosen their lover for a reason, even if it's not obvious to you.

Be careful here; I've seen friendships end over: "I just don't see you two together long-term."

Don't fret. If the real problem for you is being witness to your friend's suffering in some way, you are free not to do so. If you love your friend but don't care for their lover, try to find common ground. Often, we don't like others when we don't feel comfortable to be ourselves around them, or we change who we are in front of them. Work on that. Be yourself. Be kind, and the common ground will emerge. Remember the adage "Water seeks its own level?" If you're connected to them on any level, there is something that is resonant and a reason you are there.

Handling Deep Attractions to People Who Are Already Coupled

What if you find yourself attracted to someone who's already taken, and they're flirting back? This is where you may be inclined to use destiny as an excuse—don't. Maybe you are feeling an undying eternal love connection to your friend or family member's lover. If that's the case, it can wait. You've got an eternity.

Sometimes we have soulmate relationships in which the circumstances are meant to teach the difference between love and attraction. The deep soul love you may feel for your friend's mate may be the very teacher you need to learn respect, honor, and unconditional love for yourself or another. And trust me, those are hard won lessons that activate the deepest personal power you have.

To sum it all up: unless there is a circumstance that can result in physical harm, your friend's partner is not your business. Tread lightly on their desire for your opinion, and be willing to witness their journey with an open heart. When you master yourself and recognize that the true source of your power is unconditional love, you no longer focus on the injustice in life but the fulfillment that comes from its continual bounty.

Mental Illness and Karma

As a spiritualist, I believe all mental illness is spiritual illness first—it's been left overlooked and unhealed. Mental illness is unprocessed pain from another time. Until western philosophy embraces the hidden spiritual component of treating mental illness there will continue to be a great divide between treating symptoms and healing souls. Our culture, in general, tends to create the illusion that we must feel happy and joyful all the time—supporting the idea that feeling and expressing pain makes you weak. If you feel bad, medicate yourself and feel better.

With spiritual illness existing on both sides of my family, and being prone to anxiety and depression myself (in addition to being psychic), it always felt safer to hide my symptoms and my story. I had no interest in a diagnosis or medication. I always preferred to treat any symptoms holistically. What I came to learn from keeping my experiences to myself was that grief, depression, and anxiety are a natural part of the spiritual process of expansion. Doing your spiritual work and reconciling your karma is a profound, sometimes difficult experience that takes work, focus, and assistance.

I'm not anti-medication; I think there's a place for it, for some. For most, however, it can impede the spiritual healing process that is the impetus for emotional transformation. I am not suggesting that one should go against their doctor's orders. What I am saying is that no matter how you choose to handle your symptoms, you must get help and do the work of healing. The more you grieve the loss and pain at the origin of the spiritual pattern, it will make it easier to modify any behaviors set in motion as a response. Doing those things, over time, changes the brain and its chemicals—and its signals to you. Once you've done that, you'll have a different body, and your diagnosis may need to be re-examined. I've seen it happen several times with clients. Conversely: lifelong mental illness is karma for some.

Regardless of your choice on the matter, being informed and self-aware of your soul imprints and the spiritual dimensions around you is paramount to deepening your understanding of all things. Spiritually speaking, the point at which you are unable to be accountable for your actions, and you become a risk to yourself or others, is the point at which you must consider medication. Mental health patterns can be layered over time and are made up of ungrieved spiritual trauma.

It's a common misconception that spirituality is equated with religious beliefs. They are very different. Our society has left it to religious organizations to educate spiritual seekers, but unfortunately our humanness has gotten in the way. Many of our religious organizations have become corrupt. The real responsibility lies with each individual and the Universal Truth: what you seek, seeks you.

Those who experience mental illness karma are afflicted with spiritual patterns that are created from a resistance to embracing alternate spiritual dimensions (or the desire to understand them). Spirituality is about accountability on all levels, and taking authority of yourself and your life. For the context of the information in this book, I am making a distinction between people who can enact their own willpower and discipline to access healing for their spiritual trauma, and those who cannot. Ultimately, through multiple incarnations, a soul will find the relief it needs to ameliorate its soul-level trauma and be born again into mental balance and reason.

Many years ago, I worked with a young lady from Iowa. She had just arrived in Los Angeles to embark on an acting career, and she looked so much like Marylin Monroe, it was startling. My client was beautiful, smart, and suffered deeply from the voices in her head that amplified her low self-esteem and paranoia. She came to me for psychic readings, but it didn't take long to comprehend that the voices, in addition to some of her obsessive compulsive behaviors, left her vulnerable to people who'd take advantage of her.

I had maybe three or four sessions with her, doing what I could to help her set and enforce boundaries, but I soon found that her paranoia disallowed her to feel any element of safety and self-trust. This paranoia also put her in a position to overlook any boundaries that we had set. At this point, any techniques I had to help decipher her spiritual trauma would not be effective; she was unable to access the mental discipline to use them. I suggested that a medical professional would be better suited to help her in this phase of her healing, and I made a recommendation. Doing spiritual work is not for everyone at all times. It is for those who are able to be firmly rooted in our shared reality and have a grasp on their personal willpower—while remaining open to their soul's spiritual information needed for healing.

The Narcissist, Apath, and Empath Relationship

Although there are thousands of medical mental diagnoses, there are two personality types that are important to understand for the current climate of our world, and in particular, for empathic and sensitive people. I'd like to address them from a spiritual perspective; these are the narcissist and the sociopath.

For our purposes here, I am addressing these from my personal experience and that of my clients—again, from a spiritual perspective—and I will condense both personality types into one as they have many over-lapping tendencies. I'll use the term *narcissistic-sociopath*, or NS.

On a spiritual level, it took lifetimes to accrue the denseness of energy and lack of empathy that people with NS personality traits exhibit. It is important to understand your spiritual power with these personalities and how to set effective boundaries, on all levels, when dealing with them.

Manipulation, self-absorption, deceitfulness, and lack of empathy are just a few of the traits for a person with NS tendencies. However, in the United States, about five percent of women and almost eight percent of men present with these traits.[4] The rest of us only exhibit some form of them at different times and under specific circumstances in our lives. It should also be said that it is common for the folks that exhibit these traits to never see a diagnosis as they don't feel anything is wrong. They have no real awareness or care of their impact on others.

So, while it may feel like every ex you've ever had is an NS, it just isn't the case. However, although a person expressing several of the aforementioned criteria may not have earned an actual diagnosis, they may just be the kind of person you need nothing to do with. The behavior of the NS is abusive, diminishing to your spirit, and at times, a real challenge to overcome. Recognizing the traits and setting boundaries early and often in a new relationship can help to identify and mitigate the damage of a deeply selfish abuser.

The Signs

Risk Taker: NSs are often deeply ingrained in high-risk tasks or dangerous behaviors: thrill-seeking sports, high finance, cheating in relationships, drug and alcohol addiction, and lying. These are a few of the ways a person who lacks empathy gets any rush at all. The average person is able to connect emotionally with other people and have the experience of *feeling* connected. An NS doesn't actually connect but often is a great actor, seeming to connect. High-risk behavior gives them the adrenaline rush they need to feel something.

Lovebombing: NSs can be incredibly charming. Usually, by adulthood, a person who lacks empathy has learned how to mimic the social mores of the times. They know all the right things to say and do to make you feel like you are the most valuable, important, sexy, or whatever-you-want-to-feel-about-yourself person in the world. Early in a relationship, they lovebomb you with it. They communicate consistently and often, giving the illusion of love and support. They make themselves invaluable, either emotionally or in some physical service, like offering to do little tasks around the house or seeking to fill any void you may have. At the beginning, you can't fathom how you got so lucky.

Gaslighting: What happens next is the gaslighting phase. As you get to know someone you begin to see inconsistencies in their behavior and stories. You can even catch them in a flat-out lie, but when you call them on it, the cascade of criticism, insults, and negative focus on you begins.

Their goal is to immediately remove you from the pedestal they appeared to put you on. They criticize you for little things, insult you and your intelligence, and make sure to tell you you're crazy—they're not really doing the things for which you're accusing them. These conversations often escalate, depending on the level of control they need in the moment, from anger and raised voices to possible hostility and violence. In order to be successful, an NS needs to diminish your personal integrity and amplify your self-doubt.

The Entourage: Every narcissistic-sociopath targets specific people, usually those who have extreme empathy and care for others. Often it takes a village to con a target, and the abuser knows how important connection is to their sensitive bullseye. So, the charming NS often parades their dishonest behavior in front of their apathetic friends: the established relationships with whom they have made themselves mentally, emotionally, or physically necessary.

We call these people *apaths*. They don't necessarily lack empathy, but they stand by and witness what the NS is doing to the empath because they value what they're getting in their relationship with the NS; they don't want to experience the final phase of the narcissistic repertoire: the casting off of the relationship.

The NS will easily cast out any relationship from the circle without hesitation and at a moment's notice. They will defend their behavior ad infinitum and smear the name of anyone who steps up to challenge them.

The Queue: NSs easily have multiple romantic relationships simultaneously. I call it the queue. They can have two or three they're grooming in case the main relationship ends. They don't care about the impact to the targets, and they often have delusions about the good they're doing for everyone. They can make a public spectacle of the other relationships to create a sense of competition or jealousy for a partner. It's not uncommon for them to constantly see or speak with an ex, or continually talk about how other people would be better for them, and finally the suggestion of bringing a third party into the relationship because party number one just isn't enough.

This element usually comes in towards the end of a relationship when the empath, in spite of the beating their self-esteem may have taken, is trying to break free from the connection. It's an attempt by the NS to bring them emotionally back into the partnership and remain in control.

There is no cure or treatment beyond talk therapy and spiritual renovation for the people who function in this way. They are not diagnoses and terms to loosely throw around, and most people don't qualify. Having said that: there are a lot of folks that have dangerous levels of abusive habits to contend with.

If you've run into any of these red flags, it's important to remain calm and move on. Any sort of engagement with this type of highly manipulative personality is all they need to bring you back in and keep you reeling in confusion.

No matter how much you like or love an NS, you won't ever truly be able to reach them; somewhere in your sensitive spirit, you know that. Do your best to reach out to your trusted friends, who have no connection to the person in question, and rally support to leave the relationship. And, just so you know, this personality can't really be your friend, either. They don't have the capacity to truly value your needs.

The Slayer's Pact: I Free Myself by Accepting the Truth

We, as humans, have many truths. We have our beliefs or what we've been taught is true, we have our feelings and what we like and dislike, and we have what we know to be true for which we have no empirical evidence—our spiritual truth. We must work our way through all of those to get to the Universal Truth, the deep truth that is connected to all things—we all are created equal. That is, we all are valuable with different purposes for our value, as well as the things for which the opposite is true (which is a deeper truth): it's all an illusion and we have no value or purpose—we just are.

Seeing and accepting things as they are in the moment, creates an enormous amount of freedom—freedom to figure out what you'd like to do next. Liberation is something that you give yourself—liberation of the spirit, heart, and mind. It is when all those elements of the self are freed that the body can possibly follow suit. It is this independence that allows for the innovation necessary to create physical-world self-determination and Truth.

Your goal is to unencumber your heart, mind, and spirit by facing the burdens that exist there, uncovering one after another until they have all been revealed on every level. With every step forward, you begin to emerge from isolation, frustration, and confusion, finally connecting to the universal flow of energy that supports all of us.

I have a client who was diagnosed with breast cancer. Receiving such a diagnosis can be world-shattering in every way. Not only contending with the realization of one's mortality, but dealing with a flawed healthcare system that requires a hyper-vigilance to detail would be challenging in any condition. I accompanied her on a retreat to confront her diagnosis and to decide on a treatment plan. The plan she was given seemed excessive, common, and possibly unnecessary; she needed to decipher what was right for her body to heal.

In order to do that, she needed to get to the bottom of the spiritual presence of the cancer in her life. The first task on deck was to begin setting boundaries with certain folks who were more than happy to take advantage of her kindness. As we began to excavate her desire to help others (even when it was clear they were taking more than what was offered) we found that she lived with a level of fear and anxiety. She had done so every day since childhood—witnessing violent episodes with an abusive authority figure. The doctors in her latest medical scenario had taken the place of the unempathetic authoritarian, and her rage and grief were triggered virulently.

She had not fully grieved the childhood trauma, the multiple layers of decisions, or lack of boundaries with others on a habitual level (for the fear of reprisal) that she experienced and developed as she grew up. Now she would have to grieve her childhood circumstances, forgiving them and herself for all that had happened. Once that was cleared from her spirit, she could see what was right for her and choose a treatment plan.

The truths we carry are sometimes obvious, but mostly they are subtle vibrations of our layered past waiting to be uncovered, healed, and recycled into a new truth to live by.

Using Complete Honesty To Work Through Karmic Patterns

The truth is, honesty is the only direct path to reveal, review, and rescind karmic patterns, and there is a lot of honesty to contend with. There is the honesty about our feelings and expectations in relationships and for ourselves, as well as the value systems and beliefs we grew up with—or lack thereof—which create or diminish conflict depending on how suitable they are for the people we have become. Finally, there are the things that we know to be honest about and the things that we keep hidden in the recesses of our consciousness when we are not yet prepared to reveal them. Honesty is the key to the multivolume encyclopedia of information that has gone into creating every aspect of who you are today.

Embracing honesty requires forgiveness as well, when you have one you will eventually receive the other. Learning to face either is a courageous step forward. Forgiveness comes when grief has gone. It's one thing to say you forgive yourself, a situation, or person—feeling forgiveness is entirely different. When you feel forgiveness you are content that there is nothing more to do or to feel regarding the object of your forgiveness; you are genuinely free to move on.

Finding My Father—Finding Myself

Thus far, I think the greatest mystery in my life has been my relationship with my father. By the age of eleven, we'd established a deeply spiritual and energetic connection, mostly based on similarity, mutual respect, and a lack of emotional connection. His passing that year left me with the same relationship I'd always had with him: a spiritual presence without any way to understand its purpose and wisdom. Finally, in my adulthood, I was able to hone the skills—mainly the ability to channel a conversation with the spirit of my father without the lens of my grief or adolescent confusion—that could reveal many of my long unanswered questions.

It's been my experience, not only working with my own trauma but having been witness to thousands of others, that life's purpose is the confluence of many layers of personal events and skills. Over time, they allow us to realize who we are. Our purpose is the thread that connects all of them.

The first time I consciously understood I had shamanic abilities, I was about the age of ten. My father was gravely ill, and I'm not sure if my parents knew, but they hadn't shared it with us. One night, I was sitting on my sister's bed when I had a premonition my father was going to die.

A flash of light in my mind's eye contained the knowledge my father was sick and in his final days. I burst into tears and cried for a few hours. It was about two years from that time that my father was diagnosed with pancreatic cancer and died approximately two months later.

Although I was born psychic and empathic, and had conscious otherworldly experiences every day, the foreknowledge of my father's death was the first time I recognized my ability to perceive and understand the many spiritual realms and what it took to navigate them safely. It was the only time I cried for the loss of my father. From that point on, I cried for myself and this burden of vision I'd been given.

It's true that parents are the first emotional imprint of love and relationship in your life, whether they are present or not present. For me, this journey took a hard left on the Christmas of 1977 when my father's health began to deteriorate. It would be my last Christmas with my father and, consequently, the last happy Christmas we would have as a family for many years. Although the diagnosis was not spoken of, his cancer was taking its toll, and he'd be gone by spring.

Christmas was always a joyous holiday at my house, and my favorite. Stockings, hung by the fire with care, were complete with an apple, orange, and sometimes a pear. Always in the stocking was a Bonnie Bell lip gloss, or a bar of soap, and—to round it out—the final ingredient was a handful of Hershey's Kisses. A collection of whole walnuts, Brazil nuts, and macadamias were promptly poured into the collective wooden bowl with a nutcracker standing upright in the middle. And, as the final touch on the lighted tree, were the homemade felt ornaments my mother made with me.

The full moon was in Cancer that day, and little did I know what was slowly slipping away. Not just the loss of my father but the loss of a family as I knew it. After that year, Christmas was never again the same, nor any other holiday for that matter. In subsequent years, if my siblings, my mother, and I did gather together, the day was fraught with loss and conflict. What left that December day would take decades to recognize. Its magnitude and velocity increased with every year. The love of my life, my father, was now in spirit—and that's where I'd have to go to seek him. His love and comfort were never too far away.

It took decades for me to decipher the pattern of psychic intimacy and deep fear of physical loss that was ingrained in all of my love relationships. What appeared as my love of solitude was only my struggle to navigate the confrontation of communicating my feelings and needs, and finding a way to move forward.

Letting Go When the Relationship is Complete

One of the most difficult rites of passage in life is making the tumultuous decision to call it quits with a karmic partner. For some, it is profound and heart wrenching, while for others it is mere sport. I think people have a difficult time viewing themselves as they are and, of course, accepting others with compassion.

We spend our lives in constant cycles of self-realization, and our relationships with others will follow that pattern. The pattern of attracting a mirror (people or situations that reflect your inner experience or condition) tends to dissolve the more you accept yourself as you are—communicating your needs without confusion or shame. This, in turn, leads to the acceptance of your partner; everything else is negotiated.

Meeting a soulmate usually renders one of two immediate responses: instant love and familiarity; or extreme resistance, disdain, and judgment. Souls tend to reincarnate in groups, based on similar issues and ideals. However, that doesn't mean that we are the same. From personal experience I know that when you have an automatic affinity with someone, it doesn't always translate to the same values, experiences, or intentions. More often than not, the past-life dynamic coming forward to be healed is often one of a difficult nature, hence the extreme attraction and familiarity between souls.

Every relationship we enter has its own truth, as does each partner. The more clearly you understand your truth, the more you will be attracted to a partner with whom you can cultivate a lasting relationship. If a connection begins with a job or agenda for you or your partner, you are reducing the long-term possibility for the relationship, especially if you haven't communicated that job up front (e.g., children, marriage, sex, your happiness, etc.).

No matter how you slice it, relating to another person is work—fun, challenging, invigorating, loving work—and every relationship is only a series of choices. It is important to negotiate your relationship up front. Be honest with yourself and your partner about the work you are willing to do in the relationship, what you like and dislike, and the kind of relationship you want or expectations you have. Sometimes the point of a karmic relationship isn't to stay and fix it. Sometimes it is knowing when you can't, and to leave and let go. There are many circumstances in which trying to work through things just isn't an option, and your relationship should not be a product of your partner's conditions. Here are a few partners you need to seriously consider before you engage, or reevaluate when you have the important details. Love isn't the only thing needed here:

Addict

Addiction is one of the most profound and debilitating life patterns to grapple with, and based on where your addicted partner is on the cycle of healing, determines the possibility of longevity in a relationship. If you're going to stay in this one, you need to be three things already: self-sustaining, firm with boundaries, and compassionately patient. Make no mistake about it, this one is a job and a half. To navigate it, you must embrace with conviction that it is your choice and not just your karma.

Married

I really get it. It appears that there is a lot of upside to dating someone who is married: you don't have to pick up after them, be responsible for them, or deal with them all the time. Before you choose a relationship with someone who is married or otherwise coupled, there are three things you need to know: being an interloper in a marriage will inevitably break your heart; often, the person who will do it with you will do it to you; spiritually speaking, when you take on a person who is married, you take on the energy of the marriage, the spouse, and sometimes the family.

It takes a lot of energy to carry all of that. Trust is fundamental in any relationship and this one may never have it. While your partner is married, you may feel empowered by having all the information, but you will always be kept a little off balance.

Cheater

A person who cheats, will do so for many reasons: some people don't understand themselves, others make emotional mistakes, and then there are those that follow in the footsteps of other family members. It's up to you to decipher the situation and decide how you want to move forward.

As we spoke of earlier, the narcissistic-sociopath has personality traits that are often trivialized for our entertainment. To clarify: the person who is selfish, inexperienced, and immature is not necessarily a narcissist. People lack empathy for many reasons, and no matter how they got that way, they may not be wired to truly connect in a heartfelt way with another person and may not be prepared to do the work necessary to change.

I mentored a young man for a period of time, and in one of our conversations he mentioned he had a girlfriend—and a mistress. He told me that he assumed the women knew about each other. I was confused.

I said, "Don't you have to be married to have a mistress? I think you just have two girlfriends."

Then he was confused. I suggested he was free to have as many girlfriends as he wanted, but it was imperative he find his way to being direct and honest with all of them. Expecting they knew was not enough. This was a completely new concept for him. All the men in his family had multiple relationships while the partners didn't know or speak of it. That was their family norm.

Cruel

Both men and women can be abusers and most abusers have been abused. The numbers of people suffering well into adulthood from some sort of trauma are high and chances are you landed one of them. Some folks with the proper encouragement, resources, and discipline can overcome their tragedies and be loving, honest, and compassionate partners and lovers.

Some will never recover. If you've chosen someone who is mean, you probably won't see it up front. If your lover is cruel to you, themselves, or small animals—well you know the drill. If your partner fits in this category, you may need professional assistance. Don't be timid about asking for it.

Helping a Friend Work Through a Karmic Pattern

It can be uncomfortable to witness the ingrained monotonous patterns engaged in by your friends, especially when it comes to their love relationships. Or maybe you're the one in what seems to be a continuous loop of karmic behavior you're trying to figure out. All relationships are negotiated, and if you begin with a common understanding of what you and your friend or partner both need, either in love or friendship, then you can bypass a lot of confusion, misunderstanding, and hard feelings.

Unfortunately, knowing what you want, or being able to ask for it, takes time to develop. Being embarrassed or fearing rejection is common. If you or someone you know is working through a conflicted relationship or break-up, here are a few pointers to make the experience a little easier.

What does your friend need?

It's important to ask what your friend wants or needs from you. In your mind, they may be well served by your expert advice, but may not need or want it. A relationship—and the break-up and grief process that follows—is a karmic experience. How a person relates to what has happened is usually much more important than the relationship itself. Everyone is attracted to relationships for reasons that may or may not be obvious to you and often may be unapparent to them. The relationships we enter teach us something about ourselves every time; therefore, they hold immense value.

In order to be an expert in the needs of your friend, it's imperative that you be able to empathize with the spiritual, mental, emotional, or physical needs your friend had in going through the experience. Be willing to see it from their prospective rather than your own. Ask your friend what they need from you, and how you can best support them. Then take the time to think about what you have to offer.

Be clear about the time and energy you have for listening.

The next step is being truthful with yourself about the time and energy you have to offer someone who is grieving a loss. Grief for the bystander can sometimes be very taxing, especially if you don't understand or can't align with the situation at hand. It's easy to judge someone as having made a bad decision by entering into a relationship that you could see the end coming a mile away.

As a friend, it's not your place to judge, criticize, or belittle your companion about what you feel they should know. If these are the feelings you're having, it may be best to let your friend know that you are unable to help in this situation. Consider if there is any other way you can be supportive. Setting that boundary may be the most compassionate thing you can do. The antidote to the pattern for you and your friend may be your radical honesty. It's okay to say:

"Hey, I care for you, but I'm not able to listen or talk with you about what happened. What I can do is take you to a movie, help you around the house, or go for a run."

Or, if the truth is, you really just don't want to be around your friend—say that.

It's okay to say: "I am having a hard time watching you go through this."

Don't feel obligated to help.

A person who has just experienced rejection and is grieving a loss will do better with your open honesty than passive aggressive avoidance. Their spirit is busy finding the answers to what happened in the relationship they've just separated from, and they don't need further confusion or loss created by your discomfort. Ultimately, your honesty can only make your friendship stronger.

There is no shame in being unable to support someone how they need to be supported. It is far better to take yourself off the call roster if you're not going to answer the phone. I tend to be leery of people who say, "Call me anytime, night or day." Because the truth is: maybe they'll answer or maybe they won't. When you call, they may not be available or, in fact, may not want to be available.

Whatever the case, the emotional skin of someone who is grieving a loss and rejection will be hypersensitive to any disappointment. It's best not to set up an expectation that is not possible. If you'd like to extend this offer to a grieving friend. Say something like, "Feel free to call me, and I'll be sure to get back as soon as I'm able. I really want to speak with you about what you're going through."

This way everyone wins. You've been honest about availability, and your friend knows how much you care.

How to listen and set boundaries.

Everyone knows someone—maybe a friend, colleague or co-worker—who has a new boyfriend or girlfriend every month. With that much relationship negotiation going on, there's bound to be some fallout. As a friend or confidant to this person, it's important to be able to set kind yet firm boundaries. When someone is recovering from a major rejection, for you—as a witness to their life—it may seem more like self-sabotage or a consistent unresolved life pattern. It can become tiresome for the person supporting the loss.

This is a delicate situation to say the least. Remember, for the person experiencing the loss, the pain is very real. You, as an outsider, may have some objectivity that your friend does not have. It's vital for you to listen with compassion or be kind enough to be honest. Honesty may entail letting your friend know that you're unequipped with the time or energy to go through the grief process with them. Or, if you do spend the time and energy needed, that you are going to be honest with them on your thoughts and feelings. Most of all, make sure they know that you love them and wish them well.

Are you a friend or a healer?

A friend says what you want to hear; a healer tells you what you need to hear. There are times in our lives where the circumstances are set up for us to experience a loss completely on our own. It's truly one of the most amazing experiences to have worked through a loss or problem for yourself. When we bring others into our grief, we are sharing our grief with them; they share in processing the grief we have. It's an enormous job to put on someone but one of the greatest acts of love and trust that two people can share in any relationship.

If you're a friend, these are the things you can do to help

- Actively listen and respond with empathy and compassion.
- Offer to participate in distracting activities like hiking, shopping, movies, or a visit to the spiritual place of their choice.
- Help your friend with their responsibilities, such as house cleaning, car maintenance, food preparation, or anything else that may get swept under the rug in times of grief.
- Do something thoughtful: send funny text messages, share funny videos, get them a card or their favorite candy, or show up on a lunch break with their favorite *venti quadruple half-caff with organic almond milk, extra soy whipped cream, and cinnamon*. It's sure to bring a smile, no matter how fleeting.

If you're a healer and they want your help

- Listen, digest, reflect, and then give your opinion.
- If you've known them a long time, offer perspective on the part of their journey you've witnessed.
- Encourage them to treat themselves kindly and with respect. Times like these bring out the inner addict. Whatever you do, don't criticize. Under no circumstances is it helpful. If your friend has a tendency to self-medicate with anything, do your best to be present and offer other options like a spa day or afternoon of sports (sans beer).
- If your friend does have substance issues that bring you concern, consider where your values lie. Are you going to be involved and

invested in the relationship, or take a stand by not participating in the relationship? Ultimately, it's imperative to be honest; however, your honesty in this circumstance may possibly end your friendship for a period of time. Staying involved and offering consistent, loving, alternate options may be the way to go—depending on the severity of the situation.

Connecting with Power and Presence

It is possible to feel in power and empowered by all our relationships. Although life and duality require experiencing powerlessness and disempowerment as an opportunity for education and healing, we must learn to relate to it, not as conflict, but as a ritual of disintegration and reintegration into a better form. All things in life fall apart so that they may come together in a way better suited for our current needs. This perspective can give you the ability to address all your relational challenges with an open heart and mind—remaining where your power lies: in the moment.

The Twin Flame

A Twin Flame connection is one in which you energetically unify on all levels, a spiritual marriage. There's a lot of buzz about this relationship—people think that it's a person who has the other half of your soul, that you are destined to be together when you meet them, or that the resonance alone insists upon a long-term pairing. There is some truth to all of these beliefs, but I'd like to clear it up for you.

We don't share a soul with anyone else. We may at times share a body but never a soul. Often, when Twin Flames come together they are unable to sustain the deep spiritual knowledge they have in their union because the sexual connection is overwhelming. They need long periods of time developing themselves to strengthen their relationship on a mental, emotional, and physical level first. And yes, often a Twin Flame is a long-term pairing, but that doesn't mean there will be romance or marriage. Sometimes it is through the desire for romance or marriage, but the absence of them, that compassion grows. Ultimately, this connection is a long-term teacher of love with the possibility of many mountains to overcome.

I'm not trying to make it sound less fun, I'm just trying to clear up the fantasy around your expectations if you've not yet met a Twin Flame. This pairing takes a lot of energy and work, for sure, and I don't think everyone chooses to have this type of experience in every lifetime. The Twin Flame relationship is cultivated for healing, and to partner in the rewriting of your unified energetic code by triggering kundalini energy movement where the experience is so intense and significant that it often needs to occur within a partnership so that both partners remain safe during the quantum shift. I've had a many of these healing crises, and much of my life has been focused on the karmic patterns that pull me in and push me out of certain relationships.

One night, asleep, I'd fallen into what felt like a dream. During this experience I astral traveled (moved in a spirit-body to another locale) to a house where there were two men facing off with guns pointed at one another. They looked similar but not identical. They were both wearing white t-shirts and jeans, but one man was significantly larger than the other.

I'd arrived mid-argument, wearing a sleek black suit, turtle neck, and boots (the outfit I often showed up in my demon-slaying dreams)—standing equidistant to both. Next thing I knew, the larger man shot the other in the heart. I dropped to my knees, and holding my hands over his wound, I began to beg this gunshot victim not to leave his life, his body, his love, and the opportunity that awaited him. I begged, pleaded, and cried for his life for what felt like hours. Suddenly, and with a lightning force, I was thrown back into my body. I landed with a thud that only wailing could relieve. I cried for the next several days after and always wondered about what happened.

Flash forward five years... I was with my sister at a shopping mall when we walked past a man that caught my eye. From my sisters perspective, I'd caught his too. However, I was feeling a lot like a patchwork quilt: very disheveled in mind, body, and spirit—not interested in meeting anyone. A few months before, I'd indulged the urge to discover my Raven side and colored my hair black from a box of wash-out color. Little did I know, black doesn't really wash out. So at that point, I looked like a dingy calico cat. I finally took my beat up dry hair to a colorist and had some highlights put in, but that only embellished the patchwork effect by adding red, brown, and blonde to the mix, a look to which I'd temporarily surrendered.

My sister, however, was on a mission. She was so determined for us to connect that she took a business card from my wallet and ran back to where he was, introduced herself, and gave him the card. This was the beginning of an alluring six month affair that would that would lead to a quantum spiritual, emotional, and physical transformation for both of us. It forever changed the way I saw my world.

Mark called a week later. What was to transpire over the coming weeks and months completely awed me. One night we were having a get-to-know-you session over coffee when he abruptly and uncomfortably blurted out that five years before he'd tried to kill himself. He undid his plaid, button-up, short-sleeved shirt to reveal a gunshot scar next to his heart. In that moment I was transported back to the dream I had five years earlier.

The focal point of my memory was the young man—shot and lying on the ground—and me begging him back to life. In that moment, it all made sense. My eyes began to well up with tears, to which Mark cocked his head and gazed at me with concern. It took me a moment to regain my composure.

"Five years ago," I began, "I had a dream of you. It didn't make much sense at the time, but now I understand. Two men were facing off. They looked similar and were dressed the same, but one was larger than the other. The bigger guy shot the smaller one in the heart. I arrived on the scene in that moment, so I didn't know what had led the two of them to that point."

Mark now had tears streaming down his face. Somehow, on some level, he'd remembered me too.

"That was a very painful time for me. Well, everything up until that time had been painful, and I just didn't want it anymore. I'd gone to a friend's house, who was out of town, and been drinking tequila all day. By the time night fell, I was done. I woke-up in the hospital, a neighbor had heard the shot and called 9-1-1."

"Oh, Mark. I'm so glad you're here, that you made it."

In that moment, I saw the door to his openness, close.

"Do you really think you were there?" he said with a bit of a smirk, as he reached for his coffee cup.

As was always the way with him: he'd speak only the information I needed, at the last possible moment I needed it.

Our relationship, in general, wasn't about words. We were deeply telepathic. Even though I didn't see him often, I knew a lot about what was going on in his life on some levels. We were in constant telepathic communication, and the times we spent together were impromptu but intensely meaningful. One day, I arrived back to my apartment to find him sitting on the couch. I'd left the door unlocked, as I'd just been at the neighbor's for a bit. Seeing him, I was elated, but also uneasy.

"What are you doing in my house?!" I said.

"I just knew you were here somewhere and that it would be okay," he responded.

Normally, I'd think he was a stalker and tell him to get the @#$% out of my house, but what he said was true. There was a calm about the whole situation, I could feel he had no ill intentions. And, it really was okay; I was glad to see him. By that time in life, I was getting better at letting things be how they were, rather than grasping at how others thought they should be.

One thing about Mark—although he was successful in his chosen field, very smart, and even-tempered, I could tell he was plagued by something. The series of experiences we shared, spiritually and emotionally, had been building—but he was still holding something back.

Until one day, late in the summer, he came by for a visit. It was in the afternoon, and he said he'd been in the neighborhood and wanted to stop in. Once again, it was perfect timing for me. A client had just left, and I was having a snack.

He started with, "I have to tell you something."

Which is never good.

"I'm getting married next week."

My jaw dropped, as I took in some air. "What?"

"I'm sorry. I should have told you, but I just didn't want to give you up."

Once again, for some reason, I wasn't mad. This is exactly who he was.

"Okay," I said, as my eyes welled-up.

"I don't know what to do. I'm in love with you, but I can't leave her. I'll be with you forever, if you want, but I can't leave her," he said.

Definitely not the confession of love I was hoping for.

"Mark," I started. "I have so many mixed emotions right now, but you know I could never abide your offer. I mean, of course that's never going to happen. How could you do this to me? How could you do this to her?"

"I don't know. She and I have been together for so long, and she deserves for me to marry her."

"Humph," I said, shaking my head. "I see."

I did not know what to do with that statement.

"Well, good luck with that," I said. "I think it's best you go now."

At the door, he turned and said, "Are you sure you're okay?"

"Are you sure you are?" I said, as I closed the door behind him.

I walked to my bedroom, and throwing myself on the bed, I began to wail. All of a sudden, out of nowhere, a beam of light descended and connected to the middle of my body. The rays filled the entire room. I was lying on the bed diagonally, as if I was going to make a snow angel, and I was sobbing uncontrollably—with a beam of light extending from the sky, right through the roof, into my belly.

I laid there weeping for hours, until I finally fell asleep. When I awoke, the world looked different. Everything had a brighter hue. I wasn't sure what had happened to me, but I knew it was a healing in some form—a miracle of some sort—compliments of knowing my friend Mark.

Soon, I came to understand: it was a Kundalini activation of my second and third Chakras. (Kundalini is your life force in the body, and the Chakras are your energy centers.) It was a transformation I inspired when I said no to someone I loved without anger, resentment, or bitterness—a complete surrender to what was.

Mark and I remained connected for a few months through some intense conversations that revealed his profoundly depraved treatment as a child. Abuse for which he picked up the torch and continued in the form of self-sabotage as an adult. I never questioned why he did the things he did: how could he have done anything else?

I have no regrets and was able to be myself fully, on every level. He received me openly and without judgment—especially my honesty. It was an experience that paved the way for a life-changing spiritual transformation through which I emerged with more peace, less judgment, and no anger or resentment.

Although we cannot always be with our Twin Flames, they offer an opportunity to recognize and cultivate a deeper love and compassion for ourselves and each other. But how do you tell the difference between a soulmate and a possible marriage partner?

The Perfect Marriage Partner

Perfection is the first illusion to be released if you want a life partner. No one is flawless. The marriages that stay together keep choosing one another. One year I received a break-up text on Valentine's Day. The unfortunate part wasn't being dumped—the relationship was never going to work—the unfortunate part was the illumination of how common it is for people to relate to love based on how they feel.

Being an empath for a living, I am a professional feeler; I feel everything—if I open to it. Through my empathy, I've learned about love more than any other part of life. The feeling of love is most often the basis from which young lovers choose their partners. It is also the reason they break up so easily. The foundation of how we connect with others stems from our ability and willingness to be vulnerable. It is not always relevant who we open to and their character. Those things are road-tested over time.

I feel I need to throw in here a bit about the stereotype that men are much more capable of *just* having sex. Not true at all. Any person who isn't emotionally open and vulnerable to a partner can have sex without attachment. Someone who needs multiple partners, or cheats in a relationship, is seeking information about themselves; their real goal is self-realization.

It's true, people are emotionally open or not to one another for many reasons. It can be hormonal or bio-chemical, as a result of trauma, karmic patterning, or the two people can have an emotional dynamic in common that connects them to each other. None of those things have anything to do with love or choosing a compatible relationship. When we have an instant emotional connection with someone it will often feel sexual as well, and that's where people get their lines crossed. If sex happens quickly or if it's good sex, they may fall in love—until they find out the real deal about their partner or their own hidden motives which might be propelling the relationship.

Beyond all that, love and marriage become a choice based on your ability to be open to another human being. Choosing a marriage partner is about your willingness to be honest with yourself and committing to the negotiated lifestyle and choices you make directly or indirectly with your partner. If you're contemplating marriage or trying to distinguish between a karmic relationship and a long-term compatible one, here are a few things to consider:

- **Are you able to relax and be yourself?**

    If you haven't caught the vibe yet, getting married has more to do with your readiness rather than the character of your partner. Of course, their character has everything to do with you feeling comfortable, safe, and willing in a relationship. When you accept yourself deeply you will have what it takes to navigate anything.

- **What is your true nature?**

    Relationships endure when each partner knows and accepts their fundamental nature— so they may negotiate their needs.

- **Are you honest with yourself?**

    Relationships don't last when they aren't negotiated honestly. If you have specific expectations, chances are they won't go as you imagine. The trauma to a relationship that must overcome the fantasy you've created in your head can be significant. The future is created from every day moments that you co-create with your partner.

- **Are you self-aware?**

    Cultivating your character and setting boundaries is prime in a marriage. Recognizing how your personality, behavior, and ideals will impact your partner—and being accountable for them—is important.

Reasons to Keep People in Your Life

I've always been of the mind that everyone deserves a second chance if they have learned and changed from their mistakes. Learning from a mistake means that you acknowledge it and are willing to take responsibility for yourself. Changing because of your mistake is vital. It means that you've worked to think, feel, and conduct yourself differently. Even so, it doesn't always mean that your partnership should continue.

The reasons people come together are profound and varied, from creating a family to getting each other through a hard time—or resolving karmic conflicts. When it comes to a second chance, the choice is yours and yours alone. Others cannot possibly know, or understand, all of the variables in your deep and abiding partnership goals—just you.

The following are a few things to consider when deciding if your love might be worth a second chance.

If your partner left the relationship there is a reason

Whether or not they're honest about it, they may want to come back for multiple reasons. It's my experience that additional time will only bring them back to their original conclusion to leave in a more honest way. Karmic relationships usually start out strong and passionate, and may stop exactly the same way—several times.

If this is where you find yourself, your goal is to find peace and kindness (or at the very least neutrality) by doing what you most need for yourself. This allows the relationship to form in a new and strengthening manner. Everyone deserves love, and sometimes it's best to love from afar. Some folks just can't manage being together. Accepting that may be the very reason you came together in the first place.

Everyone wants the relationship

Mutual desire for a relationship is essential for longevity. Often times people break up because they don't feel acknowledged, appreciated, or valued. If this fits your situation, communication is your remedy. Before you say yes, make sure that both of you have spent time reflecting on your needs and communicating those needs to each other. And, whatever you do, don't say it for them.

Sometimes it's excruciating to confess the deepest parts of your heart by saying what you need and how you feel, but a second chance requires it.

Everyone has been honest

Honesty is a must—honesty to yourself and your ability to communicate it to others. If your partner demonstrates this trait, they're a keeper. Everything else in a relationship is negotiated and will take time and compromise. Honesty can take a lifetime to cultivate; one must be honest with themselves before they can be honest with you. Reconsider your love, giving it the respect it deserves.

They do what they say

Finding a partner with follow-through is the aphrodisiac to strong intimate love. It means your partner shows love and respect to your needs, and they must receive it in kind. Some people don't feel comfortable—emotionally or sexually—until they feel safe with their environmental needs being met in the relationship. Emotional intimacy is cultivated through kindness and longevity. So if you're not a jerk, and you fulfill your promises, rest assured your partner will come around. If they are able to commit to following through with commitments, they are worth the extra time it takes to cultivate intimacy.

You share the same values

In a karmic relationship, shared values aren't necessarily present, but, if a long-term partnership is your goal, shared values are where it's at. Love is cultivated, but values are given. They come from your spirit or the way you were educated, and people don't change them as easily and quickly as they might change who they love.

Understand, for a person to change their values, especially late in the game, it requires they betray themselves and possibly their friends, their family, and a culture of a lifetime of beliefs—just to be with you. Desire to do this is one thing, but facilitating and confronting it is another. So if you find someone with whom you share core beliefs, they're a keeper.

They can live without you, but don't want to

Trust me, you want a partner whose every move doesn't depend on you. If you find a partner who wants you but can survive alone, they are worthy of your true consideration.

I find that new relationships sometimes don't continue because a partner doesn't feel like they are loved and needed, just because the other person isn't always around—even when their partner continually reassures them. Unless there are other reasons to discount this person, maybe the issue is more about trust than it is the loving feelings.

Again, the more people express their most heartfelt emotions, the safer they feel. No matter your circumstance, love and kindness are the ultimate goal. Love yourself and treat everyone kindly; let yourself create a relationship with the partner who makes this easy for you.

If You Must Leave: Dignity Releases You from Karma

Acting with true dignity means considering everyone in the situation and deliberately choosing your actions and your words. Not necessarily to be nice, but to do the right thing. At times, the only way to complete a patterned relationship is to move against the waves of habit that created it. Although a karmic relationship can have many possibilities, they are destined for a new ending—one that considers everyone or just you.

Claiming dignity for yourself fills you with strength, self-compassion, and joy, as does leaving your karmic connection that is sometimes fraught with misunderstandings, hurt feelings, and pure disappointments. Allowing your dignity the final say helps to break the energy pattern that brought you together with your partners in the first place.

This is your opportunity to focus on the bold and mature behavior of being heart-full instead of hurtful. No matter how you angle it, you are not alone in the relational dynamic. Whether you entered into it mindfully or not, you owe the time and energy you invested a clean and deliberate exit. Following are a few things to consider.

- **Don't let Your Mother Do It**

    It's common to bring outside influences into the relationship and break up because of intrusions by family or friends. Remember, this is *your* karmic pattern. Learning to work through relationship issues by yourself, or with a selected objective confidant, is a sign of maturity. Of course, I'm not addressing dangerous situations or partners here; for those, the bottom line is safety—period.

- **Take Time**

    Breaking up out of anger or grief never sticks; it's like a boomerang. If you have an unruly fight, give yourself a few days to cool off. Making rash judgments that end up in abrupt actions will eventually lead you back into negotiation with your partner—in addition to doing some damage to the spiritual and emotional integrity of the relationship.

If you or your partner are one of those people who say they want to break up when they really want space, time, or things their way—stop it. Give yourself the time to figure out if you want to end the relationship, or if this is a strategy to negotiate a problem with your partner. Only time and reflection will give you the answer.

- **Be Honest**

    Do your best to stay away from *it's not you, it's me*—unless that's what you mean. Trying to save your lover's feelings makes them want to try harder to preserve the relationship. If it really is them, tell them. Use as much detail as necessary. However, consider whether or not the things that bother you are deal-breakers or can be negotiated before you have that conversation. If you definitely want out of the relationship, you don't want to leave hope for a future in their mind. It just makes it harder for everyone to move forward.

- **Be Clear**

    How you express your sentiment is important. It's best to break up in person, and if you tend to get a little tongue tied, feel free to write all your thoughts in a letter and read it to your partner. Truly, the most important thing to a person being dumped is whether you consider them and their feelings, or if you are selfish and incapable of doing so. Ultimately, a break-up is meant to create freedom for you and your partner to move forward and find new and true love.

- **Listen to Your Partner**

    If it is at all possible, the most complete and powerful thing you can do when you want to break up with your companion is to take the time and make the effort to walk through the discomfort it takes to let your soulmate be fully expressed.

    Again, a break-up is meant to give freedom to both of you, on all levels—especially freedom of mind and heart. Having constant telepathic conversations about what went wrong is no fun. Don't leave them hanging. Letting your lover fully express their feelings about your decision is absolutely the most important aspect of the process of release—that is, if you truly want things to be over. If you do, be prepared to be present for an emotional response, and after hearing what's said, respond from the heart. The fact that you are breaking up doesn't define you—your actions do.

One final thing, on the subject of friendship after a break-up... It is sometimes the go-to salve on a precocious wound of the heart—the promise of an enduring friendship. However, this isn't always possible (or necessary) for many reasons. Sometimes people in a karmic relationship come together just to make the educated, wholehearted, loving decision to walk away from each other.

Being free from guilt, manipulation, delusion, or selfishness is the heralding of a new kind of relationship for you and may not include a future friendship with your partner. In other words, a break-up is just a path to a more appropriate kind of relationship for both of you. Respecting yourself first puts you in a position of strength, enabling you to love and respect others.

Mindfulness in All Your Relations

Mindful relationships aren't really a new concept. In fact, I think it's what most people strive to have. Mindfulness is the process of being conscious of your thoughts, feelings, and reactions while allowing them to move through you without resistance. Not attaching action to them, just awareness. Let me reiterate here that the patterns we are addressing are the core of how you function. That means the behaviors you exhibit permeate any situation with all your actions towards lovers, friends, colleagues, animals, plants, and the planet.

Being mindful in your connections is applying that same awareness to your life as a whole; essentially, you're being a witness. If you can pay attention to how you treat all living beings, it may be less triggering than to solely focus on a specific relationship. I think most of us, in a heroic attempt for mindfulness, struggle with the one ingredient not included in mindfulness: judgment.

Following are some things to focus on, and a bit of perspective on how it looks and feels to be mindful in your karmic entanglements.

Accomplishment

Mindfulness of thought: it's good to have issues, great to understand them.

In each one of us is a profound constellation of interacting feelings, thoughts, spiritual and biological patterns, as well as learned impressions. Paying close enough attention to your own issues allows you to witness another's without judgment.

Determination

Mindfulness of emotion: fear and distrust leave as easily as they come.

We fear what we don't know—and sometimes what we do know. When you can witness your fear, it becomes a foreign language that you have the opportunity to decode through mastering its message. Embracing your fear in all your relations can be peaceful if you let it. Fear is not a premonition of things that won't work out, it is the presence of pain needing to be transformed through grief.

Peace

Mindfulness of desire: wanting is good; wanting what you have is magnificent.

Being mindful means that you've considered the partner you want to be. It also means not attaching yourself to this ideal. Let the acceptance of what is happening wash over you. Allow the understanding and value of what you're attracting to meet your awareness of the deeper needs that are being met. There is purpose in everything; when you no longer need something it ceases to exist.

Power

Mindfulness of reaction: taking action is good; choosing your action is fantastic.

At any given time, anyone can experience the power of their hormones surging through them. While life cycles can dictate the power of those surges, self-mastery dictates how we channel it. It is the perception and understanding we have, based on our life patterns, that drive the impetus for action or reaction.

Many times in a relationship, what you perceive as being communicated will have more to do with what you expect to receive than what is being given. The only control you will find is to cultivate acute awareness of yourself, your partner, your surroundings, and the needs that you must fulfill for yourselves. Consider that what you receive from one another is a bonus.

Synergy

Mindfulness of behavior: patterns are the building blocks of relationships, especially yours.

Relationships are the result of the combining and intersecting of spiritual life patterns between partners. For every lock there is a key to open it. Mindfulness is the natural synergy created between people when they accept their differences and begin to understand the purpose and movement of their intertwining connection.

By now, I'm certain you've gathered the theme of self-responsibility and personal autonomy as the pathway to happiness and harmony through mindfulness. Know that resistance, conflict, and struggle are just as much a part of the process. It is the repression of these dynamics that create discord, not their presence. Letting your thoughts and feelings come (and go), gathering intel all along the route, will leave you peaceful, powerful, and partnered.

The Slayer's Altar and Ritual: Free Yourself from the Opinions of Others

Eternal life is our spiritual birthright, enabling us to transmute and transform anything that causes us imbalance—complete healing on all levels. It can be difficult when contending with the stresses of engaging, understanding, and modifying a difficult relationship pattern.

Addressing the opinions of those closest to us can complicate matters. It is a natural response for your loved ones to protect you by offering advice, but unhelpful at times. You are the only one that holds all the information about what you're doing and why you're doing it. Letting go of other people's opinions is certainly easier said than done, so how do you do it?

Ultimately, all the bits of information that come from external sources must pass through the lens of your own thoughts, feelings, or experience in life. Other people's opinions are reflections of your innermost beliefs or fears about yourself, and we certainly only value them when we must deal with them face to face.

Some of us make every decision based on what others say or think. The truth is, this information gives us an opportunity to reflect on who we will become and contemplate where we are now. Your goal is to view these observations from outside sources with curiosity and a grain of salt. Allow them to teach you something authentic about yourself.

The Altar

Go to your kitchen, or the southwest portion of your house and clean and clear a space for your altar. You are creating a sacred space to call in new life and peace into your home. Cover a table or surface with any beloved cloth, then gather together the following articles:

- White seven-day jar candle
- Blue seven-day jar candle
- Tobacco, corn, or oats for offering
- Glass of water
- Any item representing specific situations or people whose opinions are troublesome

The purpose of the altar is to align your subconscious mind with the deeper spiritual and emotional meanings of the opinions you come across and how they reflect aspects of your inner world or outer behavior. Keep the altar going as long as you are doing the rituals below. Once you've completed the altar and ritual. Pour the glass of water in a houseplant or outside at the base of a tree.

The Daily Ritual

Spend 10-15 minutes a day for seven days, reflecting on those opinions of others that you've received which inspire anger, frustration, disappointment as well as joy, entitlement, and compassion. This ritual is an opportunity to understand your personal needs and empower yourself to receive them.

Next, take time to evaluate what boundaries need to be set with those closest to you—regarding their opinions.

Write:
- The name of the person.
- The opinion in question.
- Your feelings about it and what it's telling you about how you see yourself.
- The boundary you'd like to implement and why.

Explore Who You are without Judgment

A relationship needs loving maintenance to stay in balance, and your karmic connections are already infused with a dynamic that may leave you at a deficit. This easily leads to assumptions and misunderstandings that tarnish your natural psychic and telepathic connection on a personal level as well as with partners.

We shut down the subtle frequency of openness (e.g., presence, love, affection, esteem, confidence, vision) and reroute it to a denser frequency (e.g., emotion, hurt, sadness, depression, apathy, criticism) every time we have a misunderstanding or feel disrespected in some way. Contemplating the way you process information—getting all the facts or letting go of your attachment to what you don't know—clears the way for you to engage your higher self on every level.

When we lack self-awareness, it is natural to look at others with judgment—we naturally critique those things in others we embrace or resist in ourselves. The more we know about ourselves, the more we can find acceptance with others as they are.

Anywhere in the news today you can see a story of judgment, bigotry, or racism. Millions of people trying their best to feel safe and protected by seeking to control the lives of those with whom they disagree or lack understanding. Of course, it's always easier to see the folly of this pattern when someone else is doing it or focusing it on you.

Weekly Ritual

Once a week for thirty-days, take an inventory of all the feedback you've received from your environment during those seven days. Pay attention to the images and stories you come upon via social media and the news, or the words and behaviors you witness and receive from others. Is there a theme? How have they made you feel and what is your relationship to their source? Write all of this down with as much detail as possible, then sit with it for a day—going over it all again once you've had twenty-four hours to process. Evaluate how all of this information connects to you. What, if anything, would you like to embrace or change from what you have learned about yourself through paying attention to your environment?

PART THREE

UNITY

Your Karmic Relationship to Others and the Environment

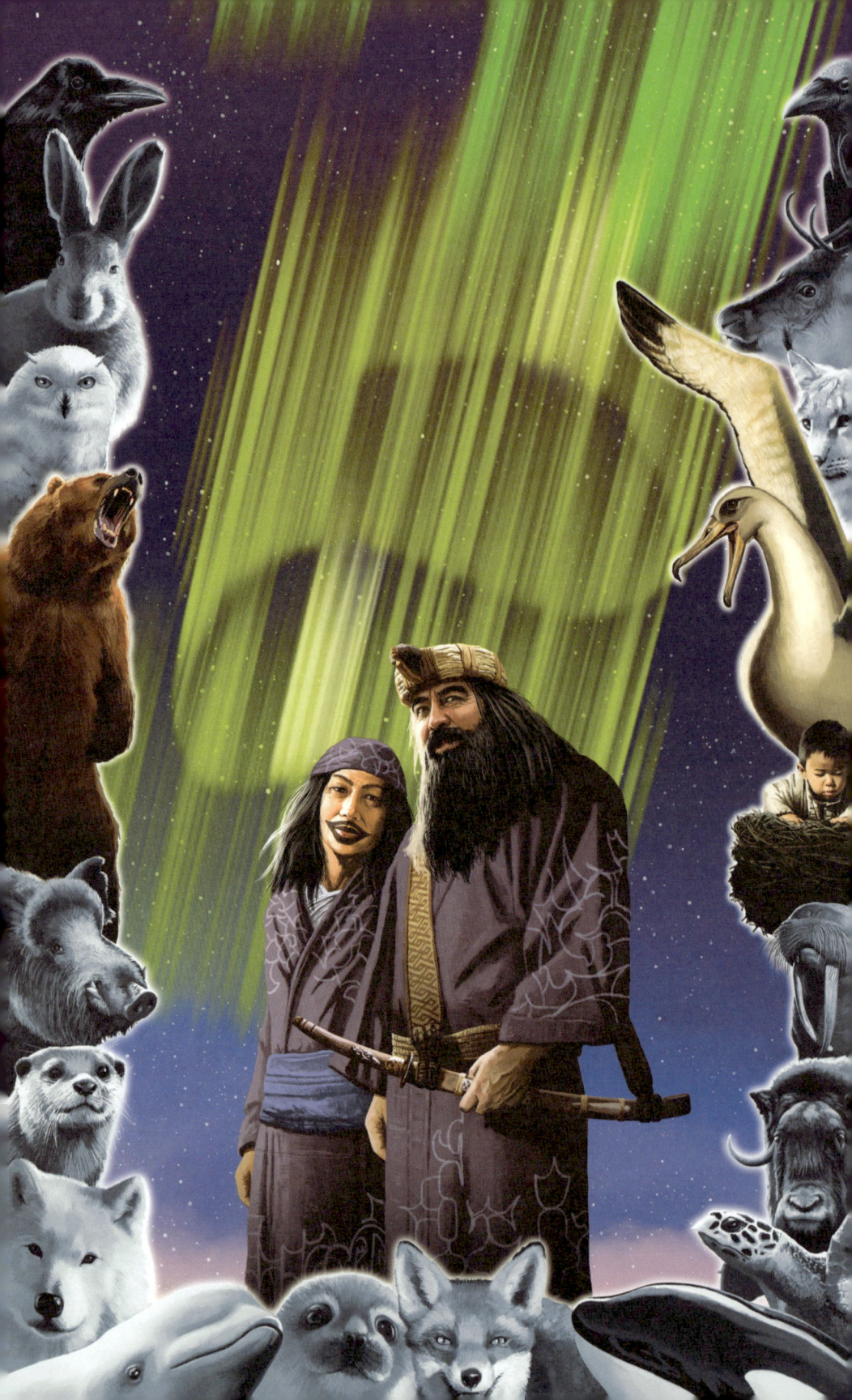

Karma Defines Your Options—The Universe is Conspiring to Expand Them

The Slayer's Weapons:

Communication, Flexibility, Flow, Ability-to-Respond, Affirmations, Angles, Stick-to-Itiveness, Compassion, Cooperation, Harmony

The Karmic Story:
The Place Where All Things Are Possible

Thousands of years ago, long before our records, there lived a proud and joyous people—the Ainu. Along the Okhotsk Sea, in between Japan and Russia, sits the magical Kurile Islands—bursting with life—where anything can happen. These first ancient Ainu were a deeply spiritual people with a connection to the land, and every plant and animal on it—a fabric of understanding woven so tight, nothing could overcome it. Their village was a place where equality was natural, and people took pride in their special contributions to society. They relied on themselves always, and others when the sum of the whole was necessary.

As the sun peaked just past the horizon, Resunotek was up and working by firelight on a new kina (mat) for the hut. The transition of the seasons was colder than usual, and she just couldn't sleep. As she sat weaving the kina, her three-year-old son had been awakened by the light and made his way to where she was sitting. Chikap had just received his name in the tribe, it meant *bird*. He had been infatuated with them since birth—all kinds. They had the power to make him happy and sad.

Chikap was a wily boy, and because he saw his mother peacefully working, he took a chance—ambling towards the birds singing near the tall grasses, hoping to find their nest. It was light now, and Chikap followed the sounds until he was so far away from his mother he couldn't see the smoke of the fire. Stopping to rest near the water, he heard a rustling in the tall grasses—then a sound he had not heard before.

With a rumbling grunt and a loud snort, charging out of the thicket was a wild boar. Chikap had never seen one, and just as he turned to giggle at this great hairy beast rushing towards him, a huge bird swooped down—catching his garment in its claws—whisking Chikap up into the sky.

The thundering sound and wind from the flapping of this white bird's almost twenty-four-foot wingspan took him by surprise. Little Chikap began to cry as he saw his mother quietly working from his airborne vantage. She was getting smaller and smaller in his sight. After being in flight for some time, the mother albatross slowly laid down Chikap in the nest with her baby, who happened to be very close in size to him. The young boy cried a few moments more.

It wasn't until the boy's father had awakened that they realized Chikap was nowhere to be found. Of course, his father was frightened, but there was no time for anger or blame. He knew they would need to use all their available resources to find their son. Soon a search party was gathered, and Resunotek had gone to see Ipetam and Kanto, the tribal leaders.

They were husband and wife, and both had certain spiritual skills. Ipetam was known all through the islands as the wailing shaman. She was a force to be reckoned with, in spite of her 5' 2" stature. Her name meant *blade*, and cutting through the fray to the truth was her strength. She would go into the wooded area and wail—piercing through the veils of understanding—calling on the information that was sought.

Kanto, however, worked another way. He was always irreverently jovial. And although he was a formidable size, almost 6' 4", he was receptive and accessible to all—easily melting any tension or fear in his midst. The Laughing Shaman, they called him. Somehow, he could see the energy lines of history, and the ones to the future as well. His laughter uncovered what people were most afraid to reveal.

Every moment was an adventure in the shamans' presence, and the people loved them. Close together or far apart, Kanto and Ipetam were in unison—telepathically communicating or using the natural world forces to transmit their messages. On this particular morning, Ipetam was still sleeping when Resunotek arrived at their door. Instinctively, Ipetam awoke in a panic—finding Chikap's mother in a dreadful state.

"Come in. Come in!" Ipetam exclaimed. "What has you in such a condition?"

Resunotek released a sigh but still no words; she was paralyzed with fear.

"What has become of Chikap?" asked Ipetam.

Resunotek began to cry, and finally, through the tears, she explained that Chikap had been right by her side; then, he just disappeared. She was afraid for him as it had been hours, and it was still chilly outside for a boy as young as Chikap. Ipetam stoked the fire to warm some water for tea.

"Do not worry, Resunotek. We will find your son."

As Ipetam added the tea to the water, she made a series of clicking noises—not once but three times. Soon, a raven appeared at the door.

"Go find Kanto," she said with another series of clicks, and off the raven flew to find her husband.

As it happened, Kanto had already turned back from his morning walk the minute he'd felt Ipetam's earlier panic. It was only moments later when he walked through the door with the raven on his shoulder.

"What is this I hear of a missing boy?"

Ipetam went on to tell Kanto the story, as she placed two cups for tea on the table. Filling each cup half full, she said, "The two of you enjoy your tea. I am going to the forest to see what the kamuy (bear) knows."

Off she went, deep into the forest, where her sacred hut was situated. It was a simple round structure with a thatched roof to keep the water out. Ipetam entered the space and sat quietly for a few moments, focusing on Resunotek's fear. Soon she was wailing. It would only be a short time before the revered kamuy arrived, and then the message would spread throughout the forest: find the young boy named Chikap.

Not surprisingly, Chikap was still in good humor; he was having the time of his life. He sat in the giant albatross nest, making faces at the baby chick who stared back in wonder. They understood one another, giggling and cooing as two playmates do.

It was the masterful kamuy who found the scent first. Down the mountainside this mama bear galloped, all the way to the tall grasses of the waterside. She saw the albatross cleaning her feathers in the water and said, "Hello. Perhaps, you have seen a young boy named Chikap?"

The albatross replied, "Why yes. He's with my baby in the nest. I came across him this morning being charged by the boars on the other side of the island. The silly boy was laughing at them; he had no idea."

"Thank you," said the bear. "I'll let the others know."

Back in the village, Kanto and Resunotek were finishing their tea, and she was just beginning to feel calm. Kanto started to laugh; laughing was how he received telepathic messages. He took Resunotek's hand and said, "Come. It's time to go. It seems they've found your venturesome boy in an albatross nest on the other side of the island."

Fearing the worst, Resunotek began to cry.

"Oh, no, no," Kanto responded. "He is safe and sound. It appears she saved him from the peril of stampeding wild boars."

Resunotek continued to cry, but now with a smile on her face. They walked quickly but calmly, and it was no time at all before they arrived. Resunotek, seeing the enormous wings of the albatross, ran until she saw the large nest giving shelter to her precious baby boy.

By now the entire island was abuzz about little Chikap's adventure. The ravens told the foxes, who told the turtles, who told the otters, and now everyone new. When the joyous news reached Resunotek's husband and the search party, Resunotek heard a loud thunderous cry from the other side of the mountain—and then laughter and clapping. Even the wild boars were a little taken aback by the story and its humble beginnings. They hadn't meant any harm.

The search party turned into an occasion for hunting and gathering; Chikap's father made sure there were offerings for everyone involved. They caught a squid for the albatross and her kin, the ravens got their favorite nuts, the bears received a stockpile of a treasured leaf, and there was a feast for the people. Ipetam and Kanto had already received their bounty: another opportunity to use their skills. All were pleased with the final outcome.

As it is with all history, when there is an accounting of the facts, mostly they're remembered through our feelings, beliefs, and hopes for the future. The people of this little Ainu village were human—at times filled with confusion, pain, and fear. But it really is about the story you choose to tell that gives you the power in the story you want to create.

Unity

Unity is the coming together of all the parts of ourselves: loved, misunderstood, and unknown. It is this unity that is the basis for our relationship to others. The harmony or chaos we have within ourselves is no more evident than in the relationship we have to our communities and environment, or how we treat ourselves, each other, and the planet with all her creatures. Our personal integration begins with understanding our current beliefs. Beliefs aren't truths; they are the bridges we cross to the Truth.

At the beginning of my professional psychic-arts career, I was in a healing seminar when the unimaginable happened. It's one thing to live with your spiritual secrets and harbor the awareness of them for others, but a completely different matter to have evidence of sharing that intuitive knowledge with someone you don't know well—while channeling simultaneously. We were a group of about five, and Diane, our teacher, was receiving a final-exam healing from the class when she began to speak another language. It was a language that was spoken thousands of years ago on this planet, and no one in the group understood it but Diane and me.

As she began to speak this ancient tongue, I naturally began to translate as if I spoke it every day. The story that came to light was of an island culture who had been warned for several years by their spiritual leaders to move inland from the coast. The coming of a great wave—a tsunami large enough to take out the entire island—had been prophesied for decades. I could hardly believe the words coming from my mouth.

The monotone channeling from these ancestors flowed for at least thirty minutes; it was almost hard to believe. At the same time, the experience was like being home. It was like a conversation with family. Diane went on to say that not many people on the island listened. For many years the residents belittled themselves with violent and angry reactions towards the message bringers, calling them names and finding ways to sabotage their livelihoods.

Hundreds of thousands of people perished when the wave came, but the few that made it to the highest points of the mountain region survived. There was no glee in their triumph. The survivors were left with the aftermath, the guilt, and the frustration of being powerless to save more. They were left with an immense anger at those who wouldn't listen and the obligation of beginning again.

It is the relationships that appear to be inconsequential that, in fact, may have the most impact in ways we have no conscious awareness—until it's too late. Unity allows us to have a more expanded vision of ourselves, others, and situations, giving us the opportunity to hear the truths of others differently.

> Unity is the coming together of all the parts of ourselves: loved, misunderstood, and unknown.

The Slayer's Path: Harnessing Your Ability to Respond

The Akashic record is the spiritual listing of every energetic imprint past, present, or future that informs the knowledge we bring into each incarnation. It is the very essence of being human and our ability to adapt to our ever-changing environment and social landscape. Even if one is living a life that feels sedentary, our lives and our planet are always fluid—moving through change after change without end or regard for our feelings.

Take it from a person who has been in hundreds of relationships—personal and professional, living and in spirit. My empathy allows me to see and understand someone in moments, when it may take others a lifetime of experiences to gather the same information from which to cultivate the compassion that comes over time in a relationship. It is an aspect to my being I have learned to accept, as it has its joys and pitfalls.

A part of the process of learning about ourselves is accessing who we are through getting to know others and our environment. Inevitably we like or dislike people based on who we think they are—until we find out who they actually are. We see others from the lens of how we feel about ourselves, until we are able to take an inventory of our karma—forgiving what we find and realigning with our highest possibility—finally leaving our judgment of others behind. This process teaches us to use our innate compassion to come to a deeper self-acceptance, knowing that judging others becomes a burden meant to help us deepen our self-compassion.

A component of how I am able to do the work I do is my paradigm of unity. I see the connections all things have to one another. There are no walls between the elements of our lives, the people we meet, or the things we come across. In general, our culture empowers certain illusions regarding separation of the self—for example, having professional and personal lives.

We are whole people with whole lives—not a professional life and personal life. All that we are, and every change we make, is made easier by embracing this idea. It is this thread that weaves together the information held in our spiritual blueprint—from our lowest common denominator to our ability to respond. Perceiving a whole life allows us to be empowered by our surroundings, no matter what they are. They are an expression of our own compassion mirrored back to us. Therefore, the people, places, and things in our surroundings can become our environmental soulmates.

Types of Environmental Soulmates

Environmental soulmates are the beings we come across in our daily lives with whom we feel a deeper or special connection. We may not see them every day, or even more than once, but when we do, they have a lasting impact. They offer us help and support, new energetic information from their presence, or challenging situations to help us set boundaries and expand our compassion. Soulmates can also be animals and spiritual beings with whom we relate on an energetic or emotional level. All these connections have valuable input to your life and development.

Allies

Allies are often people we cross paths with, whom we may or may not cultivate lasting relationships with. When we are connected with them, they will stand with us giving loving support and guidance.

I'd just moved to Los Angeles and was driving home one Friday evening when my car began to stall on the freeway. Luckily, I was near an exit and rolled off as the smoke from my engine drifted upwards from the two cracked gasket heads of my vehicle. Two guys saw what was happening and pushed my SUV into a parking lot where many young folks had begun their Friday-night hang.

I got out of my car to use the pay phone, when three drug addicts (a woman with two men standing behind her) backed me up against the wall and began to shout at me, calling me names and saying they were going to hurt me. I was caught off guard and immediately recognized the subtle chewing motions each of them displayed—caused by excessive long-term use of crack.

The group gathering in the parking lot, about fifty people, started to gravitate towards us to watch the commotion. But no one was doing anything to help—just watching.

I was in a unique conundrum. Having lived in a drug-infested area of New York City in the '80s, I'd been through many harrowing experiences. But here in Los Angeles, the warrior that I had been was gone—or at least had taken the night off. I was overwhelmed and frightened.

I was shoved up against the wall, with only my Rose Quartz and Moldavite necklace to protect me. Wide-eyed and in shock, I stood there. After several minutes of people just watching this debacle, a young woman stepped out of the laundromat next door. She was an imposing woman about eight months pregnant and probably not a day over twenty-two. Evidently, she knew the three people accosting me by name, and when the crowd parted to let her through, she told them to stop—and they did. As everyone backed away, my Rose Quartz pendant broke in half, and a portion fell to the ground (a phenomena I call *taking one for the team*: when an object metabolizes the energy of an experience and breaks).

My foes and I were acting in concert that day, as a lock and key, brought together by a deep feeling of vulnerability and lack of support. I'd been experiencing it for months—as had they, no doubt. My ally's name was Gloria. After I thanked her, she suggested I get a tow truck and leave as quickly as possible—which I did. Gloria was quite a gift that night. I never saw her again, yet she is woven into the fabric of my personal history.

Animals

Animals play a large role in our life. Whether they are the ones we choose as companions or those who reveal themselves during our day, they are considered our animal healers and totems. All are guides to us and vehicles to wisdom, if we'll pay attention.

Each creature on the planet has a purpose and a way of life. Some we are deeply familiar with and others we may never know; each of them play a valuable part in how our world works and that it does. We experience two types of animal medicine: the message bringers and the life totems.

Coming across an animal during your day can give you special insight to an event or problem, if you will seek further information about it. What it does, where it lives, and the role it plays in our ecosystem are all good questions to answer. Animals with whom we have a deeper affinity are considered our totems. We may spend a lifetime cultivating a relationship, on some level, with those animals.

Animals were the original communicators for our indigenous cultures. All the first peoples of the globe have creation stories involving animals from their specific locales, each becoming totems of expression for their tribes and lifestyles. Totems given to or discovered by each member of the tribe are guides to understanding one's self and navigating the physical or spiritual worlds.

Personally, I have several totems: horses, bears, crows, cats, and dogs (to name a few). All have come to me many times, in physical or spiritual form, regularly and during times of duress or spiritual revolution. Then there have been the temporal animal sightings: the jaguar in my dreams; the squirrel making its way from a fence to a tree, inches from me on my city walk; and the spider living in the corner of my kitchen. Each of these have been an opportunity for personal revelation specific to the experiences and events taking place in my life at the time.

Special animals can get our attention in many ways. For those folks who don't have easy access to nature and live in predominantly urban settings, our totems will follow a unique path to us. Currently, I am working with the antelope, an animal indigenous to many continents (except where I live). It came to me via an estate sale's safari room.

Evidently, the individual who owned the estate had enjoyed multiple treks to Africa and had brought back several things. I went to the sale to procure items created by my beloved Massai, a tribe with whom I have a deep spiritual affinity. I arrived early on the property to obtain a shield and staff I wanted. However, when I got there, I found a bounty just for me. This included a beautiful cast iron mask of an antelope—with a painted face and twigs for antlers.

Antelope carry the medicine of acute and vigilant awareness, adaptability with decisiveness, and clear graceful action. The antelope symbolism reminds us to focus on the love and abundance that surrounds us, trusting our instincts to make wise, purposeful decisions. Another interesting aspect of the antelope is their sense of smell; those with this totem will have a keen ability to perceive all sorts of information through essence.

One time, just after the death of my mother and prior to a Hawaiian trip, I was meditating—when I was enveloped with a flowery and sweet scent I'd never experienced. Being by myself, with no one in sight for over an hour, I was perplexed. The first day on Maui, I was wandering in a gift shop when I stumbled upon a perfume display where I found the pikake scent that had overcome me on that day. It was a foreshadowing of a deep healing I received while on the shores of the island.

Indeed, the gifts and traits of the antelope have emerged many times for me, bringing spiritual and physical world reminders of attributes I possess, and others I need to focus on, in order to walk the current path. So, when an animal gets your attention, follow its lead and receive the blessings as they arrive.

Friends

The good friends we cultivate over our lifetime are often people from our soul-group with whom we experience enough comfort, love, and trust to sustain enduring relationships. They are the people with whom we can work through conflict and transcend adversity, laughing all the way. They are the soulmates who teach us to learn unconditional love and communication—inspiring us and requiring us to be better.

I have cultivated many friendships over my lifetime and the one recurring theme within all of them is laughter. It acts as the ultimate antidote to any confusion, conflict, or disappointment. It's nice to enjoy relationships when everything is peachy. But what's better than when the chips are down and you're surrounded by folks who can make you laugh?

Enemies and Rivals

Enemies and rivals are profoundly vital to our education in regard to boundaries and the will of the human spirit. They are the soulmates that come into our lives to show us adversity and compassion. When we first meet these people we may like them, but something doesn't sit right. Our enemies offer us an opportunity to trust our instincts within the karmic pattern. They don't have our best interest at heart but require us to be self-sufficient. In truth, it is our enemies that help us decide who we are and who we want to be.

My last year in New York City was quite tumultuous. I lived in one of the many gentrifying neighborhoods that had previously been in an extreme state of dilapidation. As people moved in and started rebuilding, so did the criminals.

Every night I'd come home in a cab between one and four in the morning. Waiting for me, there were a particular group of juvenile thugs who found it entertaining to chase me into my building. They would see my cab round the corner on the one-way street and start running towards me. Knowing this was a probability, I would've already paid the driver thirty blocks in advance. I'd be ready to run like the wind from the street to the outside door. Then sprinting up three flights of stairs and into my apartment, I'd lock my apartment door safely behind me.

One night, one of the kids gained such time on me that I barely made it halfway up the first flight of stairs before he was pounding on the entry door. I got upstairs and realized I was missing my beautiful kelly-green-and-black plaid mohair scarf that I just adored. It was my all-time favorite thrift store find, and I loved it. As I looked down on the street from the window of my apartment, there it lay in the middle of the road—with my dignity. It was that night I realized how much I had changed. No longer angry, with no rage for my protection, I now understood the choice I needed to make—to live in a new way, with love. And then I thought: oh well, I hope someone enjoys that scarf.

Soulmate Groups

A soulmate group comes in many shapes and sizes. It is a set of people, large or small, found in your environment at any given interval—whether it be once or continually over time: from those you find shopping with you at the grocery store to those with whom you share a city or state. What creates a soulmate group is a common ground or interest of any sort, and we will have many in a lifetime.

Then there are those with whom we share multiple lifetimes, the souls that circle around us in different roles within many individual incarnations: the people we call friends, family, colleagues, associates, or constituents in the physical world. And let us not forget the spiritual world as well. In the spiritual realms we have beings from many other dimensions who will move with us from lifetime to lifetime as our teachers, guides, and nemeses. In addition, we have relationships with souls who have lived in a body for a time and then spirit for the remainder of a life cycle.

If for no other reason, this is why lumping people into a single understanding, belief, or vision will never be accurate. One individual has too many unique traits and resonances with multiple soul groups. Some are obvious; others, one must have the lens to see before they come into view.

Consider that those you may judge as you cross their path on the street are members of your soulmate group and might be judging you too. Or, they just might be carrying that seed of compassion that reveals what lies beneath your judgment. Following is a list of some major soulmate groups.

Humans, Animals, Spirit Beings

All beings have power and value. To exalt one and diminish another only creates imbalance for our planet. It is within the understanding of soulmate groupings that one can release themselves of the illusion of superiority. The deeper you look into an individual's connections, the more they will reveal knowledge that can't be expressed through stereotyping.

Ancestry and Ethnic Groups

Sharing ancestry and a physical ethnicity with others gives an understanding of geographic origins but will always be colored by one's culture, current geographic location, and social traditions. The DNA we share with our ancestors connects us spiritually and emotionally to all that the group experiences, regardless of our life preferences and choices.

Culture, Societies, and Tradition

This is where we begin to choose, on some level, our soulmate groups. One can be born into a culture or society but ultimately not choose its traditions, or one might have a spiritual affinity with a culture or society different from the one in which they were born.

Geographic Locales

The geographic locations we choose or are born into will shape how we live and think on a fundamental level. The countries, states, cities, neighborhoods, apartment complexes, schools, or large organizations where we spend a majority of our time will create alliances, or eventually we will be moved from them.

Interests

A major aspect of our lives is expressing ourselves through our interests: music, art, sports, nature, food, politics, cars, beauty, fashion, philosophy, and religion (to name a few). Regardless of how we are brought to our interests, they are the things in which we choose to invest our time. Connecting or disconnecting with an interest-related soulmate group can be the tipping point of our maintaining that interest.

Connections Through Trauma

Many people connect through the adversity of their experiences: illness, deaths, natural disasters, traumatic events, and so on. These soulmate groups can be vital to how one survives the worst this world has to offer.

Connections Through Social Events

Marriages, divorces, birthdays, and a multitude of other social constructs that are marked by celebrations and time, create their own soulmate groups. These links allow for people to find superficial alignment and dialogue in order to find common ground.

Leadership and Community Position

Comparison has always been a social construct through which a person or group could become self-aware. However, when comparison makes its way to superiority, truth ceases. Every individual within a community is deeply valuable, from a group's membership to its leadership. Each individual and the role they play together become the naturally occurring checks and balances of a society.

The Warrior's Hidden Motto: I Am Invisible

Feeling invisible is a phase of spiritual development that each of us will encounter at some point. I say *feeling* invisible because we are never truly invisible; there is always someone in body or spirit to be witness to who we are and to our accomplishments and struggles in life. So, being mindful of such witnesses when one is feeling concealed from sight is an awareness to be developed.

Invisibility is often the experience that comes when a person is struggling with a new challenge, necessary change, or trauma. It is the time when you feel no one else in the world could possibly understand what you're going through because they don't know you. The important thing to remember, no matter which side of the coin you're on, is that anyone who is willing to deeply empathize with you can, in fact, know and understand your struggle because they can feel it from your perspective.

We are living in a time on planet Earth like no other. It is the ending of three natural cycles of change, each approximately 25,000 years in length. The cycle of human conflict, economic growth, and climate change—all three of these natural life cycles are coming to their cataclysmic end simultaneously, and we are all here to participate.

This time on the planet has been prophesied by many cultures over the millennia. It has been prefaced with deep caution and hope as a time when human beings will recognize their individual equality, power, and compassion—and make the changes necessary for all beings to continue to reside here. In order for that to happen, we must learn to see ourselves, each other, the earth, and the cosmos as an integral part of our connectedness and survival.

Overcoming Invisibility: Namaste

Namaste is a Sanskrit word meaning *to bow*. It is often used as a greeting that personifies the meeting of two people in love and respect—the God in me sees the God in you; this is the antidote to invisibility.

Because this is such a unique time in our history, many people are having to change long held skill sets, beliefs and ideologies in very short periods of time. Families who've anchored certain jobs, expertise, or traditions in certain locations are in upheaval as the need for those jobs or skills become obsolete. Much how we witnessed changes to the city of Detroit as major car companies took an economic dive in the recent past, we are seeing this type of cataclysmic change all over the globe. The globalization of knowledge and the web, the social acceptance and deeper understanding of once taboo groups, immigration and our relationship to other countries, war and its impact on all of us, and a new understanding of the purpose of religion— are all challenging our ideas, jobs, habitats and mores.

Consider that a willingness to be seen and receive new attention to parts of yourself, which up until now have remained undiscovered or well-hidden from others, is vital to this transformation. The intense vulnerability that comes with these new revelations can feel like a door being blasted open or slammed shut. This acute abruptness can be frightening and disruptive, not only to the individual but to the family, community, or further-reaching soulmate group.

Always remember: in this destined shift of paradigm, your soul has all the necessary spiritual imprints needed for a balanced transition. Important spiritual information, along with support from the soulmate group, is activated when you move—with resistance or willingly—towards the change.

Overcoming Blame

The essence of blame has a powerful purpose within our karmic experiences. Blame brings our awareness to the origins of any spiritual or real-world trauma that we may be carrying. The stronger the desire to blame another or yourself for an occurrence, the more you desire—on a subliminal level— to grieve and move forward. When there is a need for release, if there are obstacles for you in grieving—like believing grief is weakness or inappropriate in some way, or simply feeling uncomfortable with the process—the natural path is to transfer the pain or rage onto something outside of yourself through blame.

Ultimately, we must bypass the seduction of blame and do the real work of grief. Don't get me wrong, there are times when others and their malicious or ignorant attitudes and behaviors are the cause of enormous destruction, and they must be taken to task and held accountable. However, at some point, each of us will be faced with the effects of our choices on others and the environment. Blame is costly, in either time or attachment, and must be evaluated for its efficacy in creating needed social changes.

> Trust doesn't dictate that bad things don't happen; trust paves the way out of them if they do.

Accountability

Accountability is the antidote for blame. Anytime you complete a karmic relationship, the reward is accountability. When you are honestly accountable for yourself and consider how your decisions will affect others, you are answerable to no one. And when you aren't obliged to others, you are free to enjoy their presence and be yourself with them. People like the opportunity to be generous of their own accord and are less interested in feeling like they owe others something.

When you practice accountability, you achieve honesty and compassion—and the Universe tends to respond in kind. As we've spoken of before, we are never alone or do things single-handedly; there are always others involved. The more you strive for the ease of an autonomous life, the more the Universe presents opportunities to achieve what you need and how you need it. It allows for the perfect timing to meet those with whom you can barter, to negotiate the perfect price you'd like to pay for an item or for the exact way you'd like to spend your time making the money that sustains you.

How does one practice accountability? Simply put: trust and preparation. Learning to trust the outside world is a practice in and of itself, but first you must learn to trust yourself. Learn to make the decisions that truly make your life easier, not to take the shortcuts that always end up in your doing things twice. The world outside of you will rise to your call and mimic what you do.

Now, I'm a person who loves a bargain, but unless your shopping at a thrift store, or an ultra-high-end boutique, they just don't make clothes how they used to—the kind with finished seams and linings. I recently purchased a fabulous linen blouse (a long tunic style) on the internet, and the minute I sat down in it, the back seam ripped.

So, who is responsible? How does one practice accountability in this situation? First off, I didn't spend one minute getting mad—maybe 30 seconds feeling disappointed. My criteria for ordering the blouse were: it had to be real linen, inexpensive, and I had to like the color. It was from a company I'd not heard of before; so, frankly, I was just glad to receive it. When it arrived, it was linen. I had no idea that linen could be so thin, but it was linen. I could have returned it, but the company was in another country; I'd probably pay as much shipping it back as I paid to get it. The truth is, even damaged as it is now, I like the blouse and the color. So, I'm going to fix it...or wear it with a long coat.

In order to place blame and hold others accountable, it's important to consider what the cost will be to you and those you love. Sometimes your karma dictates walking away from a situation even if it feels incomplete and the situation warrants punishment or resolution that does not come. Holding onto anger and resentment towards another will not make them be responsible for their actions, but it will keep you attached to them indefinitely—until you are able to grieve and move on. Only you know the best course of action for yourself and the ones you love.

The fact is, mishaps and unfortunate events are common occurrences. When they happen, giving them power over our feelings and actions never creates a better situation. What often comes about is that we take the frustration, anger, and resentment we have regarding other events in our lives out on these petty situations where we feel justified and somewhat anonymous. We do it to compensate for the experiences we've had when we've not communicated what we needed to someone we know or care about—or other situations left unaddressed, in which we have been intentionally victimized.

The key concepts for being accountable:

- Consider others and then trust yourself to make choices you're willing to back, even if they go sideways—forgiving yourself if they do.
- Be honest at all times with yourself and others.
- Be courageous enough to stand up to the people who have truly hurt you.
- Have compassion and grieve your losses.

In a world where frivolous lawsuits and other social mayhem are at an all-time high, give yourself permission to put your fight where it can actually make positive change. Only you know what that is for yourself. For sure, you'll know in your heart if you're seeking revenge, responding in anger, or being spiteful (by the disparaging mental and emotional impact your attachment has on you). And if it appears that way? Promise to reevaluate the circumstances; grieve to let go and move forward. Showing yourself compassion by giving up an ill-considered or untrue conflict is the definition of strength.

Getting in Flow with the Universe

There is a divine matrix that includes all life and traverses all dimensions of energy. Like any home, it has joists and beams to hold up even the heaviest loads, windows through which to witness magic, and doors that open to invite you into a new idea and close when you've stayed too long in one place. There are winds of change and rains of celebration, thunder to announce a new way and lightening to show you where it begins. This beautiful home doesn't need us in order to continue being what it is—we need it in order to continue being who we are.

The minute you take in a breath and embrace a profound reverence for Mother Earth and all she provides to you, you can recognize the extraordinary opportunity you have to be here, now, during such a prolific time on the planet—exhaling any confusion of who's actually in charge of the ground that steadies your feet. It is then that you become quiet.

Once you become quiet enough to hear the flow of the Universe through your own beating heart, and hear your heartbeat with conviction and clarity, you connect with all the other hearts within the matrix. Now you're in flow with the Universe. It doesn't take any special meditation, just a moment of breath, reverence, remembering, and quiet. Your heartbeat connects you anywhere, anytime to your Universal home—the interconnectedness of all that is.

The Slayer's Dilemma: Becoming Visible

If the warrior struggles with feeling invisible, then the slayer must learn to be at peace with visibility—standing in their rightful place, wherever it may be, and being seen for who they are and who they are becoming. It is true, however, that being witnessed brings revelation. When we are viewed by others, our self-consciousness kicks in and begins to shape our imaginations to what others may be seeing.

Humans tend to spend a lot of time on how others may be seeing them, rather than how they see themselves. If you'd like to be seen fully for who you are, you must first look at yourself. What do you like or dislike? What are the aspects of your life for which you have compassion? Pity? Joy? Frustration? Do you love yourself?

Being able to look deeply at yourself and others is a learned skill and requires empathy. It's an emotional investigation of the soul, using your feelings and emotional body to reach out to another in compassion. The spiritual aspect of being seen is dictated by the aura, the multiple layers of energy that surround the body. It is your auric field that makes first contact with others, and it is where invisibility and visibility begin.

Thoughts are energy that vibrate in your auric field—your truth out there for all to see. So, unless you are a master of disguise, others can and will perceive how you are really feeling. They will experience it before a word is spoken. I say this not so you'll try harder to hide, but because there is no shame in whatever you feel. Embrace it, so others may see and embrace you.

Visibility Exercise

Playing dress-up was one of my favorite childhood pastimes. I loved wearing things that weren't in my normal repertoire. Sometimes in life we are looking to become invisible and other times we need to become visible, so whichever you find yourself doing now, here's an opportunity to do the opposite. The most important thing is not what you wear but the energy you intend to gin up with your presentation. It is your aura that people see before they see what you are wearing; essentially, they see you—what you deliberately want them to see or what you are unaware they see. There is a magnitude of power in how you energetically communicate with others, and this needs only a modicum of attention, intention, and awareness on your part.

Become Visible

To become visible, first of all, consider what you'd like to communicate to the world? Write out a list of five important things you'd like to get across to others. Once you've done that, think about what kinds of clothing express those things for you. It's important to know that it's not the clothes that get attention, it's how the clothes make you feel and what they bring out in you when you wear them. Choose three different outfits and wear each one of them for at least two hours in a public place like a mall, on a bus ride, or any public establishment. Take notes of wearing each outfit and how others respond to you in them and how it makes you feel. With each outfit, become more and more specific about what you intend to communicate—like feeling sexy, smart, happy, powerful, helpless, or fearful. Consider that you're not just seeking to experience something different, but also to understand the power of what you project with your intention. Take notes on how it feels to be visible in the world in a new way.

Become Invisible

To become invisible, you will do the same as above, but this time focusing on why you'd like to become invisible and five possible things you'd like to achieve from the experience. You'll choose clothing that makes you feel quiet, grounded, and unseen. But, again, it's not about the clothes you wear it's about the energy you extend into the outside world. Take a few minutes to practice imagining the energy field around your body, and that it extends ten feet outside of you on all sides. Then, imagine pulling back your energy body to approximately 1 foot outside your physical body. Consider what it would feel like slipping in and out of public spaces unseen. The purpose is not only to understand the power of your intention but to heighten your awareness to the subtleties of how we express ourselves and communicate with others through our energy body. Take notes on how it feels to be invisible in the world.

The Spiritual Purpose of Self-Pity

Intense feelings are your way of digging into your soul for information and then using it for self-realization—especially self-pity. It's a sharp arrow, powerful enough to pierce the absolute heart of the matter. Experiencing pity for yourself means that you are recognizing, empathizing, and commiserating with your sorrow, which is the prerequisite for compassion.

Self-pity brings an extraordinary focus to where you are wounded and the attachment that holds you in that state of emotion. It's a valuable process to become clear about the people, places, and things that trigger you to feel sorry for yourself. There is always a deeper message in connecting the dots to your sorrow.

Overcoming Self-Pity and Other Overwhelming Emotions

Self-pity is what precedes grief in the transformation of emotion, but it can often become a placeholder instead of grief. Remember that all your strong emotions have intended messages for you, but it takes the movement and release of the emotion through grief to fully comprehend the communication.

When we consider overcoming uncomfortable emotions, what we're really speaking of is grieving them. There is no way to overcome your feelings without experiencing them. Setting them aside will only postpone the inevitable and create energetic blocks in the body. Allowing the movement of energy through the auric field and down through the brain and physique, activates the process that initiates the cascading of chemicals in the body that promote antidotal feelings of safety, balance, and peace.

The Slayer's Motto: I Flow with a Changing World

Getting in flow with your environment is necessary to survive in today's changing climate. But to do that, you must begin to understand the people and dynamics at play in your outside world. Not just how things are, but more importantly, how they got that way. When you can visualize the process or path something or someone took to get to their current state or condition, it becomes natural to find a solution to what ails them, or a new path for projects that have stalled.

Everyone's heard of a midlife crisis—it's the point in anyone's life where a dramatic change is wanted or needed—and in previous decades it commonly occurred between the ages of 40 and 50. Today, there are less and less people working for companies for long periods of time, and the corporate structure that was typical in other times is less desirable for people today. In this climate of entrepreneurship, the new midlife crisis is the constant change in jobs and work environment that has become the norm. So, instead of just one job and one major life change, people today are sure to have many.

Fields of work that have been independently run are disappearing, and many jobs have or are becoming obsolete—if not completely, at least in part. People whose families have done the same thing for centuries are finding themselves in a unique position to no longer have a daily structure created for them to rely on. Today, while anyone who wants a job can find one for themselves, there needs to be a fundamental shift in one's thinking about work. There needs to be an acknowledgement that if you or someone you know finds themselves in this position of making an unsolicited life or work change, you (or they) will need to grieve the transition and can expect to feel many emotions such as: anger, sadness, self-pity, depression, confusion, and fear.

In the karmic cycle, everyone will be a leader and a follower at some point. Followers become leaders when they can no longer tolerate the climate they find themselves in and desire to forge a new path. They are the transformers and courage builders that initiate new ideas and ways of living. Two things are vital when creating a new work opportunity or environment. First, look towards the tasks in life that bring you the greatest joy. Second, be mindful of inclusivity. Any project, no matter what it is, will need others to move it forward.

How inclusive are you of others in your environment and in the world at large? Naturally, the more acceptance you have of all people, the larger the pool of people the Universe has to call on for your assistance. I find that people with smaller ranges of inclusivity stay in heavier emotions for longer periods of time.

Again, anyone in transformation will experience these emotions. They are the spirit's natural process of helping the body and mind to access information and transmute the old outdated habits, beliefs, and experiences. This process naturally includes other people (known or unknown) for help, inspiration, and support. Being in flow with a changing world only requires that you put yourself in new environments; be open to the new ideas and opportunities as they flow your way.

Group Karmic Contracts

Spiritual contracts aren't directly negotiated written agreements. They are often unspoken commitments that either come together pre-incarnation or within an energetic dynamic between individuals or groups of people. Everyone who participates in or experiences an event is a karmic group member, with the contract being their presence at that very time and place.

There are many types of group karmic contracts, from the entire audience of a winning World Series to everyone involved in a mass shooting—every time a group of people congregate, such as the patrons of a restaurant or movie theater on any given night. All of these clusters of people resonate with one another, for whatever reason. It is in these seemingly random group formations where ideas are exchanged on the subtle-body level.

Download at the Smoothie Counter

One day I had gone to the local health food store. I'd ordered a smoothie and was waiting for it to be made when a man walked up to the counter. He caught my attention from across the room. He was tall and in spectacular shape. I had two thoughts: he was a pro-athlete and he would speak to me. He placed his order and then turned in my direction, walking over to me as if we knew each other.

That day, I wasn't feeling particularly social. I was there because I'd been considering changing my fast food diet to something that would give me more energy; frankly, I felt a little lost with the overwhelming proposition. So, when this athletic man walks over and launches into what he'd eaten in the past day and a half, and what he was thinking about for dinner, it was music to my ears. These were exactly the ideas I needed.

Coincidence aside, as he spoke, I felt this energetic shift in my physical body and auric field. It was like the healthy eater in me was being activated. He continued on for two more recipes, never gave me his name, received his order, wished me well, and left the building. I laughed and thought, *I'd never been so turned on!* I walked over and took my smoothie from the counter where it had been sitting. I felt like a new person, and from that day forward, it was no longer a confusing struggle to listen to my body about what nutrition it needed.

The following week, I was standing in line at the neighborhood liquor store waiting to purchase a pack of cigarettes (a coping strategy I used, for a time, when I had extreme anxiety), when another good-looking athletic man stood in line behind me. As it turned out, he was an athletic trainer. We walked out to the parking lot together, and he asked if he could contact me. I gave him my number.

During this time, I didn't have a traditional sleep pattern; I was used to receiving calls in the middle of the night from distressed clients. So, when I received a two-in-the-morning phone call from this guy, I wasn't shocked. He asked if I'd like to go for coffee right then. Normally, I would have considered that this was some sort of booty-call; however, for some reason it felt different. I met him at the nicest restaurant I knew to be open all night, a place where the staff knew me and I felt safe. When he arrived, he was wearing a suit and looked very handsome. I was very intrigued about whatever this little adventure was.

We'd been sitting making small-talk for a few minutes when he broke out a manual he'd written on living a well-balanced life, complete with work-out and nutritional tips. I had to laugh. The Universe was really supporting my desire to make change with all of these unconventional unplanned events that completely suited my lifestyle at the time. My new acquaintance and I had a cup of coffee and some fresh fruit, continued to speak for another hour or so, and then left. I never saw him again.

Whether or not it is obvious, the places we go, the people we see, and the things we do have a deeper impact and connection that changes everyone on subtle levels. Sometimes it's for the better, and sometimes it's not. Paying attention to your subtle feelings and thoughts can give you indications of the common denominator of the energy in the group and the main energy line of connection.

Changing What I Do Doesn't Change Who I Am

The awareness we have of the subtle connections to others and our environment gives us potential power in any situation—if we will harness it. No matter your situation or circumstance, there is an option of ease to making necessary change, regardless of how daunting. You have only to be open to the possibility of effortlessness. This is the lesson karma seeks to teach.

Jobs, places of employment, living spaces, activities, and hobbies don't define us. They simply give us an opportunity to inspire and express who we are. When we are required to change any of them, it can be difficult and deeply tumultuous, especially when we perceive these long-held circumstances as extensions of ourselves. These life changes will offer us the circumstances to become better.

Take a few minutes to write down these things from the past five years, and how they express an aspect of your character.

- Jobs
- Places of employment
- Living spaces
- Activities
- Hobbies
- Entertainment choices

Walking Away from a Long Career

The kind of loyalty—or at very least, attachment—that is inspired through spending forty hours a week doing the same thing with the same people is potent. So when you must walk away from a long standing career—regardless if you are fired, pushed out, laid off, retiring, invited somewhere else, or flat-out quit—the lens through which you look is paramount to your ability to move forward.

The idea of our work life ending at a certain age is a cultural one and does a profound disservice to living a long and healthy life. Today there are approxi-mately 500,000 people over 100 years old living on the planet, out of the estimated 7 billion here—that's a substantially low rate. Spiritually speaking, death does not exist, only transition and transformation to other planes of existence. It is my experience in working with death, dying, and the dead (again, all concepts of the physical realm) that people at some point, consciously or unconsciously, choose to continue living; the work one does in the world is a an important factor.

When you consider this expanded vantage point, it offers the opportunity to discontinue looking at life as something that happens to you and open to the idea that it happens for you. Every change and challenge you transform is a karmic clearing that offers you the freedom to create a life you feel good about every moment of every day.

Often, in my line of work, I see people relate to the karmic wheel as something that we endure: incarnation after incarnation, suffering on planet Earth, all until we finally graduate to live in some other magnificent dimension where there's no pain.

I experience the purpose of karma as the structure we are offered within which to learn that true power is only something we're given when we are able to respect it in others. Pain is the process that teaches love, compassion, and awareness. The key to living a long life, then, is how you relate to and embrace compassion, power, and equality while living on planet Earth.

Transforming your life always means an upgrade in some way. The Universe has a way of breaking things down that aren't working to their most basic elements; it is in order to rebuild them in a new and better way. Even though this perspective may appear obscured from view, remember: the life you have is a result of your spiritual history, your current environment, and your present circumstances. You are empowered by your awareness, and choices regarding all three of them.

The Slayer's Pact: Harmony is Inevitable

As I was contemplating harmony, two things came to mind—music and math. Harmony occurs in music when two pitches vibrate at frequencies in small integer ratios. The Chaos Theory describes a system's process over time, where any small change that occurs in that system can have a large impact down the line.

Now, I am not a musician or a mathematician. In fact, I had to beg my senior math teacher to give me extra-credit work so that I'd have the opportunity to change my F to a D-, all so I could speak at my commencement ceremony. Though I didn't have the wherewithal for math equations, both math and music are deeply intuitive and are lenses through which viewing human relationship dynamics between individuals and groups makes sense.

My math teacher's decision offered me an opportunity to fulfill the honor of speaking to my fellow classmates—it changed my life. Rather than feeling the shame I experienced from failing so miserably in math, it allowed me to focus on something I was good at. It was the small change in my life that is making a large impact now.

There is nothing more influential in human relationships than either harmony or chaos. One small decision can create a lasting irrevocable change in ways the one who makes it might never know. To achieve harmony, one must be able to flow in a way that feels like complete disintegration; all things in life fall apart so that they may be rebuilt in a way that will suit the changing individual, group, or community.

Ultimately, relationships are a series of choices we make and the mastery we possess to facilitate those choices—at times, under duress. The latter being our ability to be present with ourselves, each other, and the environment—enough to intuitively consider all of them—in the moment an irrevocable action must be taken.

Understanding the Karma of Culture and Tradition

How things begin and what they become are often unique. Cultural customs and traditions have been the storytellers for centuries past, the guides to offer those who follow them insights on history and ways of living—from fairy tales, creation stories, songs and dances to media outlets, television programs, radio shows, and the internet. But what often begins as a vehicle for well-meaning education becomes a method to embolden those who seek power in attempting to control others, whether it be justified or not.

The history books I learned from in first through twelfth grades referred to some of our First Nations as savages—as commonly as one would drink a glass of water. However, if a person stands their ground and protects their home or property today, we consider it acceptable—even when it ends in murder. If I hadn't been born with the spiritual background that I have, I might have believed what I was taught.

Living Multi-Spirited

I, like many living today, was born multi-spirited. I incarnated into this life with multiple souls attached to me—in addition to my many past-lives and spirit-guides for which I gained automatic awareness from being psychic and empathic. I tell the full stories of some of the incarnations and attached spirits in the first two volumes of this series, but in short, all of my spirits were multi-ethnic from different times and places—China, Africa, North America, South America, and the Caribbean Islands to name a few. In fact, I arrived in this pale body having a deep understanding of what it meant to live in a brown body in the culture of the Americas over the last 5000 years.

The experience was different than just having empathy for someone. I saw through their eyes and witnessed my life through their understanding, as well as feeling what they felt. When things around me would happen, I'd experience it through them as well as myself. Although I knew I was different, I felt right at home with all my people. There was never any separation of personalities, and I always felt in control of my faculties; although, as an empath, and being multi-spirited, I grieved every day. Sometimes it was about the tumultuous world, but often the grief I carried was for the generations of others who were unable to grieve for themselves. And, of course, I told no one.

Now, we are seeing the spiritual liberation of millions of human souls who have experienced marginalization in some way in their lives on the planet.

We bear witness to this through the grief of the empaths and multi-spirited. They help souls process their unexpressed grief from the trauma they experienced during the incarnation in which they lived. There are millions of people who've been born multi-spirited in the last three decades as the three planetary cycles come to an end. The dynamics which created the spiritual trauma must be grieved for healing to take place for all of us. Empaths and the multi-spirited are here to assist in healing the deep cultural wounds that exist—some for thousands of years.

What It Takes to Heal Cultural Wounds

Understanding, empathy, and grief is what it will take to heal the cultural wounds that exist today. Many people are haunted with the daunting task of repairing the spiritual, emotional, and physical damage done by the victimization of their ancestors and the cultural aftermath that perpetuates those injuries. There are many levels to address.

The first thing to consider is that there is a difference between soul memory and DNA. No matter the body you were born in, it is the soul that carries the ancestors and their memories—it is they who must find healing. Making an assumption about who people are from their physicality is ignorant at best. It will be necessary to use all your faculties, learning to feel who people are, their intent, and your connection to them.

The second thing to consider is that everyone who comes into your view in your world vibrates at a frequency similar to you. That means that you are connected in some way and can empathize, possibly through experience, culture, upbringing, career path, sexual orientation—something. There is no more of *our kind*, there is one race with billions of people going through the same life as you, no matter how it appears. So, get on board. You are all *my kind*.

The third thing to consider is that healing takes place through the process of grief—for everyone. If you've been taught that grief makes you weak, you've been taught wrong. If you're afraid that if you start grieving you'll never stop, it's not true. The only way through the darkness is to grieve in the light for all those who lived but could not grieve for themselves: those who were abused and shut-down, those who died in trauma, and those who lived in an environment where it was not safe to grieve.

Not every human is equipped to do the work of long-suffering. But make no mistake about it, if you aren't the one who is grieving, then someone is grieving for you. Find a way to have compassion for the role that you and others play, witnessing the difference and stepping in with support where you can. Embrace the idea that grief integrates a disparate soul and brings all the pieces together into the whole.

The final thing to consider is that the world may never go back to how it was. So while we can restore love, dignity, joy, sobriety, and wisdom—and certainly restoring those things will create a world that we can all share—it will never again be the *old ways*. It can only be a new version of the old ways, or just new ways. Now is the time to review your cultural customs and traditions, and transform what no longer serves the greater good for everyone on the planet. Some things won't change, but many must transition.

Racism and Bigotry

Everyone experiences or perpetrates racism and bigotry on some level. Whether you're describing the black girl over in the corner standing with the white guy, or making an ethnic joke, or even using the pronouns of *they* or *them* to describe an entire group of people (as if they all share the same attributes). The other day I heard a man say, "I'm Asian; I know a lot of doctors," as if being Asian was a prerequisite to knowing a lot of doctors. All of these are the little ways we express racism.

We are all individuals and—when looked at beyond the surface—a plethora of descriptors come to mind, if we will take a breath and the time to really look at someone and maybe even empathize. The goal here is to recognize the ways you think about people, and your preconceived beliefs about them, in order to shift how you communicate to them and about them. There is no shame involved, just the opportunity to think, feel, and communicate with compassion towards others and yourself.

I received a powerful letter from Amber Coleman, a woman who described her experience with racism beautifully. She wrote:

> "I really resonated with a statement in your article about drama addiction where you said, 'Anyone who has experienced racism or bigotry is going to be very sensitive to disrespect.' I'd never heard it articulated that way. As a black woman, living in Los Angeles is a very triggering experience overall. While I've been living here, I've been working in professions where I am constantly mistreated. The culture of this city is severely low in its integrity, and I want to transcend it all somehow. I'm sick of being offended. It's justified, but it doesn't feel good. How do you not live in denial but not live in anger?"

I responded:

> "I'm glad you reached out. Whew, Los Angeles is rough. I know. I find the racism here more passive-aggressive than in other cities, which makes it essentially harder to address.
>
> "The answer to your question is a multifaceted one, and requires many things be examined deeply, not just other people's bad behavior or your anger. How we feel is directly related to the lens through which we look at life. This lens can have many origins and anchors, and we can't underestimate ancestral scars. I find there is a lot of room for transformation once we've allowed ourselves to acknowledge our circumstances or condition (the lenses) and then grieve them.
>
> "The real journey is to forgive—yourself and others—deeply. You will then transcend the illusions of race, gender, and cultural stigma. You've got to see in yourself first what you feel other people do not.
>
> "Having said all that (in a completely oversimplified way), achieving it happens one step after another—starting where you are. Every small accomplishment has its reward that motivates you to continue on the path of freedom.
>
> "It is absolutely possible to not be in denial *and* not be angry. The link between those is through communication—and communicating in a new way takes practice. While you're doing that work for yourself, it's productive to remember that racist people have deep-seated ungrieved trauma and aren't actually in the position of real power.
>
> "Thank you for giving me the opportunity to delve into this a little more with you, it's a deep and abiding topic that desperately needs new revelations and discourse."

> The real journey is to forgive—yourself and others—deeply. You will then transcend the illusions of race, gender, and cultural stigma.

The point is to expand your knowledge of others and make efforts not to stereotype and lock them into a pigeonholed grouping in your mind. While for some, there are cultural similarities; even so, no two people look alike, act alike, or think alike. As far as who you like, that's completely up to you—but be honest and upfront. When you are clear with someone that you do not enjoy their presence, they are free to adjust their behavior accordingly and not feel bad about it. Communicating your feelings with grace and without shame allows you to accept people as they are, so that you may keep moving forward.

Learning to communicate peacefully comes by having grieved through your anger, and with a lot of practice. Rehearse what you'd like to say and how you'd like to say it, over and over, until it feels natural. I had a boyfriend who was deeply manipulative; every time we had the same argument: he always found a workaround to what I was feeling, never fully acknowledging my viewpoint. I realized that each time we had the conversation, my lead-in to his workaround was, "I feel...." I would say it every single time, and that's where the conversation would turn into an argument. I left the conversation feeling defeated each time. My anger made me understand I wasn't being heard. In recognizing this, I finally set out to write what I wanted to say. Finally, reading it aloud, role-playing with a friend until I felt confident in the discussion.

I had an enormous amount of anxiety when the day came to have the same conversation with my boyfriend (yet again), but I was prepared. For the first time in my ten-year history with him, we were able to have an exchange that required him to acknowledge me and recognize his own actions. Consequently, it was the last talk we had for several years. I was elated on all accounts.

In order to transform racism and bigotry we must come together, understanding that there are those of us who must transition our ways of thinking. These conversations aren't about the color of our skin, our gender, or our condition in life; however, we cannot underestimate the effect these elements have on our ability, sense of righteousness, and confidence to express ourselves. Learning to have uncomfortable conversations and address the real dynamics of power at play are paramount. It takes time, honesty, and dignity to have truthful, from the heart discourse on how and why we feel the way we do—and to set and respect boundaries without fear or shame.

Karma of Politics and Religion

Karma dictates that every individual will have the opportunity to cultivate a deeper understanding of themselves and others, that means understanding life from all perspectives. Some people will do that over multiple lifetimes and others will traverse many perspectives in one lifetime. The more religious and political experience one has, the more difficult it is to choose ideologies that exclude others.

Religion and politics are societal constructs that we use to help us become familiar with the initial concepts of personal mastery: how to treat people, how to respect ourselves, how to break down and conceptualize the spiritual world, and how to understand the intrinsic power-structure in both systems that support or deny all of us in some way. At some point in the multiple lives we live, we will be empowered or disempowered within or by both, leading to our eventual independence and esoteric spiritual revolution. This is where we learn to be accountable for every aspect of our mind, heart, body, and spirit—becoming aware of the energy we generate and contribute to the reality we share.

The Karma of Dignity and Respect

Some would say that finding true dignity for yourself and respect for others releases you of karma, as most of us relate to karma as something harsh and binding. It certainly can feel that way. The truth is, your karma is what you've made it. On a personal level, It is your inherent reactions over time to your choices, thinking, and behavior. Acting with dignity and respect creates higher vibrational waves of energetic response.

Does that mean that everyone becomes dignified and respectful around you? While you certainly have a choice about who you continue to spend your days around, you can't control others, and your karma will—at least for a while—dictate where you can be the most helpful, either to yourself or others. Living with dignity and respect is something that you do for yourself, not because there is a pay-off.

Dignity and respect are like a salve to an ancestral scar—day by day, removing layers of pain, grief, disbelief, and confusion that you may not know you have. Honoring others and their insights can become a paved road instead of a rocky one, allowing you to deeply understand you and your karma—and eventually others.

"BECOMING A LEADER IS THE MOST CRUCIAL CHOICE ONE CAN MAKE—IT IS THE DECISION TO STEP OUT OF THE DARKNESS AND INTO THE LIGHT."[1]

– DEEPAK CHOPRA

The Karma of Leadership

Each of us has a leader somewhere inside that seeks expression. The expression builds as we begin to live in a respectful way, organizing and leading our own lives (being directed by our soul's connection with the Universe). A true leader does not search for followers but understands the wheel of fortune—life's inherent ebbs and flows and the natural position of power in each.

Power-seeking is not leadership. If one is searching for it, they are compensating for feeling inept or isolated. Natural leadership comes when one has become so full that all they have to offer must now flow out into the community, allowing others to be exalted in their own personal contributions to the whole. This kind of leader is accountable for themselves and committed to others, helping them to find their place within the group.

Making the decision to lead while understanding its intrinsic responsibility means becoming a conscious leader. All of us will be asked to step into this position at an appointed time and place: leading a friend, colleague, or acquaintance through a profound moment; guiding a family, company, or organization through a transition; or shepherding a group of strangers through the darkness. No matter the journey, the gift of true leadership is the path that leads you to conscious commitment and responsibility.

The Karma of Corporations and Big Money: Profit at the Expense of Others

Learning to communicate with our environment is paramount to our survival on the planet. When you take time to quiet the inner chatter of your mind, you can hear the subtle whispers of your seemingly static surroundings; they have a lot to say. Listening to your habitat is the same as listening to your own body and paying heed to what it needs to thrive, to heal, and to endure.

The other day I purchased three red tropical anthurium flowers. I was having a gathering and planted them in a pot to adorn the table. The next day, after the party, I'd forgotten to bring them out of the hot afternoon sun. I was sitting inside when I felt a subtle pain in my gut and heard a loud screaming in my head. It was the anthurium. It was over 90 degrees and they were in direct sunlight. I ran outside and brought them in; many leaves and flowers were completely burnt.

I apologized to them and gave them a little water and placed a few different crystals and minerals to ease their pain. I left them a few days to regain their balance, and then I asked if it would be okay to prune some of the burnt leaves, to which they agreed. Every few days I pruned, until all the burnt flowers and leaves were gone; each time I went back, there were new beautiful leaves.

We are living in a time of unprecedented damage to our planet, our plants and animals, our water, and ozone layer. The karma of companies profiting at our expense will not be in some other lifetime. The response is here and now in our present time, and it is affecting all of us. Can you imagine having no water to drink?

I've been considering what will happen when there literally is no drinkable water. You can't go to the store and buy it, there are no natural springs left unharmed, and we don't have purification systems powerful enough to undo what we've done. We've allowed chemical companies, oil companies, and pharmaceutical companies (and plenty of others) to destroy our water tables, rivers, and oceans.

Some of our communities are already in this predicament, placed there by politicians who looked the other way. There is no better time for you as an individual to step into your natural leadership position and bring your skill set to the problem. This is an all-hands-on-deck situation, and we must all do what we can to forward a cure—not only for the planet, but for the insidious sickness that has a hold on those who have perpetrated these crimes.

What Are the Lessons for Disruptors?

A disruptor is a generic term for anyone or anything who causes a disturbance or problem. However, it also establishes an opportunity for comparison. This duality is the creator of awareness. It is the light revealed by contrast that illuminates both sides of anything. Once you can see opposing aspects then you can bring into your awareness the multiple dimensions of cause, effect, purpose, and understanding. So, what is the karma for disruptors? What becomes of the people or souls who incarnate onto the planet solely to indulge in chaos at the expense of others?

The answer is not so clear-cut, but rest assured, one way or another they will at some point experience what they have caused. One's extreme greed will ultimately pendulum to poverty, or their cruelty to others will be visited upon those they love the most. Consider, that this process may take the soul on a journey of a thousand years and multiple incarnations. In order for a person to be impacted by the vibrations they put out into the world, they must be able to feel them. That's why it often appears that the disruptors of our society rarely experience backlash or consequences—why some criminals never get caught.

To be a disruptor teaches the illusion of power. Power, in the beginning, is exciting and inspires great kinetic energy, but for humans, constant motion is not sustainable. Then, add to the mix the spiritual, mental, and emotional dynamic of selfishness. Self-centeredness is generated by need and lacks self-awareness. Many disruptors are insecure and selfish, ultimately with needs that are insatiable. They cannot get what they aren't open to, or don't understand what is truly required to fill the void they experience. The feelings generated by power can be a short-lived substitute for self-esteem, until the inevitable adrenaline crash and subsequent depression.

Disruptors are no more than manipulators of your perception, capitalizing on your fear, anguish or confusion. All of which you control with your self-love, determination, and education. Not the love, courage, or knowledge you receive from others but the truth you follow in your heart and soul. It leads you to seek out the information that inspires understanding of yourself and the role you play in the world in which you live.

It doesn't matter if you are an involuntary disruptor or one at the hands of a mastermind, the only benefit of this position is the guilt that one carries from their ability to feel the emotional resonance of the impact of their actions in the same body from which the actions are committed. That guilt leads them to remorse and hopefully restitution.

The Art of Getting What You Want

The idea of getting what you want, in this new context of integrity and inclusion, becomes a completely different dynamic. As I mentioned earlier, being able to language your desires accurately is a phase of the manifestation process. It is important to understand, when you've hit bottom, things don't get worse than they are, they become clearer than they are. You may not have been seeing them as they were, on all levels. Your ability to manifest experiences you want are based on energy flow—how easily you receive and how quickly you can let go of what does not serve you.

Allowing conscious ebb and flow of energy in relationship to the things you want also changes how you get them and is a skill that takes time to cultivate. For example, if the job you have doesn't bring the kind of money you want, makes you unhappy, or doesn't make you feel better about yourself for doing it, you'd think that letting go of it would be easy. In fact, there is a lot more to letting go than just letting go. There is a grief process inherent in releasing our attachment to things, including ideals and philosophies—like being a lawyer because you think it's prestigious. For many, it is the saying goodbye to what you believe your target will bring you that causes the grief response, and the mourning process of shifting your motivation to something that is sustainable.

Keep in mind, anything is possible in its natural progression, but being able to feel comfortable acquiring, having, and managing well all you possess is what keeps your universe providing more. If you want more love in your life, focus on receiving well the love you have and being loving to others. For instance, if all you think about is wanting love, what you feel is angry and lonely; what you do is isolate yourself from others and judge them. The Universe receives this as you saying, *I'd prefer to be by myself, thank you*. Which then translates in your life as attracting selfish, judgmental, or cautious people whom you don't trust or want to be around.

The Universe multiplies what you do, not what you say. Now, this is where your thoughts become important. They lead you to every action you take. It goes as follows: your spirit contains emotional images and patterns that lead to your thinking; the more you become aware of your thoughts, the more deeply immersed you'll be in your emotional expression of your thought patterns; this then leads to your choices. We do this every moment of every day, whether or not we are aware of it. So, being conscientious of others and your impact on them is paramount.

Creating in a Conscious Way

Learning to create in a conscious way is the act of including others in building your ideals. The spirit of collaboration is infectious, and it will be those connections you make with others that will add exactly what you need to go to the next level in all your relations.

To call down Universal Life Force, there must be a physical world conduit that can manage all the energy, hopes, and lofty dreams you can imagine. Sometimes, there is too much energy for just one person, organization, or society to handle; that means we must be able to connect with others on deeper levels more readily, in order to metabolize the life force that responds to our call.

It may seem counterintuitive, but navigating negative energy in any form is often easier then managing energy that is positive. We learn very quickly in life how to tune out those things that bring us discomfort—not feeling the negativity or grounding it in some other way (via addictive tendencies or otherwise). However, positive energy or *lightness* can create an adrenal, emotional, and mental response of repulsion until we can learn to function in that faster energy resonance. It requires us to grieve, and surrender to everything the lightness represents.

Making New Connections

I have a philosophy regarding connecting with new people and others that share your interests: whoever comes to the idea first starts the conversation. It's fairly simple and game-free. Getting to know people in today's immediate gratification and networking culture is unique and unlike any other time. People make connections for very specific reasons and expect pointed results. So letting go of your agenda allows for the creation of a relationship without a particular job. Regardless of why you'd like to connect, being open to other people is a natural form of support.

Every relationship has an alpha persona. Feel free to be who you are, and if you're the one who knows what you want, go after it. You don't need a reason in order to make a new connection or share a kindness. Create an opportunity—without calculation—to get to know one another, establish boundaries, and witness each other's natural spontaneous temperament. Now, let's take a look at what happens when you do reach out.

- **Make Someone Happy**: Reaching out first shows that you are genuinely interested. Who doesn't want to know or feel that someone is genuine in their interest? Beginning a new association with good will, certainly brings good fortune.

- **Create Clarity**: One day, I had a conversation with a gentleman on the above subject. He must have gone on a twenty-minute rant about why he was always the first to reach out. He went on to say that it made him angry when people reached out but just said hello.

  "I mean, why couldn't they just ask me a question? Why am I the one expected to ask all the questions?"

  He was none too happy when I questioned him further on his thoughts. I find this to be a common feeling people share when getting to know one another—an ultra-awareness of the work involved in making connections with others. A person whose sole focus is the meeting ritual and not the person at hand has more important things to be focusing on within themselves.

- **Reduce the Power Struggle**: Every relationship, at least at the beginning, goes through a time of establishing boundaries. Many people experience this as a power struggle. If you're serious about being open to others, this phase has got to be approached with an open heart and a mature mind regarding the boundaries and battles you'll choose. If it creates conflict for you or your new friend to be the one to say hello first, you'll never make it to the values that actually count in an enduring human connection.

- **Face Rejection**: If the real issue around why you don't reach out more is that you fear rejection, then face it. The more people you connect with, the more opportunity you'll have to meet others with whom you share values and can embrace a meaningful connection. At some point you're going to hear no, and that is just fine. It's a great way to let go of or work through any issues you may have with sensitivity or attachment. If someone isn't interested in communicating with you, it's best to know it upfront.

All in all, fraternizing with others is supposed to be the fun part: relaxed, joyful, and free. So let that be your guide. Focus on being yourself authentically. If you'd like to reach out, do it. Take the actions and say the things you'd say to your best friend. Somewhere in that pile of meetups is the person who needs to see exactly who you are today, right now. But they need for you to feel safe, secure, and loved by yourself first.

Determine Your Motivation for Having Relationships

In today's immediate gratification cyberspace-culture, long-term friendships may be harder to come by. You may find it difficult to cultivate relationships for many reasons or need to set boundaries in the ones you have. The goal of any relationship isn't to meet the needs of either person, but to be willing to witness each other and create life experiences.

The traditional model for any relationship has typically been a vehicle through which you get your needs met, whatever they may be. The idea of a good husband or wife, networking with specific groups, or visiting trendy places—all with the goal of meeting people to provide what you may require. As we've examined before, having a job for people before you've even met them, isn't a good idea. It's hard to feel comfortable and be yourself with others when you are concerned with your basic necessities.

How does the world relate to you when you are self-sufficient? A natural response to an independent person meeting their own needs is having a milieu that shares the same values of independence. We attract what we do for ourselves or to ourselves in our social environment. Here are a few things to consider about your independence and relating to others:

- **Self-motivation, or lack of trust?**

    Do you ever find yourself thinking: I just can't depend on anyone? Making the decision to invite others into your life is an impactful one. Relationships take time, energy, and emotion. Sensitive people are deeply affected by those in their environment. It's important that you make the choice to get to know others based on what you have to offer instead of what you're hoping to receive.

    It's common to lose interest in your connections when you see the only purpose for them are their usefulness. Being let down by a community member can embitter you, embroiling you in a tit-for-tat relationship— or worse, discourage you from participating in relationships at all.

Letting yourself get to know another from an authentic place of genuine interest in them rather than what they may be able to do for you, releases you from the debauchery of expectation.

- **Career-minded and ambitious, or fear of intimacy?**

    When you break down your personal or cultural idea of gender roles and friendship, giving yourself permission to be who you are instead of who others need you to be, many new doors will open. It's true that a romantic partnership can sometimes be a full-time job, but—from my experience—time isn't usually why people choose a career over love. If you don't think you can have both, maybe you fear the emotional connection that inevitably comes from a major time investment with someone. After all, it's not the good times that sidetrack us.

    The only remedy for managing discomfort with intimacy is communication. If you've been too busy to interact with others, take the time to reflect on what that's about. What you want is valuable, but what you don't want becomes even more valuable here. Write out on a piece of paper your top ten *I Don't Want This* list. Somewhere in that mix, look for what's underneath all that ambition.

- **Power struggle, or Incompatibility?**

    Our biggest struggle is discovering and expressing ourselves truthfully—knowing what we like and what we don't, and then knowing what we'll do with that information. Often, in relationships, we get the idea of compatibility confused with liking the same things or being similar. The two aren't necessarily connected. Communication is what builds true compatibility. Liking something because it's what your new partner likes, only lasts for a short period of time. Choosing to join your partner in things they like because they like them, is authentic care.

    Now you see that choosing a relationship is never about your independence, but in our culture today, that can be a plus. Never underestimate the ways that love, connection, and support can help you recognize and anchor who you are as an individual in this profoundly mobile and ever-changing world. Compatibility, then, is a series of choices you make in celebration of your companion, not the obligation to change who you are or how you are, just for the opportunity to love.

Renew and Reset for Love and Peace

If you're not living the loving peaceful life you desire, it's going to take a resetting of the daily habits and rituals that have created the life you have to make a new life happen. Actually, the reset is most of the fun. It's easy to be intimidated or distraught at the idea of change, especially when we need to make big life-altering changes. But when you break down into phases what you'd like to be different, piece by piece you transform your life. If you don't quit, getting what you want is inevitable.

Overcoming the Impulse for Conflict and Struggle

Struggle and conflict are an inherent part of the duality of being human—the navigating of spiritual and physical realms. Conflict is the dynamic that helps you transition your idea from a spiritual realm to the physical plane. When you feel in conflict, it is the struggle to resolve and the inevitable results that solidify the dimensional transition of your idea. So, learning to be loving and peaceful will require that you think of conflict and struggle differently.

Adding compassion to the mix is key. When you have a specific all-encompassing belief about anyone, you must first honestly evaluate why you think or feel that way. Figuring out where your beliefs begin and then questioning their current value is the next necessary step.

One afternoon, I was working at a makeup counter in a department store, doing makeovers, when a customer came up to the counter. The sales gal I was working with was a delightful young lady: smart, gentle, well put together, with a great sense of humor. She also had a strong Jamaican accent and brown skin. She approached the customer, saying hello and asking how she could help. I happened to be standing a couple of feet away, behind the counter, when the customer asked if I could be the one to help her. My colleague and I gave each other a *mmm-hmm* look, and I stepped over to help.

The lady went on to tell me that she was afraid of black people because of a recent mugging she'd experienced. I told her that her honesty was brave, and I asked what she needed from the counter. We completed the transaction and she left. I told my colleague what she said, and she too had empathy for the woman. Then we moved on. You cannot change how people see the world, but you do not have to meet their expectations of the world.

Welcoming Love

The three most important principals for opening your mind, heart, and home to love are: cleaning and clearing the way for it, welcoming it, and harmoniously embracing the object of your love. Love comes to us in our lives in many ways, subtle and overt. The more we recognize the subtle ways love comes to us, the more harmoniously we will embrace the overt ways we engage in the giving and receiving of love.

Believe it or not, human beings need to give love more than we need to receive it, and the mind-trick here is that receiving love is a natural response to having given it. The more you give love freely, the more it finds its way back to you. Keeping that in mind, here are the changes to make to manifest more love.

Receiving Love

The most important thing to do when you want to have more love in your life is to create space for it, literally. Getting rid of clutter, cleaning out drawers, and having as much surface space in all the rooms of the home, but especially the bedroom, is vital. Once you have cleared all that space and have had a garage sale, it's time to clean.

Start with the bathroom and kitchen. Those two rooms in the house are where energy is piped in and released all day. You really want to scrub the baseboards and walls, all of the appliances and fixtures, and keep the lid down on the toilet as it is a major point of energy release. Take my word for it, there is nothing sexier than a clean bathroom.

Giving Love

A person's preparedness to give and receive love is always evident in their home, if one really looks. Take a moment to take your own inventory. How much extra space do you have? How clean is your environment? Do you have past memorabilia up everywhere, or is it concentrated to one area? On a scale from one to ten (ten being ready), how prepared are you? There are quite a few enhancers you can add to your home to support love and relationships in your life.

Chances are that if you have a lot of past relationship memorabilia, you're not really open to a new encounter. So, it's important to mark the heralding of a new time for love in your life. Some of my favorite ways are: planting a lime tree in the southwest sector of your garden; placing pictures of peonies, or a pair of something (flowers, animals, or whatever resonates with you) in your living room and bedroom; hanging a vision board (a collage of photos from magazines that create a pictorial of your relationship of life's desires). These are all symbols of a happy connection.

Creating Love

It's true, your heart radiates harmony to all you come in contact with. If you have the relationship you want with yourself, you will easily be able to live with the new love that you draw to you. I believe the meaning of eternal life is our human and spiritual birthright to transmute and transform anything that causes imbalance in us, so as to completely heal on all levels.

Some of the most impactful blows to the integrity of any relationship are the sometimes daily feelings of disregard we might receive from our partners or the ways we may be subtly neglecting them. Examples of this might be: the way your friend spoke to you when she was disgusted with something else; or when your lover made a joke and didn't notice that it wasn't funny to you and was, in fact, slightly hurtful; or maybe your boss, during a stressful day, spoke sharply to you. Any one of these seemingly harmless gaffs, over time, can add up to frustration, resentment, and unexpressed grief. This leads to distrust, bitterness, withdrawing of affection... I could go on and on with this list. Suffice it to say, every relationship we have needs loving maintenance. This includes friends, lovers, colleagues, and (of course) ourselves.

Consistent self-reflection and taking your own inventory about your thoughts, feelings, and actions can really help. We may not be perfect but it's really important to be self-aware. Every time you reflect on your actions, and then strategize on what you can do and say next time to include everyone, creates more space for love.

> Compatibility, then, is a series of choices you make in celebration of your companion, not the obligation to change who you are or how you are, just for the opportunity to love.

Trust Yourself and Your World

Remember, having compassion for others, in addition to yourself, is the goal; whereby, there will begin to be a cultivation of your own self-trust. The more you trust yourself and your own integrity, the more you are able to accurately discern those who you can deeply trust.

You may find that not every relationship will end up staying in their current position in your universe. Some people we can trust, others we know better than to trust. Either way, what's most important is our self-honesty.

Creating more space for love, and cultivating awareness of yourself, your environment, and others, will allow and promote a loving flow in your life. When you have flow, you will gain trust in the world around you, helping you to find new and conscientious ways to express and receive love in your life.

Living on Purpose

Living on purpose means doing what you mean and meaning what you do—being present to everything you engage with in your life. It means, if you're needing to reconcile any portion of your past, you do it with all the focus, joy, and energy that you have right now. When all your energy is available in the moment, you are effective and accomplish your goals.

The first thing to understand to become present is the five primary levels of focus we have: spiritual, mental, emotional, etheric, and physical. Spiritual focus is the unseen world. Mental focus is all the thoughts and ideals you carry. Emotional focus is becoming aware of your feelings, past and present. The etheric body is a layer of energy vibrating outside your physical body; it's the energy that holds your physical habits in place and what causes the internal struggle you may experience when you begin to change them. Finally, your personal awareness of how your physical body works and how it communicates its needs to you is paramount. Understanding yourself on each of these levels allows for presence in everything you do.

Every minute you put towards knowing and accepting yourself more deeply not only helps you act deliberately in your life but can give permission to others to do the same.

The Slayer's Altar and Ritual: Changing the Way You See Your Environment

What You'll Need:
- Orange seven-day jar candle
- Glass of water
- Old magazines or newspapers
- Scissors, glue, poster board (any other fun crafting item you'd like to add to your Vision Board)
- Completed Vision Board (or picture that represents how you'd like your world to be)

Defining Energy and Vibration

For our context, energy and vibration are like a moving car and the speed it's going. Our physical body is matter (very dense energy), and our energy bodies (aura) are made of many layers of higher frequencies of that same physical energy. All frequencies are purposeful.

When we speak of raising our vibration, what we're really talking about is becoming self-aware of our emotions and thoughts. For example, feeling grief, anger, depression, vengefulness, disappointment, or jealousy are lower-vibrational emotions; whereas, feeling safe, joyful, content, peaceful, and curious are higher-vibrational emotions.

It is a natural part of the human experience to traverse all frequencies of emotion. It is through the expression and release of the lower-vibrations that we discover how we feel—revealing our inner truth and innovating our options for resolving conflicts or manifesting the experiences we want.

Raising Your Vibration to Attract Your Desires

What you first need to raise your vibration is to focus on radical honesty. Be truthful with yourself about who you are—your life, the people in it, and what you have. If you are experiencing any negative emotions, their presence is an indication of a topic that needs some self-honesty and deeper understanding—usually pointing to some unresolved trauma. Once you grasp the new information, you can allow grief to help you move forward. Grieving helps you raise your vibration.

Next, become clear about what you want. Clarity paves the way for you to open your mind and heart and begin to imagine the reality of having what you say you want.

Finally, imagine what it would feel like to have the object of your desire within your sight. Often, we think we want something but don't want all the elements that come with it. So, in actuality, we don't want what we tell ourselves we do. Taking yourself through the feelings of already having something, helps you to determine if you have any unconscious reservations to all that comes with your desire, thereby allowing you to manage or respond to those aspects. Once you've done that, you're free to receive what you wish.

Do One Thing of Service for Another—Every Day

One of the most powerful things I've done for myself over the years, whether I've been in a happy place or struggling through darkness, is to do one act of service for another. It's easy to be impassioned for life when things are feeling good. But what can you do when they aren't?

It's natural to struggle to control the details of your life when times are tough, but spiritually speaking, that usually doesn't work. Trying to control your environment or others in stressful times often causes more stress. It's the way we attempt to control ourselves but end up creating a lot of drama in the process.

Drama is the buzz word we use to describe what appears to the superficial eye as another's irrational behavior. What I like to do is substitute the word trauma every time I use the word drama. Spiritual wounds are the most deeply buried and often remain hidden from view, even to the ones who carry them. A dose of compassion can go a long way. It can be as simple as speaking well of someone, saying a prayer, holding the door, or a bit more demanding like offering them your time and resources.

One morning at a local coffee shop as I sat waiting for my coffee, a guy walked in and he seemed so sad. It wasn't just the 5:30 a.m. blues; I could tell he was burdened by something more. I noticed he was wearing a uniform from a pest exterminating company. I could see the company patch on his uniform but couldn't see his name. I stepped towards him and made a remark about how early it was, to which he turned just the amount I needed to see his name. He shrugged a half-smile.

In that moment I decided I wanted to do something nice for him, and hopefully, it would be completely unexpected. A few hours later, I tracked down his company office where he'd be arriving later that afternoon. I called the local florist and had a delightful happy bunch of flowers delivered before he arrived back to work. That act of joy kept me going for days.

Doing good deeds for others doesn't necessarily need to be as altruistic as you might hope for, but they possibly may be a way of staying engaged in life and taking the focus off ourselves for a while. We all need to feel as if the world we live in supports us. Giving what you have to others creates a bridge to new energy for everyone.

Create a Vision Board for the Altar

A Vision Board is a visual journey of your hopes, dreams, and desires, in which no dream is too much to accomplish. The Vision Board is to inspire you to think outside the box about what you want or feel you can have. Think big. Gather the magazines and newspapers together and cut out any pictures, words or phrases that represent what you want to have, be, or do in your future. Paste them on the board adding any other form of craft you'd like to enhance the story of the board. It's your vision and can look any way you'd like. Place the completed board on your cleaned altar area.

Now, get your journal and spend fifteen minutes a day contemplating and writing about what it means to raise your vibration and being of service to others. Light the candle during each session. Pay special attention to your subtle thoughts and feelings during the week, and make note of any experiences you may have with other people and your environment. Once you've completed the altar and ritual, take all your notes and burn them in a fireplace or firepit, and empty the glass of water outside at the base of a tree.

PART FOUR

MASTERY

Your Karmic Relationship to Authority, Fear, Hate, and Death

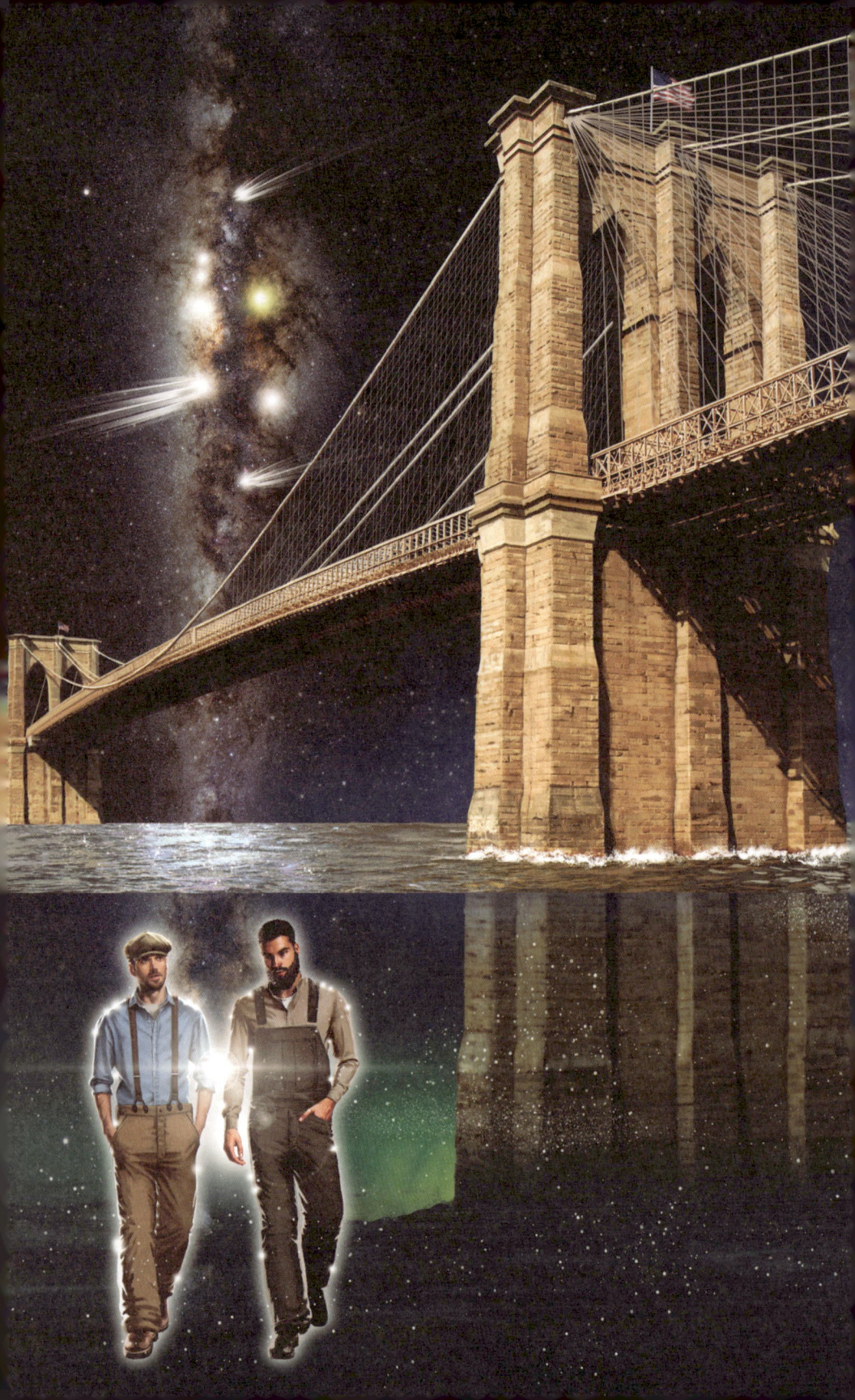

Karma is the Great Equalizer—Teaching Us to Embrace Our Power by Including Others

The Slayer's Weapons:

Discipline, Control, Surrender, Love, Rigidity, Flexibility, Eternity, Transcendence, Innovation, Freedom, Cooperation

The Karmic Story: Building Walls and Bridges

A tale of erecting America out of steel and grit, and the bridge that connected them.

The year was 1877, and by the time politician Boss Tweed was caught, he'd stolen almost $45 million from New York City taxpayers and the Brooklyn Bridge project. Political corruption was at an all-time high, as was the divide between the haves and the have-nots. This was the year that Jebus Stroh fell to his death while working on the Brooklyn Bridge.

For Jebus, it wasn't the widespread corruption that created his inner divide...

Jebus Stroh was a fine young man, tall and lanky, with sandy-blond hair always hiding underneath his brown wool cap. He wore that hat every day, even as he began working on the bridge. Jebus was twenty-three years old and the son of Jethro Stroh, a German businessman, who spent his time traveling up and down the coast from New York to New Orleans.

Jebus lived with his mother in Brooklyn. He had no siblings to speak of but a gaggle of friends who for the most part stayed out of trouble; he led a generally happy life. He'd been working on the bridge for just a few months, learning the ropes and hoping to find a task at which he excelled. Jebus' nervousness made him a jokester, and he quickly discovered he wasn't the appropriate personality type for the caissons.

The caissons were the two boxes made of wood and steel that'd been lowered into the East River all the way down to the hard riverbed. This allowed the workmen to dig out rock and rubble, ultimately replacing the shale with the massive 90,000 tons of granite it took to build the towers at each end of the bridge.

Jebus was prone to anxiety, which quickly escalated into panic on his first trip down into the river boxes. Eventually, being mechanically minded and surprisingly not afraid of heights, Jebus found working on the suspension portion of the bridge was where he was most comfortable.

Jedidiah Stroh (or Corneille, as he was known by his mother's surname) was born into slavery in New Orleans, Louisiana in 1839. His mother worked in the home of a business colleague of Jethro Stroh's where she and Jethro met. Within a year, Jethro moved her and his baby, Jedidiah, into a home he purchased in the Creole neighborhood of the 7th Ward—near Frenchmen street. Although Jethro's young wife from New York only visited once, she couldn't help but notice the obvious; she was haunted by a look she recognized in Jedidiah's eyes.

It was the same look she saw in her husband—every day. She never said a thing, but neither did she go back to New Orleans again.

Jedidiah, on some unspoken level, always understood the complications around meeting his half-brother Jebus, but longed for it just the same. He knew about him from the photographs that began popping up around the house, shortly after Jebus was born. He saw something familiar in his little eyes. Sometimes, when the others had gone to bed, he'd spend long hours by candlelight looking at the photographs and wondering about his baby brother. Would they ever meet?

Jedidiah hadn't spent too much time within the city limits. He worked shoveling coal on a riverboat that carried cargo up and down the Mississippi River. Some days he wished he could hop a clipper ship, just once, and sail all the way to Brooklyn to meet his brother, Jebus. One day, he found a map and studied it the best he could while no one was looking. Jedidiah knew in his heart: one day they would meet.

Jebus, on the other hand, had no idea about his half-brother, Jedidiah. He considered the dreams he would have about a Negro on a boat as night terrors. He didn't know how to make sense of them. He would wake up in a panic every time; he didn't quite know why. He'd had anxiety as long as he could remember and hadn't gotten any real relief, until he started working on the great bridge trestles. Upwards of 120 feet above the water—somehow—was where he felt at peace.

In May of 1877, Jedidiah was working on the docks of the Port of New Orleans when his leg became entangled in a rope and he lost his footing. A steamer dragged him down in between the dock and the boat. He lost his leg a few days later and succumbed to an infection within forty-eight hours of the amputation. Finally, Jedidiah was free to roam. His spirit was unencumbered by his body, yet his heart was weighed down from his unrelenting desire to meet the brother he wished he'd known.

Jedidiah hadn't spent much time with his father. And his mother, with whom he was close, died two years before his accident. He thought, when his time came, that surely his mother would be there to meet his spirit at the pearly gates. Instead, he felt his soul transported to the Brooklyn Bridge.

Working on the Mississippi, he'd heard people talk about the *Eighth Wonder of the World* but couldn't really imagine its magnificence—until his spirit was walking its planks and discovering the concrete filled caissons deep in the East River at the base of the towers. Somehow, this work of art drew him in.

Jebus, waking up with an excruciating amount of anxiety on this morning, made his way to the bridge for his shift. While he was making his second trip across the footbridge towards the top of the Manhattan-side tower, an enormous gust of wind blew the wood and rope structure—swinging it a solid three feet, side-to-side. Jebus quietly tripped and slid down the wood, catching a rope with a loose grip, briefly, before plummeting over 200 feet to his death in the water below.

He died instantly from the impact, plunging deep into the river near the base of the tower. As his body lost oxygen, it was sucked down deeper into the water by a rip current, and no one on the bridge seemed to notice. Jebus was stunned, but his anxiety was gone. Now in spirit—his awareness intact—he looked over towards the base of the tower and saw a brown-skinned man standing not more than ten feet away. He was just standing there peacefully, submerged in the water with him. Jebus was confused.

Jedidiah had seen the man plunge into the East River, just near where his soul stood. Then he saw his eyes, and he knew. It was his brother Jebus, and all he felt was love. He walked over to him, extending his hand, beckoning him to come closer.

"I'm sorry, youngblood. You didn't make it. Your body is already somewhere downstream," he telepathed to a still bewildered Jebus.

"What?" Jebus responded. "Who are you?"

Then, like a stroke of lightning, he remembered the man from his dreams—but this time he wasn't frightened. Strangely, he felt lighter—and safe—comforted by this man before him.

"I am your brother, Jebus. My name is Jedidiah Corneille. I was born of your father and my mother, fifteen years before you. My body died several months ago, but I have been here waiting for something. Now I see that it is you."

"You are the man from my dreams," Jebus responded.

"I am not surprised; I've always felt connected to you, too. Please, come with me."

Once again, he beckoned Jebus to the light of a new dimension. The two souls wandered alongside the East River, laughing and talking about the plight they shared—not yet knowing what their deaths and their new lives had in store. They stayed for a while, sharing and reconciling the secrets of their parents and trying to make sense of a time and society that sought to keep them apart. Finally, a few moons later, Jebus saw a ray of light, and woman who had his mother's face; he knew it was his time to move on. He bid farewell to Jedidiah. And in a flash, he was gone.

On the Banks of the Mississippi

The story began for me when spirit called me down to the banks of the Mississippi River, to a place in downtown Baton Rouge on the levee. I was there one morning a few years back on an annual work visit. On work-trips, I'm always ultra-aware of the spiritual needs of the buildings and the lands through which I travel. So much has taken place over time, in and on them, with no one left to remember or tell the story of the spirits that still linger.

On that beautiful crisp sunny morning, I walked down to the levee and sat on a bench for a while until I spied a large piece of driftwood that looked like a wooden leg. I went to investigate, and the closer I got the bigger it looked. When I got to it, it was over six feet long—with the soul of a man attached. I was certain he was the one who'd called me over.

I could see the spirit of this man in my mind's eye. He too was over six feet tall and dressed in the garb of a post-Civil War laborer. The rich, deep-brown tones of his skin glistened in the heaven he was in. I can't completely explain it, but although this man had both of his legs, I was compelled to take with me the *wooden leg* I'd found there on the bank of the Mississippi.

Off the three of us went, as I struggled to find a way to manage the driftwood. Halfway to the hotel, walking with the wooden leg was becoming heavier and more cumbersome each step I took, but I was delighted for the company of my new friend. He told me his name was Jedidiah.

It's always interesting to experience my world so clearly, all the while knowing others don't view it the same. The folks at the hotel didn't seem phased I was walking in with a six-foot log, and of course, no one saw the spirit of my new friend, Jedidiah.

I must say, it was a little awkward inviting a man I didn't know up to my room. He seemed to be enamored with the glistening white mosaic-tiled shower, which was extra-large and designed to allow a wheelchair. I placed the wooden leg in the shower for a rinse. *What was all of this for?* I thought. Jedidiah was fairly quiet, and soon my friend Faith was coming to pick me up for the final journey to New Orleans, to spend a couple of days before my flight home.

Faith arrived and laughed as she pulled up, seeing the bellman's cart with my bags and the wooden leg.

She asked, "Where'd you get that?" with very little surprise in her voice. (We have a history of finding large items and carting them home by any means necessary.)

"Down at the river. Look! It's shaped like a wooden leg. Oh, and we also have another passenger. His name is Jedidiah."

"Okay then, welcome, Jedidiah. Tracee, were you thinking of taking that leg on the plane with you?"

"No, I was hoping we could stop at FedEx to send it."

Still, there was no sense to be made of these shenanigans. This morning, I had gone to the levee to pray for those lost, calling forward all whose spirits were ready to ascend to the rightful place of their soul's origin. But the only soul I came across was Jedidiah, and he wasn't interested in leaving. Faith and I drove around New Orleans with Jedidiah and the wooden leg for the next two days, eventually leaving the driftwood with Faith and boarding my flight home.

I still had no idea what it was all about, and it wasn't for several weeks before a dream came. In the dream, I was standing at the water's edge with the sun just rising over the horizon. I was in the same place I'd been before with Jedidiah. Only now, it was different: there was no levee. Jedidiah and I were with a crowd of around fifty wandering spirits. All of us standing there joyfully, with the Mississippi up to our ankles.

Jedidiah was the conductor of our spiritual railroad, leading these souls to their salvation in the dimension of light. He was connected to the light and I was anchored in the physical realm; together we created a bridge on which the souls could travel back home. Jedidiah and I met several more times in the astral, before he finally revealed the recent life he'd lived in a body and about his brother Jebus Stroh.

Hidden truths inspire dissonance within us. It is a part of our spiritual need to reveal the secrets that our shame, confusion, anguish, and anger withhold—seeking revelation and peace—these truths persist as long as it takes to receive the whole story, and the healing that knowledge provides.

The Slayer's Path: Surrender To What Is—The Only Control You Have

When we talk about surrendering to what is, we are speaking of current physical world facts. Spiritually speaking, all dimensions of energy are the illusions we create and perceive—good, bad, or neutral—that support us in our human expression. Until we accept what's happening in the physical, we cannot make any change to it. So, while we can receive information from all spiritual dimensions, it is surrendering to the truth of the real world that is paramount.

Once you've surrendered to accepting things as they are, you can receive the spiritual information on how to change what no longer serves you—whether it's working through fear, addressing the truth, or innovating in some other way. This doesn't mean you can change others and their beliefs, but you can find ways of stating your case with a method that promotes listening, or you can move away from the situation altogether. Either way, surrender is the only path forward when you're up against a wall.

The Four Walls: Building Spiritual Bridges to Overcome Them

The industrial revolution and the massive development wave of the last century has changed our world in ways that are irrevocable by humans—an important thought to contemplate for each individual who'd like to continue living on the Earth. But with every bridge or building raised in the name of progress, the spiritual karma created from the devastated lives caught in the wake of this evolution is powerful.

From colonizing the lands to commandeering acreage in the name of eminent domain, one might think of the millions of untold stories of those who have died in the pursuit of expansion. The truth is, those disquieted spirits remain in the ethers haunting the paved roads, cleared forests, massive condominiums, and oil wells and pipelines that dot the planet.

When beginning to understand one's karma and the spiritual purpose of emotion, it is necessary to focus on what I call the four walls: authority, fear, hate, and death. The four walls are merely viewpoints, not truths. They center your attention on what is unmoving in you (authority), what you'd most like to avoid in yourself (fear), your deepest attachment to your self-loathing (hate), and your resistance to life (death).

The karmic patterns created through lifetimes of recurring life-diminishing beliefs or actions will eventually create one or all of the walls—intended to transform and reroute the old pattern to a new life-giving opportunity. The common ground that each wall shares is an intense, cohesive, seemingly hard to move and dense vibration that can feel daunting when faced directly.

It is in the life arenas that are most in need of expansion where one finds a karmic wall. These walls are often expressed via the following emotions or states of consciousness: rage, anger, righteousness, superiority, deep-sorrow, grief, shame, self-pity, emotional paralysis, anxiety, apathy, and feeling overwhelmed. The reverse is also true: the presence of these states of being, and the things that trigger them, are indicative of the existence of a karmic wall.

In the last few days of my stepfather's time on the planet, he was in and out of consciousness. During this time, one night he came to me in a dream. He and I were sitting in a concrete room with no doors or windows when he said to me, "I don't know how to get out of here, Tracee."

You see, he'd been a drinker most of his life and had no conscious spiritual relationship to anything that could help him with safe passage to the other side.

I told him I understood and took his hand, extending my other hand outward and calling for Jesus to come to us—which he did. Jesus stepped in, taking both of our hands and completing the circle; the concrete walls immediately began to disappear. My stepfather was humbly overjoyed and grateful. He thanked us both, and I awoke. The next day, he died.

When one has a prohibitive pattern, in this case drinking, it creates a wall of self-loathing that disallows for expansion in any form. The presence of Jesus, who represents self-mastery, is the antidote to attachment—transcendence.

Understanding Your Relationship to Authority

The authorities that govern us throughout life are mirrors of our spiritual blueprint of karmic needs. They give us outer or inner structure and guidance to, through, and around the elements of our karma. The powers that you come across, whether positive and supportive or abusive and diminishing, are the motivators for you to fulfill your spiritual promises to yourself.

An authority isn't necessarily a person, it is anything that commandeers your emotions, focus, or power. For my stepfather, alcohol became his authority and ultimately the reflection of his own self-hatred. Any authoritative leader—such as addiction, obsessive emotions, or defeatist belief systems in general—are the daily motivators, or subjugators, that make us dig deep within ourselves to find the life-giving resources that help us rise-up to what our world requires from us.

Often—places, times, or dates that trigger our grief can take charge and become our authority. The death and birth anniversaries that we experience—and the expectations we have for them—or the times and places where trauma has occurred can easily trigger grief, that if avoided, becomes the authority of that time and space until the grief is acknowledged.

I worked with a client Gino, who, almost every night like clockwork, would go into a delusional fit of rage and self-pity at midnight. He would begin to drink alcohol earlier in the evening so that by 11 p.m. the slow train of self-pity would pick up steam on its way to rage and conflict. During this time, he would drunk-dial friends and family members to cry or pick fights—in addition to doing the same with his partner—all of which ended in the conflict that ultimately alienated everyone in his life.

During a session with his partner, Janell, who was struggling to deal with the dynamic of her own enabling of my client's behavior, we discovered that the pattern was a product of Gino's continual sexual molestations and assaults perpetrated on him by his grandfather, every night at midnight, for many years of his childhood until his grandfather died. This abuse had gone unaddressed by other family members, and while Gino acknowledged what had happened to him, he had not fully processed his grief, instead seeking to subdue it with his drinking.

This vehement denial of the grief related to his abuse led to his nightly behavior. He often blacked out, and had no recollection of the conversations and rage he would perpetrate on those closest to him through emotional cruelty and temper tantrums. Unfortunately, Gino did not want to address this issue, even as all his friends began to refuse contact with him. The power Janell had in the situation was to set boundaries with Gino—expressing her love and doing her best not to participate in the behavior.

Whether our personal ideals help us to join together with others in their experiences, beliefs, and causes, or supports us in acknowledging a need to move away from another individual's behavior or ideology—they are the teachers that demand our commitment to stand up for ourselves. It is only through taking a position in a conflict that we can access the needed information to help us resolve the problem.

Our memories from any life experience—past or present—can also become one of our authorities, causing fear and anxiety as a reminder of their presence. No matter your command of the situation, inherent in it is the opportunity to expand in wisdom and grow in confidence—to do first what is right for you and, eventually, what is right for all of us.

The elements that create the totality of our relationship to authority are many. We are born with a predisposed relationship to it. How we are nurtured by our parents and other people in positions of power contribute to that connection as well. Our cultural traditions, and the reactions from the society they occur in, are also part of the mix. These all make up the complex dynamic of an individual's relationship to power.

Understanding Your Relationship to Fear

Fear is the alarm system we have that connects all the levels of our awareness with the physical body. Fear activates our endocrine system, which promotes our ability to fight or escape in any situation. It can also connect the subtle energy bodies (spirit, thoughts, and emotions) to communicate any possible intrusion to the central nervous system. The purpose of fear is to keep the body alive and intact—to quickly process and survive any threat.

However, in our culture, fear has become a weapon—a tool people use to expose, manipulate, intimidate, and control the vulnerabilities of others. With fear comes the enormous responsibility of knowing and believing in yourself; it is your confidence that allows you to make fear your ally.

Humans spend a lot of time processing fear around things that might happen. The depth and focus of this worry can be an indicator of the spiritual imprints within a soul and the karma to which they are beholden. It brings an acute focus and awareness to any situation so as not to miss any important detail. It is this detail that brings to light the dynamic to be re-evaluated, and a new decision made on its necessity. This is the spiritual understanding of post-traumatic stress.

Any intense event or ill-timed death from a previous life will cause a post-traumatic response in a subsequent time or life. The experiences that trigger fear are arrows pointing you in the direction of the deeper wound to be healed. Once the energy has found resolution, fear around that topic or experience will be muted.

Understanding Your Relationship to Hatred

Hate is a buzzword our global culture uses liberally to describe anything from a strong dislike to a deep and abiding malevolence. However, true hatred consists of layer upon layer of embittered attachment to the hater's object of focus. This passionate dislike will eventually become dehumanizing, and can easily pave the way to some form of inner or outer destruction.

As well, we cannot overlook the connection we naturally make between hatred and evil. As a spiritualist I have spent a lifetime studying the nature of evil and its effects on human vulnerabilities. Demons are real and have power in our physical world vectored by hate. Though not every human will have a direct connection with these dark entities, we can all witness their works of chaos—and those who hate become susceptible to their impact.

Without entering into a discussion of justice, I don't believe humans are inherently evil. They are—at times—dense, delusional, vengeful, and open to demonic support. It is the force of the darkness that wields an inhuman chaos that causes destruction. However, human beings are culpable for any action they take as they have a choice—consciously or not—to allow the spiritual support the dark entities provide.

For me, hate isn't a word I often use, because to hate anything keeps it attached to you. Your hate becomes a contract to work out the miserable relationship between you and the thing you hate. If I have a passionate dislike of something, I look to find a peaceful resolution of my issue so as to let go of whatever it is completely. If you hate, that which you hate stays with you.

Understanding Your Relationship to Death

To fully comprehend death, one must also consider rebirth. They are inextricably linked. The eternal nature of energy requires that when one thing ends another begins. Energy changes forms; it does not disappear. This is where we begin to understand the nature of death.

The next thing to consider when pondering death, especially the expiration of animals and loved ones, is that culture, tradition, and religion often play a large role in one's initial beliefs—especially if one has never actually experienced the loss of someone close. We spend an enormous amount of our life in denial of death in many ways. The movies we watch let us believe that death is instant, or when illness comes, death occurs only in hospitals with professionals offering care. The truth is people avoid death, and therefore pain and grief, like a stampede.

For now, I'd like to look at death as an incredibly vital and powerful process of transition from one state to another that is life affirming for everyone willing to be its witness. When someone begins their ascent out of the physical body, there are many phases to their inevitable journey—whether their death is foreseen or the product of an accidental, or otherwise spontaneous, mortal event.

I have witnessed the death process begin with people taking care of their personal effects, completing relationships with final conversations, or reconciling long-held resentments, beliefs, or conflicts—in advance of their demise—all to create a peaceful transition, whether death was expected or sudden.

One can, in fact, begin the *death march* years before they die. It is the ability of the person in transition, and their loved ones, to witness what's happening by recognizing it as the beginning of a process—a process of learning to let go of the physical realm. This objective viewpoint allows for feeling empowered in the process rather than feeling victimized by it. Ultimately, our relationship to death begins with our karmic experiences, then how we are educated about it in our developing years, and finally on the conclusions we choose to investigate as adults.

> Surrender is the only path forward when you're up against a wall.

Soulmates: Your Karmic Authorities

Karmic authorities are the people we come in contact with that require us to set boundaries or respect limitations that are set for us. We will always be required to take a side when it comes to these soulmates. We will either join them in their crusades and beliefs, or we will be forced, in one way or another, to take a stand against them.

Lessons of power are what these soulmates teach. The ability to communicate effectively and learning how to empathize with others—seeing and weighing each point of view—are the fruits of your labor in these relationships. Often filled with conflict, experiences with these soulmates will help you see where you can take responsibility for yourself in life—being accountable for your own actions.

Dictators, Warmongers, Political Leaders, and Celebrities

People in positions to lead others on a grand scale have a special karma. No matter the work they do, they directly or indirectly invoke groups of followers to move in thought, emotion, or action. They become the receiver of intense psychic energy generated from the public, either positive or negative.

Often these people will become icons or personal metaphors of the energy dynamic for which they have become known to the public. Imagine what it's like to be the recipient of the psychic energy of millions of people and their opinions. That's but a glimpse into the karma of one of these public soulmates.

Criminals, Predators, Murderers, and Victims

When it comes to adversarial soulmates, there is a lot to consider. For each of us to receive the karmic understanding of victimization, there must be criminals and sociopaths to create the situations of learning. This idea doesn't specifically condone bad acts, just recognizes that in a dualistic society both elements are teachers of wisdom and mastery. Karma dictates that, ultimately, both victims and perpetrators will know a position of dominance or submission.

When it comes to our most loathed criminals, such as pedophiles, it's important to understand that the karmic purpose of such a condition isn't to perpetuate continued depravity. It is an opportunity for everyone, in each situation, to overcome their predilections—mentally, emotionally, and spiritually—and to become accountable for their actions.

The spiritual contract between a victim and a perpetrator is a bond that can continue over lifetimes until forgiveness has occurred. The spiritual and emotional attachment between these two soulmates will be strong and must be considered, regardless of the apparent relationship, if there is hope of completely reconciling the conflict.

For example, a child who has been sexually molested will struggle with their loyalty towards the perpetrator as they begin to recognize the degree of subliminal and direct intimidation and disempowerment that occurs during the pedophile's process of grooming their victim into submission. Deceit and betrayal, which occur in the process of grooming, can look like affection or protection.

Often, the boundaries in these relationships can be tenuous at best. I worked with a woman who'd experienced sexual abuse by her father and other family members from the age of two until she was twenty-one. She was around sixty when we met, and she had lived a life of profound suffering because of the abuse and all the pain and turmoil it perpetuated. She came to me to do a past-life investigation in hopes of finding some understanding. We worked together about a year, and in that time, she recalled multiple past-lives during the regressions.

The most potent of these was a memory of a previous life in the 1700s, on a farm in North America. She was a widow and mother to a son. After the death of her husband, she'd begun a sexual relationship with her son, then a ten-year-old boy, which continued until he killed her some fifteen years later when she refused to let him marry. Her son in that life was the soul of her father in this lifetime.

My client grieved for days after this spiritual recollection but expressed a sense of relief and forgiveness for herself and her father. It didn't justify his actions, but it allowed her to pursue the knowledge she needed to forgive herself for the original violation. It was a life-changing realization, and it was instrumental to her finding peace—truly moving out of feeling victimized and moving forward in this life.

First Responders, Police Force, Military, and Counselors

These are some brave soulmates who make a conscious choice to train for an opportunity to help others. These mediators-of-crisis hold life and death power in their hands, which calls for impeccable self-awareness and mastery. A tough requirement for any of us. So, while we are eternally grateful to these people who help us through the emergencies in our lives, we don't necessarily look forward to our meetings with them.

The fraternal bonds forged in this sort of work dynamic can endure for lifetimes. Conversely, to hold one of these positions can be a lonely experience for some. The suicide rate for first responders is approximately twenty percent higher than all other demographics.[1] The spiritual patterns created from a lifelong dynamic of service can be thankless and easily corrupted—therein lies the karma. Everyone making this life choice will be challenged on all levels with transforming the fight-or-flight response to fear, while simultaneously learning about self-care.

Also, as a part of this karma, is the lesson of discipline and trust for authorities. All these people must follow the orders of their superiors—even when they don't agree. If a superior is wrong in their judgment call, a subordinate runs the risk of being disciplined or losing their job if they disobey a direct order. The karma, however, is divided between the subordinate and their superior. Ultimately, on the karmic wheel, it is common for those held in subordinate positions to, at some point, seek power over others. When we attempt to train any group of people out of their own presence, instinct, and observational decision-making power, there is a high risk for error and irrevocable tragedy.

It is this unique and powerful group of soulmates that will teach us all the lessons of peace, trust, and the value of making decisions by considering everyone directly involved in the moment.

Doctors, Priests, Teachers, Coaches

Again, we find another category of service-oriented soulmates. These are people that can make a lifetime mark on your psyche, as they often show up predominantly in the developmental years when setting and following limitations is necessary but often difficult. They can wield a lot of power over their patients, congregation, students, and players.

It's important to remember that people, no matter their position of power, have their own set of personal issues and human foibles. So, when you are meeting these spiritual leaders as an adult, embracing your own personal power and confidence is paramount. We are all students and teachers in this giant maze of give and take; learning and offering cooperation is the synergy that makes things work. That's the big take-away from relationships with these soulmates.

"RANK BELIEFS NOT BY THEIR PLAUSIBILITY BUT BY HOW MUCH HARM THEY MIGHT CAUSE."[2]

- NASSIM NICHOLAS TALEB

The Warrior's Hidden Motto: What I Don't Understand Will Hurt Me

Paranoia is a deep-seated form of fear that comes from past trauma present in previous lifetimes. The emotional body is always on high alert for possible intrusions or conflicts on any level, perpetuated by the belief that *what I don't know or understand, will hurt me*. When this thought presents itself early and organically in life, there is often a karmic connection.

It is the hypervigilance of paranoia that trains the possessor to pay attention to the small details. It is this detail which becomes the beginning of conscious spiritual, intuitive, and empathetic development. Cultivating strength, then, becomes the focus of paranoia. What is this strength, and how do you nurture it?

First, we'll start with what it's not. Strength is not intimidation, bullying, shouting, warring, or any other sort of manipulation within a situation. True strength is quiet, deliberate, firm, and considerate of everyone participating in the dynamic. It takes time to cultivate your ability to master your reactions, balancing out any fear-based responses to occurrences for which you are unfamiliar.

It is essential to experience some fear and anxiety as a part of learning new things; it's the mechanism that promotes focus. However, once you accept that everything in the world is built using a blueprint or process, you can learn to walk through fear with awareness. Strength is built through learning to use this awareness to recognize the subtle vibrations of information that are available from every person or situation.

The Slayer's Dilemma: Viewing the World with an Open Heart

The slayer's dilemma is to begin reading these subtle vibrations with an open heart. And by open heart, I mean without expectation—truly being open to seeing what is actually happening or what is really being said, rather than what you're afraid is happening or being said. The truth is, fear can ignite your delusional vision, which is a creative state of mind that forms a bridge from your fear to your experience or the event you are witnessing in real time. This may give you a perspective that is closer to what you fear than reality. We see it happening more and more today, as in the story of a white woman who was sure that a young black man had grabbed her at a local store, so she called the police. Upon their arrival, everyone looked at the store's security footage. It was clear that as the young man passed her, his backpack touched her, not the boy. He was oblivious to the whole event. The woman's fear created a reality in her mind using her delusional vision.

An experience such as this can be further ignited for others when someone who has a fear misinterprets a situation and communicates it to those who have been victimized, or systematically disrespected in some way, and are they themselves fearful or angry at it happening again. It is through the energy of a delusional vision that one makes the leap to reacting to things that have not yet happened for fear that they might happen.

Our willingness to see people or events as they are—good, bad or indifferent—empowers us to address them with honesty and compassion. This is the antidote to fear.

Learning New Things

Why is learning new things, or discovering truths about ourselves or others, so difficult for many of us? We are imprinted with the concept that gaining new opportunity means the loss of other things in our lives. Give one up to gain one (which is spiritually true if the new thing and the old thing hold the same place).

You've got to give up the old job to make room for the new job, or the old husband for the new husband, or the idea of marriage to have two boyfriends, or your belief that we are all separate and disconnected if you want to not feel isolated. The list can go on and on. Essentially, with every new gain there is a loss of some sort. Instead of focusing on what we're getting, we focus on avoiding the grief of losing.

Daily Anxiety: Managing your Time and Energy

In today's culture, it's easy to be busy. Having so many things to get accomplished in the 24 hours we have, anxiety and worry become the motivator for all that is not yet done. More than half of the anxiety we experience is from thinking about what we need to do, rather than doing it. Not being present in the moment is a time stealer and an energy raider.

When it comes to being productive in your life, learning to be present is the most important education you can give yourself. People use time as an excuse not to do something. The truth is, they don't want to do it. Using phrases like, "I'm just rippin' and runnin' today," and, "I wish I had the time," or, "I'd really love to, but…," these are usually gentle ways of saying, "I'm not interested in what you're proposing."

How you speak about your world is the shape your world will eventually take. Be gentle and specific. Here are a few things for you to contemplate:

- **Don't Believe the Hype**

    Being busy is a state of mind. A common issue I help clients work on is anxiety and time management. The place I start? Having them write down five thoughts they have about time. My momma used to say, "If you're early, you're on time. And if you're on time, you're late."

    Those are the words that motivated me all of my childhood and most of my adult life. Eventually, I had to give them up because they created a subtle anxiety underneath everything I did when it came to being timely. It really worked well in keeping me on track and mindful of other people's time, until my own time became of value to me as well—then, the only thing that was helpful was the art of saying no.

- **Be Realistic**

    Do what you can when you can. When summarizing the tasks at hand, be realistic and honest with yourself. If a task takes two days to do, then it takes two days. Don't tell yourself otherwise. The more truthful you are with yourself and others about your capabilities creates a bond of trust. If others trust you, they will choose you again and again. Being realistic allows you to cultivate a deeper awareness of the universal process that governs all things. This recognition enables you to accurately assess your personal timing while strengthening your confidence in doing what you say you will do.

- **Respect the Flow**

  Everything has a flow to it—a rhythm. That process takes everything you know and all the things you don't know, and can't possibly plan for, into consideration. Trust that the divine presence of your accomplishment (the time and place where the thing you're doing is already done) knows exactly the steps you need to follow in order to bring it into manifestation. Once you get in the rhythm, you garner and wield the force of the universe and all things become possible.

- **Beware of Bullies**

  Don't let anyone or anything talk you out of being truthful. A popular tactic some people use to get what they want from you is to gaslight you into believing something doesn't literally take the time it does. They'll use the threat of loss or the gain of money to enhance your belief. The truth is: the closer you get to being accurate about your skills and abilities, the more efficient you become. No matter what anyone says, that does not change; everything else is just crazy-making.

- **Say No with Firmness and Grace**

  Learning to say no without guilt and with joy will become your best friend. I know a lot of folk that don't want to say no for fear of hurting another's feelings. But the truth is, someone's feelings will surely be hurt when you say you'll do something, and you don't. Your friend then has to deal with the possible consequences of you not showing up—the time, expense, disappointment, or frustration you saying no could have avoided.

Always remember, you are the master of your universe—not others. Your world contains specific obstacles and restrictions that are there to guide you to the most efficient process of accomplishing whatever is at hand.

And, most of all, your universe is never against you. It is always conspiring for your greatness, your love, your well-being, and your success. All it wants is your acknowledgement, and it will give you everything you need—including time.

> What is within our conscious perspective, we are empowered to choose or change.

The Three Steps to Managing Panic Attacks

Panic attacks are an acute version of anxiety and are indicators of deeper wounds to be healed. You'll find panic creeping in when you are shallowly breathing and confronted with the trigger to a current or past-life emotional wound, or when you are embarking on doing something you don't want to do. Resolving a panic attack means taking control of your body and the situation in the moment. Deep breathing is the key to dialing down your panic or averting it altogether. If you experience frequent anxiety, take note of your breathing. When we are worried or fearful, we tend to hold our breath instead of taking long, deep breaths.

There are three steps to follow when you're having a panic attack that help you to take control of it when it's happening.

Step One: Calm Yourself

- Pause what you are doing in the moment. There's a good possibility it's causing your panic.
- Take control of your breathing. Breath in through your nose and out through your mouth—deeply, slowly, and deliberately.
- Reevaluate the situation and decide how you're going to move forward.
- Say no, or stop the activity altogether if you need to.

Step Two: The four hand mudras that create well-being

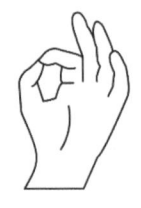

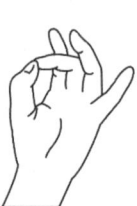

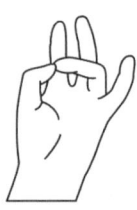

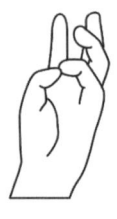

Gyan Mudra	Shuni Mudra	Prithvi Mudra	Bhudy Mudra
Grounds, Calms, Improves concentration	Improves being present, Improves patience	Increases energy, Fosters stability and self-assurance	Improves feeling and intuition

Hand yoga is a way to calm yourself and reroute your energy to resume a natural flow. These simple hand positions, in combination with your deep breathing, can be used anytime—in all situations.

Start with the Gyan mudra and continue with Shuni, Prithvi, and Bhudy in that order for two breaths a piece until you feel calm.

Step Three: Heal Yourself

The third step is getting to the deeper message the panic attack seeks to convey. If you've had a panic attack, debrief yourself by asking four questions.

- What was I doing or thinking during the five minutes before my condition shifted?
- How was I feeling five minutes before my condition shifted?
- Why are the first two answers important to me?
- Ask yourself directly: why did you have the panic attack? Write down the thoughts that come to mind.

Panic at Chicago O'Hare

I was in the Chicago O'Hare airport waiting for a flight, when I picked up the newspaper sitting next to me for a little entertainment. It was my first trip home after moving to New York City. I was still a teen, and I was suffering intense post-traumatic stress from having been raped a year earlier.

My eyes glossed over the paper until I saw an article that caught my eye. It was the story of a woman who'd been raped in her early twenties, and now in her fifties, she still had panic attacks and trauma responses from her sexual assault. Reading that, I began to cry. It had been a rough year of constant anxiety, and I couldn't imagine reliving my trauma over and over for the next thirty years.

I got up from my chair and headed towards the gate. I began heading down a long hallway that was lined with a bright lime-green neon lighting design all along the walls, and just as I was about midway through the hall, the panic attack hit. I was thinking of the woman's words from the article: *it will never be over.* This grew louder and louder in my head until I couldn't breathe. I was crying and gasping for breath while people rushed by, basked in green neon.

On the flight home, I had an epiphany. I panicked because I was conflicted by the idea that I would have to continue to suffer for the rest of my life. This was the common belief of mental health professionals at the time pertaining to the emotional recovery from any assault: you cope and do the best you can.

I was in complete resistance to this idea, because it wasn't my truth. I was not going to just cope; I was committed to doing anything I needed to heal.

Phobias from A Spiritual Perspective

Phobias, from a spiritual perspective, are connected to the spiritual karmic imprints that we carry, and I've worked with numerous clients to resolve them. Every time, it has led to the discovery of past-life memories that include a negative or fearful relationship to the object of their fear.

One client who had an intense fear of crickets and other insects (orthopterophobia) carried a past-life imprint of being buried alive. Another who had an extreme fear of cats (ailurophobia) died in a previous life in a house overrun with them. There was also the person who refused to go near the ocean for fear she'd drown in it (thalassophobia), as had happened in a previous life.

But even with all the interesting stories I've heard along the way, the one that sticks in my mind is an experience I witnessed before I was working as a psychic. Back in those days, only a few select people knew of my abilities.

I was waitressing at a little diner in Venice, California, when I sat a table of six in the outside patio where a large painting of four Clydesdale horses pulling an old fire carriage hung. This family had a two-year-old that we placed in a highchair at the head of the table facing the painting. This poor girl had been crying for almost ten minutes by the time I'd come to the table again to serve coffee. I asked if she was okay, and the mother responded that she had no idea what the problem was. She'd been in good spirits all morning.

In that moment, in my mind, I saw a young girl in a grassy field being stormed by a band of wild horses. It took me a minute to put together that the two-year-old wailing before me was the girl in my vision. Interestingly, until that moment, I hadn't paid much attention to the painting, but it was clear she was terrified to see those horses.

I then suggested to the table that maybe it would be best to move the girl's chair against the wall where she wouldn't be directly facing the painting. Once moved, the little gal didn't make a peep and was giggling as usual. The mother asked me how I knew to do that, and I responded, "Those horses are pretty scary." She smiled.

Almost all phobias can be resolved if you're willing to go back in time as far as it takes to get to the origin of its making. Any fear we have that doesn't have an obvious or reasonable cause in your current life experience always has roots in the spiritual domain.

When to Let Go of Fear

In the self-help and therapeutic industry, we do a lot of talking about letting go, but what does that mean? I'm referring to changing your relationship to the object of your healing (that which you are supposed to let go of) or surrendering to its presence. Both of these dynamics allow you to move forward. This is the requirement to healing and is the *letting go* I'm speaking of.

Fear exists to assist us in quickly assessing a potentially dangerous situation and to take any necessary action. Feelings that are a derivative of fear, such as dread and anxiety, are emotional alarms making the presence of spiritual intrusion known, and both forms of fear are necessary. However, how we relate to them is up to us. Think of fear as your security guard; get to know it.

The other day, my friend and I were walking my dog. Living near the mountains, we have several coyote families that have moved down into the residential areas, and sometimes, when they're hungry, they run the streets in groups of three or four looking for food. This has the community up in arms; people experience a lot of fear around them.

As we walked down a busy thoroughfare, we came across two of the coyotes. As they slowed to look—as if they wanted to play with my husky—both my friend and I stopped. Looking around, she saw an orange traffic cone. She walked over to it, picked it up, shook it at them, and said to the coyotes, "No, go the other way."

And they did. My friend displayed no fear, all business. I noticed that both of us had a slight rise of adrenaline in our guts, but because she had moved into action so swiftly, I just stood with her and waited until our wild friends had moved on. The entire event took less than a minute. We continued our morning stroll without interruption. My friend's composure impressed me.

Now when we speak of the idea of letting go of fear, the actual process consists of four steps: witness what's happening, accept what it is in the moment, assess the situation, and take whatever action is necessary. There will be a slight adrenaline rush in the background, but learning to breathe deeply under duress is the key.

Change is Inevitable

Learning to walk through change is something at which you must become proficient. Whether it be clearing the path with fear by your side or discovering in yourself the things that trigger fear for you and researching them on all levels—you will do it every day, in one form or another, until you have transitioned your fear from foe to friend.

Several times in my life I've been involved in relationships that have ended for one reason or another, all justified but painful nonetheless. I noticed that every time, usually months in advance, there would be this moment when I would experience an awful psychic emotional dread. Usually, it was when my partner was energetically pulling away from me. At the start, I didn't quite understand the feeling was the beginning of the end, and I resisted by grasping at the relationship (or at least the idea of it). This was a dynamic started from the premonition of my father's death so early in life.

After a few of these experiences, I came to accept the feeling and its meaning—allowing me to grieve the inevitable loss. When the dread came, even when the relationship seemed to be going well, there was usually some form of deceit, dishonesty, or imbalance with the partner I had chosen that hadn't yet fully revealed itself. Dread and I became good friends; it was my protector for a period of time. It taught me about life cycles.

As we experience recognition of these often negatively perceived emotions, they and their messages become less scary—allowing more wisdom into our hearts and minds and letting us move forward effortlessly.

The Slayer's Motto: I Am Stronger than I Know

Vitality and resilience are the forms of strength we are looking at here, and in order to fully understand these two dynamics we must uncover a truth about our emotions. Our feelings are the most powerful tool we have, and they can take an enormous amount of physical energy to run. They are the way we read our inner and outer worlds through instinct, empathy, and intuition.

Resistance is the harbinger of change: what you resist is a spiritual message of what's coming to you. The pain and grief associated with change are the bridge from one condition to a better one. Although someone may not be in the position to perceive their grief as creating or heralding a better opportunity for them, it is always the case. Grieving will allow physical relief, emotional release, and spiritual wisdom the path to enter your heart and mind—completing the process of transition.

To be mindful of this process—identifying resistance, reducing it, and locking onto the flow of the change—cultivates a vitality and resilience that will support you in every way.

The dynamics of dignity, peace, and grace are activated when you cultivate strength through resilience and vitality. You will learn to respect yourself and others through your personal awareness, producing a more compassionate view of all things.

Acknowledging Your Inner Authority

Nobody makes you do anything, ever. People can make requests, manipulate and bully you, incentivize you, and victimize you, but ultimately you are the one to take the action. This is the lesson of karma. No matter the complex confluence of circumstances that lead to a choice, you are left, at some point in time, with the responsibility of understanding all that led you to the action and the impact it had.

Remember, karma is the accumulation of the energy of all your actions and the responses to them over time and space. The Universe doesn't judge the ways in which you were victimized or inspired to act, only that you did. It will give you all the time you need, through reincarnation and other spiritual dynamics, to understand the process that led to each one and the impact of them from each viewpoint.

It is this spiritual information that becomes your own inner authority—the internal message that suggests your direction or gives an indication of possible consequences to a proposed action. This energy can also be experienced as your instinct or intuition, but it is often distinguished by giving a hard no or a definitive yes to a choice. Your instinct will let you know if the choice is safe, and your intuition will give you additional information concerning your choice from outside sources.

I also think it bares mentioning here that being victimized in any way is the onset of learning about your inner authority. It doesn't take the trauma out of being victimized, nor does it make being victimized anyone's fault but the perpetrator of the crime. It is merely an objective understanding of the purpose in all things and how they are created.

Transitioning Conflict and Struggle to Learning and Transforming

Everything is manifested through a process of change. How we learn and become aware of these inherent patterns in all things is through our conflict (subliminal recognition of the pattern) and our struggle to overcome it (conscious recognition of the pattern). This element, the interplay between conflict and struggle, doesn't change—only our relationship to it.

To overcome the impulse for conflict and struggle, you must find peace in every step of the process. That means embracing your resistance of something as the phase in the process where you are learning something new, accepting and receiving this new learning, and finally, putting it to use or not.

For almost a year, every time I spoke with a client—whom I'll call Shelly—she complained about how tedious her life was. She was an attorney, but she was convinced she was intended for bigger and better things. The people she worked with didn't understand or appreciate her, but one day she was going to end up in a glorious job that commanded the respect and adoration of everyone.

However, each time I would suggest an action plan to begin changing the dynamic of the work she was doing towards what she wanted to do, she would say things like, *I can't do that. No one will listen. Now is not the time.* So instead, my focus became why she felt the way she did and how she'd like to feel on a daily basis. To which she responded, *I am happy. I feel fine. I am not the problem.*

Finally, after a year of the push and pull—when we met for our weekly session and she started again by complaining and then fantasizing how it would be someday—this time I looked at her directly and said, "That will never happen. Ever."

She burst into tears.

After letting her cry for a few minutes, I asked, "Why are you crying?"

She replied, "I knew it! I knew it was never going to happen for me."

We sat for a few minutes more, and then I responded, "Well, it looks like our time is up for today. I'll see you next week at the same time?"

I have to say, that out of all the uncomfortable things my job calls for, leaving someone to manage their own emotional distress is very difficult for me. As an empath, I was feeling what she was feeling. But it was more valuable not to intervene, to allow her to process the grief of believing she could never have what she said she wanted.

She needed time to realize that she wasn't going to have those things she said she wanted until she began to take steps towards them, not because I said so or because some outside force wouldn't allow it. And while she was in her grief, she could have never heard that portion of the discussion.

When Shelly arrived the next week, she looked lighter and happier than I'd ever seen her. I told her she looked great and asked how she was doing.

She answered, "For the first time in years I feel free. I realized that I don't really want a job that gets me more attention than I already have, let alone a job that puts me in the public's eye. I would hate that. I thought I needed it to feel important, and then I realized: to everyone whose life I impact, I am very important."

I responded, "Whew, I am glad that's over!" And we both laughed.

> "BE FORMLESS, SHAPELESS — LIKE WATER. NOW YOU PUT WATER INTO A CUP, IT BECOMES THE CUP; YOU PUT WATER INTO A BOTTLE, IT BECOMES THE BOTTLE; YOU PUT IT IN THE TEAPOT, IT BECOMES THE TEAPOT. NOW WATER CAN FLOW OR IT CAN CRASH. BE WATER, MY FRIEND."[3]
>
> – BRUCE LEE

Fluidity is Strength

Everyone, in any situation, has a position of power. The dynamic of a predator and their prey is a point of view, or belief that elicits a response of dominance or submission—it is not the truth. When one fully acknowledges and embraces their circumstances at hand, it allows them to become fluid in the situation, responding and rising to the specific needs to be met in order to achieve the best outcome.

I worked with a client at one point, who for a period of time, indulged in getting angry every time something unforeseen occurred in his daily schedule—a colleague didn't make a deadline, the bathroom toilet broke, there was a traffic accident on his morning commute. With each unexpected event he became more and more disgruntled until his frustration and anger began to steal almost all his attention and focus.

Every week he would speak about how untenable his life was and his disappointment in his own performance. He began to ask why this was happening to him. The response I offered was this: "Life is not meant to be controlled—we are empowered to control ourselves by surrendering to the flow of life."

He looked at me with an irritated gaze, to which I asked him a question.

"What do you need to make your life better?"

"Time," he replied.

"Well then, surrendering to the flow of change will give you that time," I said.

It's common to feel that controlling your circumstances controls your use of time, but it does not. The component in power here is the element of emotion in play. The one thing my client did not have a cognizant awareness of was the time his anger and frustration cost him. His desire to focus on the elements he could not control—his colleague, the plumbing, the traffic—ginned up his frustration and disempowered him to make any other decisions to mitigate his losses of time.

If you find yourself in this position, know that when you follow your intuition and the flow of circumstances, everything that can be accomplished will be done so in the order that supports the highest efficiency possible. However, what appears to be resisting this divine order is a path in and of itself. The appearance of wasted time, enormous frustration, and missed opportunity are the vehicles through which we cultivate patience. Any opportunity meant for you will surely come around again.

Trust

Learn to trust that the Creator has your highest intentions in mind, even beyond your ability to recognize them, and that there is a path that exists to a life that allows for your contentment—if you will listen. Depending on where you are right now, there is a series of optimal experiences that will lead you to heal, repair, transform, express yourself, and thrive.

Trust is the dynamic to be cultivated and will become the most valuable skillset you possess as it has the power to change outcomes. When you trust that your world will take care of you, that it will provide for you all you need, you begin to activate the vibration of that sentiment in everything you do. It's like a beacon to your environment, giving you first what you need and then what you want.

I worked with a man who came to me asking how he could make more money. After the first couple of weeks of exploring this in the spiritual realms, his life seemed to deconstruct—piece by piece. He lost his job, left his wife, and moved out of the house he'd lived in for twenty years, all within a month's period of time.

He came to me again, this time angry that somehow, because he wanted more, he'd destroyed his life. It took us some time to break down the important elements of his situation in order to understand why things had to fall apart in order to be brought back together in a way that strengthened him.

The reality was that his wife was a functioning alcoholic. She made most of the money, and he often chose jobs that were time consuming and low paying, just to stay out of the house. Now that he had moved out of the house, and let his wife deal with her condition, the low paying job had gone away.

After some rest, repose, and reflection, he opened himself up to some jobs for which he was perfectly qualified and paid far more than he'd made at any time while with his wife.

Could he have made all those changes while remaining in his relationship? Possibly, but each individual in a relationship contributes things that are obvious and others that are less so. The impact of her lack of responsibility for her addiction matched his energy of doing less than he was capable of for himself. This dynamic enabled both not to be accountable to their highest possibilities, which he didn't realize until he moved away.

Dealing with Outer Forces

Addressing the outer forces in your life begins with your acknowledgement and understanding of their impact on you. Answering all the questions to follow will give you an idea of your current level of empathy and trust. Until you can accept the ways in which the world impacts you, you will be powerless to change it.

- Do you feel better about yourself or less so, when in the presence of the people in your life or at your job?
- When someone is angry in your midst, do you become irritable yourself?
- If someone is speaking loudly or yelling at you, are you able to remain focused?
- Do you believe the world outside will take care of you in a pinch?
- How often do you experience a crisis in your personal world?
- On a scale of 1 to 10, how safe do you feel doing day-to-day activities?
- In general, when running personal errands, do you meet people who are pleasant or unpleasant?
- When you cross paths with someone during your day who needs help, on a scale of 1 to 10, how likely are you to help?

When evaluating your sensitivities to people outside of your normal realm, it's important to think of it in terms of managing your emotions and boundaries. When you are overwhelmed by the energy of others and have a difficult time setting and enforcing boundaries, it makes sense that you are less likely to intervene, help, or connect with people you don't know. This form of isolation leaves you naturally less informed about the outside world and less prepared to deal with it; therefore, it significantly reduces your trust of it.

Creating Cooperation and Mutual Aid

In order to cooperate there must be an observance of mutual trust and a willingness to release beliefs around lack, and the first step to creating mutual aid is to become self-aware—understanding the impact you have on others and being accountable for it. There are many systems in our society that seek to train us out of our instinct and encourage us not to trust ourselves. This is the natural defect of a capitalistic society: get your competitor to question themselves while you take over the market, because there can't possibly be enough for everyone.

The way to illicit cooperation and mutual aid is to transcend society by doing business with the Universe and competing with yourself. It requires full self-trust, faith, connection to your environment, and complete loyalty to the flow of energy that knows all things. This concept allows for inclusion and success for everyone in a way that suits them.

The Slayer's Pact: Face What's in Front of You

All of us have things that make us uncomfortable, embarrassed, indignant, and fearful that we need to face in ourselves and in this world. We live in a society that would, more often than not, prefer us to avoid discomfort at all costs. It offers a thousand different ways for us to medicate, confuse, or distract ourselves. Retraining our habit of obfuscation is a worthy opponent. One that will inevitably require a lot of attention if it is to be overcome.

When facing the foibles and frailties of the human condition, take these things with you: humor, compassion, and honesty. You'll need them. This trip is often long and you're going to run out of gas. That's where compassion and humor come in.

Facing racism, bigotry, misogyny, and corruption take a special kind of integrity. But what about those topics that feel a little closer to home, like a fear of confrontation or a general inability to communicate how you feel? What about your difficulty with empathy or understanding other people's problems? How do you deal with your own personal losses and depression?

Owning up to these things can be exhausting on all levels, but did you know that avoiding them will cost you so much more than weariness?

Ignoring or dismissing your own values and disrespecting the values of others can only create conflict and strife in all facets of your life. Standing up for the wrongs that are being done and grieving the ones that have past are the only ways forward.

Social Justice and Self-Governance: A Global Cry for Healing

We are experiencing a unique time in the evolution of social justice and self-governance. The cataclysmic conflict emerging from all human demographics, right now, is indicative of the karma created from the multiple industrial revolutions that have occurred over the last 10,000 years on the planet.

Every time a group of people has sought to explore and expand their borders, building under the guise of wanting a better and more efficient future, other groups of people have been subjugated, enslaved, and sometimes murdered in the name of that progress. Today, energy on the planet is processed by her inhabitants more quickly, and the impact of these revolutionary patterns appear instantly for some.

The millions of people on the planet living with deep cultural wounds caused by war, enslavement, genocide, corruption, and victimization have no other option but to begin to restore themselves by breaking away from the tyrannical beliefs and insidious patterns of oppression that created the conditions they find themselves in. It is what we are seeing worldwide—a global cry for healing.

It is through this lens that we must take a comprehensive look at how we police and govern ourselves, personally and societally.

Communicating About Racism and Bias: Listen, Learn, and Let Go of Shame

There are a few fundamental elements we must understand, accept, and forgive in order to communicate about racism and bias effectively. We are all racist or biased at some time, in one way or another—all of us. Usually, this is because we don't understand the deep cultural system of racism and bias that exists in the U.S. and other places on the globe. Therefore, it's easy to overlook mistakes of racism and bias because they are considered normal by societal standards.

If you live here in America, we know that you live in a system of racism and bias promoted by socio-economic status, skin color, and gender. No matter your beliefs, our white and male dominated society still generates a spoken and unspoken hierarchy through which people of color are demoralized, diminished, and invalidated—openly and in secret—in all walks of life.

If you are resistant to hearing that statement, it's more than likely you benefit in some way from it. It makes no difference if you participate directly or indirectly, the goal here is not to judge any of us for this quagmire of unprocessed grief, fear, and systemic oppression we find ourselves in. The goal is to accept that it exists and to begin to make inroads in repairing or changing the system—until it recognizes all of us equally.

The white, male dominated system is evident in politics and government, education and standardized testing, gender discrimination for equal pay, and sexual power. Although many of the younger generation have a shifting relationship to the world they live in and don't feel that other people control their destiny, many of us are left to overcome the emotional reality of transcending some sort of sexual, gender, or cultural bias.

While the 116th Congress of the United States is the most diverse in history, the mix still favors white, Christian men. Out of the 535 members of Congress, women and minorities each currently represent less than 25 percent of the total.[4] For years, statistics show a strong disparity in the results of standardized testing based on socio-economic status and opportunity of different cultures, in addition to the tests themselves showing some form of bias based on opportunities to which not all children are exposed.[5] And in many places, most notably Hollywood and the world of professional sports, women are still fighting for equal pay in spite of, and in some cases, generating more sales.[6] In addition, the *#MeToo* movement has highlighted a long needed change to the sexual power dynamic in the workplace.

While it will take generations to reconcile the ingrained dynamics of racism and gender bias for everyone, we must find the courage and the language to begin to acknowledge racial, cultural, and gender miseducation and ignorance—openly and honestly—every time we witness it. We must learn to master our guilt, shame, and anger pertaining to these biases. It's important to be receptive and willing to trust ourselves to begin the work of having the necessary conversations that create compassion. Learning to listen, hear, and validate another's understanding—by accepting the needed reeducation without defense and with gratitude. This dynamic will inevitably become a part of our everyday norm.

Until we have a baseline of cultural understanding about the nuances of racism and bigotry, for all of us living in today's world, we cannot begin to comprehend the complexities of the individual karma that creates deeply intricate and unique viewpoints on racism held by each individual. Only through bringing out and acknowledging our similarities, will we begin to cultivate the trust required to live honestly—so we may all grieve for our collective cultural scars. It's imperative to know another person's experience by hearing it from their perspective.

As a striking example of this, the author Elia Winters wrote one such communication responding to another author who was inquiring about writing dialogue for her African American characters—using the words *educated* and *uneducated* English to describe a way of speech, here is Elia's response:

> "Linguistics ahead! You're not talking about 'educated' vs. 'uneducated' English. You're talking about using a Standard Academic English (SAE) dialect vs. AAVE, which is African-American Vernacular English. AAVE is a dialect of English, not 'bad English'. Like all dialects, it's internally consistent and has grammatical rules of its own...Many Black people are bidialectal and switch between dialects based on circumstance and community. Like many aspects of writing marginalized characters, you're taking on issues of power. The fact that we even think of SAE as 'correct' English and all other dialects as 'bad' English is about issues of power. As an author, you can technically write whatever you want, but writing a marginalized group asks for a higher level of research and understanding, and awareness that you're in a position to do harm (regardless of intent). The fact that you're asking this question is a good step. Go easy on writing dialect, study the linguistics of AAVE, and definitely hire some sensitivity readers before you publish."[7]

Helping others to become clear that what is normal languaging for some is diminishing for others, isn't rude; it is an opportunity for all of us to show respect, compassion, and a willingness to understand the experiences of everyone with whom we share this planet.

> "I THINK SOMETIMES I GET ANGRY INSTEAD OF SAD, I THINK IT'S A DEFENSE MECHANISM TO BE STRONG...I HAVE TO BE STRONG, LIKE LIFE DOESN'T REALLY GIVE YOU AN OPPORTUNITY TO SHOW VULNERABILITY. LIFE DOESN'T REALLY GIVE YOU A CHANCE TO LET YOUR GUARD DOWN."[8]
>
> – LIZZO

When the White Lady Cries

I have a unique experience regarding racism. As I've expressed earlier, I have the experience of being multi-spirited and cognizant of my past lives, but I didn't really get what it meant to be a *white lady* in our culture until I was thirty-five, when the last African American soul I'd carried in my spirit—my entire life—left and was delivered home. You see, up until then, I'd lived with myself and many other spirits in my body (in addition to multiple other past life imprints and spirit guides).

The most longstanding and influential were: Tracee the empath, Nguvu Jabari (African tribal leader, approximately 1000 BCE), John and Adele Battle (African American husband and wife, born into slavery in the 1800s), Nina Broussard (African American, born in the 1900s), Xiao Xin (Chinese, Qing Dynasty, 1800s), Marie Dessalines (Haitian 1700s), Chief Running Bear (2nd Chief of the Oglala Sioux 1800s), and Jasmine Lilywhite (French American, 1900s). I addressed all of them equally, in relationship to their individual emotional power and expression, and spent over half of my years experiencing life through their eyes and their emotional responses based on the triggers of their lives' challenges to the outside world.

Although I struggled with communicating this dynamic to others, I was never confused about who I was—I identified and empathized with everyone. I was at peace with having to encompass such a diverse spiritual-ancestral heritage, the wide range of cultural understanding it brought, and the gift of grief it bestowed upon me; I was proud of my birthright. In my twenties, I just considered them my posse in spirit and went about the business of my life-purpose.

For the most part, I've always lived in and been immersed in ethnically diverse neighborhoods, including my childhood; however, in those years, I was also consistently placed in environments with many white folk. As a response to the racist commentary I came across, I was compelled to engage in conversations about racism with anyone who wanted the discourse, and often with those who didn't. Both of my parents were deeply committed to transforming the racism they grew up with, both leaving their systemically racist homes by the age of sixteen and forging their ways in the world.

I only know this from witnessing how they lived their lives and treated others, not from conversations we had. It wasn't discussed as a rule, per se, but disparaging language was not used in our house towards other demographics, sexual orientations, or anyone for that matter. The only thing my mother ever said to me about racism was when I was in the seventh grade: "Just know there are people out there who don't see things as you do."

Gender bias? Well, our house was steeped in that. While my mother was never directly belittled in our household, much of what she wanted in life was set aside in order to become the wife and mother that society expected of her. She did a fine job, holding her tongue and keeping any grief-filled emotion to herself. This was the women's legacy in our family—keeping grief bottled up inside—until me. As an empath, I've cried every day since birth.

When my father died, it changed a smidge for my mother. She began to express anger, instead of grief, not only at the loss of my father but at the loss of her integrated family unit. Everything changed for us: our emotional cohesion and our socio-economic status.

> "THE TERM WHITE TEARS REFERS TO ALL THE WAYS, BOTH LITERALLY AND METAPHORICALLY, THAT WHITE FRAGILITY MANIFESTS ITSELF THROUGH WHITE PEOPLE'S LAMENTS OVER HOW HARD RACISM IS ON US...ONE MANIFESTATION OF WHITE TEARS: THOSE SHED BY WHITE WOMEN IN CROSS-RACIAL SETTINGS."[9]
>
> – ROBIN DIANGELO

In Robin DiAngelo's book *White Fragility: Why It's So Hard for White People to Talk About Racism*, she speaks about something commonly known as *white tears*. The book is a deeply needed reference to move us forward in the reeducation of our systemically white-centered culture. It deals with the subtle nuances of racism that many white people aren't aware of, don't know, or have forgotten the history of, regarding white entitlements that aren't doled out to non-whites so readily—such as the safety of emotionalism.

Having said that, my many cross-racial experiences discussing racism with male and female people of color always included tears. Let me preface that the conversations of which I speak were, for the most part, with deeply intimate longtime relationships in private social situations. Many of them occurred in my twenties, when I didn't yet have the intellectual understanding of the exact spiritual heritage I carried, and therefore, I couldn't communicate to others the multi-cultural lens through which I experienced life.

What I did have was a deep understanding of the grief we shared, the need to grieve, and the compassion I felt for my friends who I truly did not see as being people of color, as I didn't view myself as white. Of course, I saw the paleness of my skin, but I did not have a relationship to what that meant for others viewing me. I experienced many of the same emotions of anger, frustration, and disgust when viewing racism and injustices perpetrated by white people, not in the *raise-the-fist* social justice way, but with the quiet, internal rage I had witnessed in so many of my friends.

One Christmas when I was probably around six years old, my grandmother was visiting for the holidays. At one point, as we were all gathered around the television, she asked me to pass her the bowl of *nigger toes*. Immediately, and without conscious thought, my eyes welled up with tears as I looked to my mother in horror.

"She's asking for the Brazil nuts," my mother responded.

There was never any conscientious discussion around correcting her language, and when thinking back on my grandmother's racist request, I still feel sick to my stomach knowing that sort of thinking—the illusion that we are different—is still prevalent. The only thing changed for me today is that my personal karmic grief is gone.

Another time, I'd gone on a spiritual retreat to Sedona, Arizona, with a white female friend. While passing through the town of Prescott, we stopped for a bite to eat. Upon entering the local saloon, the lack of diversity was obvious and made me feel uneasy.

As we sat ourselves at the only available table, I noticed there were no other people of color in the place. (I didn't, and don't, identify as a person of color, but at the time, I was carrying multiple multi-ethnic spirits with me. And that was the exact thought I had.) I felt isolated and nervous. I overheard a table of white men not far from us use a racial slur. It wasn't just that they used it, but they used it expecting that everyone around them felt the same way; it made me angry.

I expressed this anger to my friend. Her response was, "Don't worry, just relax!"

At that, I experienced an almost uncontrollable rage course through my body, mind, and spirit. I turned to her. Raising my finger to her face and breathing in deeply, I said: "Don't ever tell an angry person to relax."

The tears began to roll (my trusty stopgap for the overflow of rage). My friend looked at me confused. She apologized, and we turned our attention to the menus.

It wasn't until years after, filled with many conversations like these, that I experienced the emotions created in a past-life as a slave—during my death from being lynched. Witnessing the shock and awe of my abduction, split-second hoisting of my body from a tree with a noose, and the subsequent release of my soul from that body—now, one hundred fifty years later, I experienced the devastation and grief I could not express in that lifetime.

Because of this lack of mutual understanding, many times in these cross-racial conversations I triggered the rage of my friends from my insensitive claims that I had some understanding of their experience. I offered this as a morsel of support, prematurely. I didn't have the ability, yet, to express where my complicated education and knowledge originated.

This culminated in one such conversation with my friend George. When the discussion escalated, his irritation and anger—and my grief (tears rolling down my face)—got to be too much for both of us. He donned the low dulcet tones and slow drawl of the voice of a character—an old Southern black man sitting in his chair on the porch.

He said, "I don't know how a snowflake, such as yourself, could possibly know what it's like for a black man like me."

To which I responded, "Mm hmm."

And we laughed; it was an honest communication for both of us. On the surface we were making fun of me. But on the inside, it was our unspoken way of acknowledging the spiritual ancestral heritage we shared—living with it from a 200-year-old paradigm—while also honoring his experience expanding into modern-times. The comments and the laughter were exactly the salve we needed.

While I didn't yet have a way of communicating about the multiple spirits residing with me or my multi-cultural understanding, George and so many others must have understood on a subliminal level—we trusted each other to share and hear our individual truths. We are friends to this day.

I'm not sure if I cry because I'm white, or that I *can* because I'm white. What I am sure of? I cry every day in this life because I've lived a thousand years of life—bucking up my emotions—eventually living to see them spill over the top into this one. I brought all this candor with me so that I could grieve—at some point. We must all process our losses.

Imagine in your house a basement two-stories deep. One level down, there is the reality that people of color in our society are subliminally or explicitly required not to show the emotions they feel, much of the time, for fear of retribution, judgment, or criticism. The second level down is the karmic need to grieve. All those who have lived incarnations of human trafficking, oppression, tyranny, war, psycho-spiritual warfare, and genocide must eventually grieve for those losses—of time, dignity, self-love, trust, peace, self-expression, and life itself.

Many of the souls who endured those conditions also died in them. Leaving behind, in that time and space, unexpressed grief and raw unfettered loss. That energy must find its way to expression and transformation, either through new incarnations of those souls or any soul prepared for such long-suffering. It may take a soul multiple incarnations to prepare for such a task to be carried out; traditionally, these are our artists, actors, empaths, mothers, spiritualists, monks, and nuns—to name a few.

Long-suffering can be expressed or triggered in multiple ways: grief, short-term or chronic disease, congenital defects, mental illness, trauma, and accidental events. What is most important to remember is that our power comes with the spirit, not the body.

Each of us, individually, must first spiritually integrate, heal, and awaken all the dormant spiritual imprints and retrieve all the pieces of our soul left in the recesses of our collective spiritual matrix. Only when this happens to many of us can it happen for all of us, and then an expression of a unified community, society, and world will begin to emerge. This is our eternal work.

> "TRUST THAT THERE IS A SPACE INSIDE YOUR HEART WHERE THIS INFORMATION LIES DORMANT, AND THE ACT OF GRIEF ACTIVATES THIS KNOWLEDGE AND ATTRACTS TO YOU EXACTLY WHAT YOU NEED. YOU DON'T HAVE TO GO OUT AND GET IT. IF YOU WILL CREATE A SPACE FOR IT, IT WILL COME."[10]
>
> – HEAL YOUR SOUL HISTORY: ACTIVATE THE TRUE POWER OF YOUR SHADOW

Don't Fear the Conversation

While grief is a powerful portion of the healing transition, it is necessary to understand equality as equal *value*—not the illusion of being identical people, as so many treat the idea of equality (as if those who are not like us should get less or be treated differently). By doing this, we will transfigure our world and system of social justice to one that serves us all, and we will learn to speak openly, honestly, and without reservation about the inherent social biases we carry while learning to understand their origins. Each of us have these reservations, but instead of feeling bad they exist, be grateful it is within your power to change them.

Sarah and Mavis in a Cross-Racial Conversation about Racism

Here is a conversation between two people that illustrates the inadvertent assumptions we can often make in cross-racial communications. The discussion is between two college students in New York City and is told by Sarah.

"I had a friend in college, Mavis, who like myself, put herself through school and faced numerous challenges in obtaining her degree. One, being that she was a single working mother with a ten-year-old daughter and little to no family support. She was a few years older than me, and we both had deep respect for each other as no-nonsense hard-working people. The difference between us was that I was poor and white, while she was poor and black.

"One day we were bitching about a variety of things that overworked students are prone to complain about, and I mentioned a ridiculous conflict that happened in my anthropology class between the biracial female teacher, who was a thirty-something Asian-Hispanic, and a young black undergraduate male.

"The anthropology teacher gave extra credit questions once a week during the semester as a way of allowing students to raise their grades. The questions were usually based on supplemental materials like documentary films or other audio-visual materials that would be watched in class. Students could receive three extra points based on how well they answered the given questions.

"The disgruntled student I spoke of only received one point on the questions he'd turned in, and he was upset. The Professor tried her best to have him speak to her in private, but the outraged student would not be subdued. She then told him why he received a *mercy point* as she called it. Apparently, the student hadn't taken any notes on the information given in the documentary. He had just given opinions about the tribal customs without fully realizing the questions he was being asked or the customs being documented.

"It was his opinion that watching films with the lights out was strictly for entertainment value and no one should be required to take notes in the dark. He accused the teacher of having it out for him because he was the only black male in class, and he gave a whole litany of reasons why he was going to report her for harassment to the chair.

"The other students were stunned by his accusations. They told him he was full of excuses and always had an axe to grind about everything. I did not know him personally and remained silent, using the wasted lecture time to finish an assignment that was due next class. When I relayed the story to Mavis, I accused the student of playing the race card.

"Mavis calmly advised me to rethink my choice of words. She told me the undergraduate was using the willfully ignorant card, and the race card was too loaded a phrase to use.

I got defensive about my choice of jargon and went immediately to, 'Are you telling me I'm a racist?'

"To which she calmly replied, 'Not intentionally, but you're using a very loaded phrase that's a smoke screen to the real issue at hand. I don't expect you to understand how what you just said shuts down the conversation.'

"I remember feeling really upset, defensive, and completely mistaken for someone other than who I thought I was. My face was burning hot and my mind raced through all the ways I was against racism. Mavis and I decided to let it go when we both saw it was becoming a circular argument.

"It wasn't until months later, after sitting with a whole host of bad feelings, that I could finally understand what she was trying to say to me. Just because you're not a bigot doesn't exempt you from participating in language and ideas meant to keep African Americans diminished with semantics that keep them in metaphorical chains. I am so glad that Mavis remained calm and firm while reprimanding the language I was using to describe the dynamic between the student and professor, because I learned from the experience."

In this interaction between Sarah and Mavis, or in any conversation where we learn something new—especially when we thought we already knew everything about a particular topic—feelings of guilt, shame, embarrassment, and humiliation can arise. This is a spiritual and emotional indication that the new information is accurate and confirms that a change of thought is necessary.

However, often, when having these exchanges, we can be prone to using inflammatory language as a subtle power-play, such as Sarah's use of *ridiculous conflict* and *wasted time* (referring to her fellow students expression of his anguish) and *reprimanding* (referring to her friend Mavis's attitude or intent, but more accurately as an expression of her feelings of humiliation). Using such language passive-aggressively dilutes, distracts, or dismisses the uncomfortable conversation at hand.

Drama equals trauma: people naturally transfer their unexpressed feelings of pain onto situations that, to them, feel the same or in some way resonate with the original trauma. Despite their behavior or your ability to set boundaries within it, a person's trauma is real and can be validated without changing your boundary.

It is imperative in cross-racial communications about racism that we remember it is not our fault we were born into a system of racism, but that we are empowered to change it. This simple reminder can shift the automatic and subtle impulse to hold our breath. Restricted breathing can lead to subtle feelings of panic, which can amplify the feelings of embarrassment, anger, humiliation, and—ultimately—the grief we may be feeling. Just taking a moment to focus on breathing deeply will calm the dynamic for everyone in the discussion and create the space for empathy.

Many times, in cross-racial conversations, there will be the situation at hand countered by the subtle presence of the energy of a power-struggle inherent in each occurrence. We recognize it by the choice of words we use. These are often ingrained automatic responses that have become habit in our culture.

Everyone will go through a process of denial and defense, anger and frustration—as well as humiliation, anguish, power-seeking, and eventually grief. In Sarah's case, it took several months for her to receive Mavis' full meaning and purpose for the conversation, and to begin to consciously process all of the subtle emotions surrounding the betrayal she felt while beginning to become aware and empathize with Mavis' experience. Going through a spiritual transformation such as this can lead to mutual understanding.

As an empath and having dedicated my entire life to grieving, I feel slightly hypocritical saying that crying must be excluded from the equation because, ultimately, grief is a necessary goal. What I can say is that whatever tears you have, unless you are by yourself, it's imperative to be self-sufficient in your expression of them. This means that you don't bring your emotion into the conversation by bringing the attention to yourself or needing assistance. Both of these take the focus from the needs of others back to yourself, and usually shut down the conversation.

Be sensitive to the needs of others in the room by comprehending that, especially when it comes to cross-racial communication, there are many ways that some communication considered normal in white America is offensive, dismissive, and rooted in the illusion of white supremacy, and is intended to disempower people of color. All of us need to adjust—creating mental and emotional freedom for ourselves through our inclusion of others in our dynamic.

> Energy must find its way to expression and transformation, either through new incarnations of those souls or any soul prepared for such long-suffering. It may take a soul multiple incarnations to prepare for such a task to be carried out; traditionally, these are our artists, actors, empaths, mothers, spiritualists, monks, and nuns—to name a few.

Some Common Racial Assumptions We Make

Here are some ingrained ideas regarding racism and some thoughts to challenge those assumptions:

Racists are bad people, therefore I'm not a racist.	Racists are people, often making racial assumptions out of ignorance.
Racism is personal prejudice.	Racism is a social system deeply rooted in our culture.
It's rude to point out racist assumptions and behaviors.	It is generous and trusting to correct a racial assumption.
If the discussion is uncomfortable for me, you are being hostile.	Discussing ethnic assumptions is uncomfortable for everyone.
If I don't see it or understand it, it's not real.	Trivializing a person's views is an assertion of power. You don't have to validate someone's experiences for them to be legitimate.
I have friends of other ethnic backgrounds, so I can't be racist.	We are racist when we dismiss the subtle and often systemic ways that people of color are marginalized in our society.
There's nothing I can do about my racial bias.	Accept that you were born into a system that you can now change. Be willing to reflect on your words and actions (not your intentions) and their origins. Forgive humanity.

Here's the good news: no matter what others do or say, it does not change your value. Ultimately, the art of grieving is a skillset that we will all inevitably learn, but crafting truthful discourse about the ethnically and socially biased lenses through which we share our experiences takes hard work, which may take a lifetime. Starting the dialogues necessary to find common ground, by beginning to recognize the ways in which we contribute to the systems that perpetuate racism, is something we are all responsible for.

What is White Privilege?

You may be asking yourself, what exactly is *white privilege*? It's an important question. White privilege is subtle, and frankly, not every person who is white experiences or understands what it is or feels they receive it. White privileges are the built-in advantages that white people receive based on the color of their skin in a societal dynamic distinguished by ethnic inequality, bias, or assumption.

The goal for us here is not to ignite a great debate on whether it exists, but rather to contemplate it fully from everyone's perspective. The truth is, each of us have our own constellation of physical, mental, emotional, cultural, and spiritual views and experiences that make us unique, and other people may never completely know or understand us at this depth.

What we can begin to do is unearth the system of racism (ethnic bias) and bigotry that does exist and was built into the foundation of the America and world we now live in. People migrated from all over to North America to give themselves certain freedoms, but have taken those freedoms from others in order to do so. Our charge now is decolonization.

First and foremost, we must give up the idea that there are *multiple races* within the human race. What we do have is *one* race with multiple ethnicities—based on their geographic location of origin, and the cultures and traditions that express them. Next, we have to distance ourselves from the ideas that different people deserve different things and it's up to us to decide what they should have. And finally, surrender the idea that we are separate from the Earth and from each other. You don't have to like or understand others, or their culture, in order to recognize your similarities or connections to them.

Here are some common experiences for you to contemplate that are easy for some but leave others disenfranchised. How do you experience these things?

Emotionalism: the right to grieve or express feelings of rage, anger, grief, or sadness and not be judged or considered out-of-control, or crazy. How often do you withhold your true feelings, or experience resistance if you do express them?

Entitlement: the experience of feeling that anything you want, you can have. How hard would it be for you to achieve or acquire the number one thing on your wants list?

Freedom to Travel: the idea that you are free to go anywhere in the world and are welcome where you go. Certainly, a new level of awareness regarding this privilege has surfaced with usage of the internet (and the availability of global knowledge). Where would you like to go, and do you feel free to go there?

Fear of Violence: waking up every day fearing violence in your neighborhood, home, or community in general—especially from those in authority positions. The privilege is not having to contemplate violence daily. How often do you think about being involved in a violent situation?

Being Believed: imagine waking up every day not only with the fear of impending violence, but add to that the possibility of being abused and not believed. Have you experienced not being believed about such an important matter?

Confidence: we gain confidence in many ways in our lives—from our parents, from our socio-economic status, from our friends and environment, and from a society that includes and supports us equally in its vision of success. How confident are you in your environment?

Fear of Blame: imagine being blamed for something you didn't do because of the color of your skin, your history, or simply another person's bias or deflection. Unfortunately, this happens all too often.

Patriotism

It's almost impossible to believe in something or someone who has fervently betrayed the ideology and trust of the people it represents, and it's hard to address patriotism without letting politics muck it up. This seems to be the task at hand for all of us.

I have always had a love affair with the United States of America and have considered myself a patriot. It was a life goal for me to visit the Liberty Bell, in the region where many of my ancestors settled after arriving on American shores. However, when I traveled to Philadelphia and the surrounding areas of Carlisle and the Civil War battlefields of Gettysburg, I was disheartened on so many levels.

Many times, as I travel to different places, I rely on spirit to offer me the topics on which I write. The theme of my sojourn into patriotism in Pennsylvania was about our nation's first people and the trials and tribulations many tribespeople experience to this day. I was surprised to learn that Pennsylvania is one of a few states with no legally recognized native tribes.[11] *How could that be?* I thought, in my naiveté. This seems to be another situation in which keeping things unclear, postpones progress.

It got me thinking about clarity. I grew up in New Mexico and attended grade school where the history books referred to the indigenous of our country as savages, which just did not make sense. I remember sitting in my seventh-grade history class and learning minimal indigenous history—yet sharing the classroom with many Native students—knowing in my spirit that so much Native history was missing, and the rest struggled with truthfulness. While some of the facts may have been accurate, they were incomplete and from a viewpoint of entitlement.

Karmically speaking, none of us can move forward from a trauma that is propelled daily into our modern life by untruths still circulating as education to the youngest members of our communities, in which many are excluded or marginalized in that history. Unless and until we can see where the trauma originated—and view it as it truly was for everyone—we cannot grieve and mourn our losses.

We can never truly be free while our systems of commerce, governance, industry, and status—isolate or marginalize any of us. We cannot undo the past or the damage that has been done from those who came to this continent looking for a better life, but we, as a society, can stop the daily abuses and oppression that occur in our communities, one by one, creating the space for everyone here on the planet to heal. This is a humanitarian pursuit that can no longer be set aside as someone else's problem. We must each, individually, be willing to recognize how we contribute to the system of oppression and make those changes in our own hearts first, and then our homes, and eventually in our societies at large.

Terrorism from an Energetic Perspective

People have always protested or rioted—fighting for their rights and to impress the value of their beliefs onto others—however, the idea of random senseless violence has become a bourgeoning expression of power that has escalated into arbitrary acts of terrorism. No matter what delusional idea drives the acts of terror, consider there is a deeper influence at play in the event: a spiritual force that plants the seeds of chaos into people who are vulnerable to such spiritual intrusion and already feel powerless in the life they live.

In the spiritual world there are entities whose entire existences are formed around creating disruption and chaos. Regardless of your beliefs about them, they do exist and can influence the world around you. These entities do not incarnate in the human realm and live a restricted life of domination in a militarized caste system within their own dimension, until at some point, they are invited into the human domain.

It is when this dense vibration connects to a human in the same condition as they, that anarchy and destruction are set into motion. A person who feels disenfranchised, rageful, isolated, nationalistic, and zealous about their religion, and—additionally—one who experiences enormous self-doubt, or has learned to set aside their instinct to lean on the understanding of others, is most vulnerable. All of these factors are present and can contribute to a human being who causes terror.

Using Telepathy to Change the Outcome

Essentially, terrorists are spiritually haunted by energy constructs of ideology, malicious entities and the spirit of destruction. The latter being an energetic component that also makes them vulnerable to spiritual and telepathic intervention. There are constant stories in the news of terrorism being committed by someone whose neighbors, friends, and loved ones didn't see it coming, exclaiming, "He was such a nice quiet guy!"

It is the spiritual component that is the malleable factor in the equation. When people are experiencing extremely dense or low vibrational emotions, they are susceptible to influence from outside sources (other humans' or entities' focused psychic energy), either to bring them lower (many suicides occur because of this) or to offer a positive possible outcome to a dilemma.

It is the same concept we often see in the outpouring of thoughts and prayers after a tragic event—this differs in that it can be used before or during an event to shift the outcome. Instead of expressing fear, it is the telepathic injection of courage, confidence, strength, or faith from the prey to the predator—to stop the action of terror in the form of a directive. For example: *You don't need to do this*, *You will stop this*, or *Doing this won't make your life better*. Injecting love into an equation of lack and desperation by telepathically stating, *You are loved*, can change the outcome. You are lending your confidence of hope to someone who has none.

To be clear, you're not trying to *light and love* the criminal out of their choices; you are psychically intervening on their thought process and focus. This is in order to stop their momentum long enough to get out of harm's way, or for other options to arise that will stop the act of terror altogether.

I've lived in Los Angeles for a couple of decades, and at one point, I spent many hours driving in my vehicle. When you spend a lot of time on the street you see plenty of road rage. One day while I was waiting to turn right at a light, two cars waiting to make a left, in the lanes crossing in front of me and cater-cornered to my right, were feuding. The driver of the truck in back threw a full soda can at the car in front, just as the first car was making the left-hand turn. As he completed the turn, and passed just behind my location in the opposite lane, he stopped and got out of his car (he couldn't have been more than twenty). He proceeded to lunge into the back seat as if to find a weapon. I could see the gun in my mind's eye and could feel the young man's rage.

There were a few people directly in front of my car, standing on the corner, who were also witnessing what was happening; simultaneously, we all began to duck as we were in the direct line of fire. That is when I set my gaze on the young man, seeing him in my side-view mirror. I began to telepathically speak to him: telling him *I loved him* and that *he had many people who loved him, nothing good could come from completing the action he was in the middle of,* and that *he didn't have to do it.* I was speaking these words directly to his image in the mirror, when all of a sudden, he pulled himself out of the back seat, and looked around as if he didn't remember what he was doing. He shook his head, got in his car and drove away at a normal speed. Consequently, my light turned green, I made the right-hand turn, and I burst into tears.

Believe me, I know how hokey this sounds, and if I hadn't experienced it multiple times, in many types of situations—from telepathically telling a mugger, *I am not the one*, and watching him change course—to startling a man who walked up to me on the street while raising his hand to hit me in the face, and stopping him in his tracks with one simple word: *no*. Those responses changed the moments just long enough to get away from the criminals.

You're not trying to change a whole life in the moment, as much as you are changing one very important irrevocable moment in which many lives would change.

Sex and Power

In this section we will be addressing a specific dynamic that is perpetuated in relation to sex, death, and other people's money—that is, power. The journey to understanding the dynamic of power versus force in relationships, communities, and culture is prolific and never-ending. We use sex, threats, intimidation, and money (power) to reinforce our own warped sense of value.

If some among us can manipulate or commandeer sex, choke out life-giving systems that others need, or use money to control outcomes—they feel powerful. Only by understanding how it happens can we change it.

Sexual Assault is About Dominance

Groping, sexual assault, and rape aren't about sexuality; they occur in response to a perpetrator's sense of powerlessness, habits, or entitlement—whether it's a hardened criminal or your uncle Hank. We have more authority over giving our power away than a criminal does in taking it. Whether they are an abuser, manipulator, or con artist, there is a process to the dynamic of victimization, and we must all learn it.

I want to be clear here by stating it outright: we are not placing blame or fault on anyone who has been victimized, only the perpetrator. Healing from a sexual trauma will teach a person the process or circumstances, on every level, that made them vulnerable in the first place —be it physical, etheric, emotional, mental, or spiritual. It is this process I'd like to put on the table in hopes of eliminating the possibility of sexual assault for some.

"To be wronged is nothing unless you continue to remember it."[12]

– Confucius

Body Consciousness

Body consciousness is our awareness of our own physical body, our feelings about it, and our ability to own the body we have and the space it claims, in order to set boundaries with others. Many years ago, I was a chaperone on a field trip with a group of about thirty inner-city nine and ten-year-olds. We were traveling to a pumpkin patch, forty-five minutes from the school. That bus ride changed my life. As a spiritual medium, I am clairvoyant; seeing this particular group of children and the energetic sexual dynamics I psychically witnessed between them was tremendous. Several of these children didn't seem like children at all. I could see their potential adult sexual dynamics beginning to emerge. Two of the young ladies in this group stood out to me. I could see the spiritual imprinting of their vulnerability to being sexualized long before they were ready. There was a group of about six boys focusing on them at different times on the bus ride.

At first, the boys were picking on the first young lady, grabbing at and snapping her bra. The more she got upset, the more they did it. She was in tears, when finally, one of her friends came to get me to handle the situation. I walked back to where the boys were and told them to stop, and they did. Then I asked, in an easy tone of voice, how it might feel to each of them if a group of bigger boys began doing the same thing to them—poking at their genitals in the same way they were poking at her? I looked each young man in the face and waited for his response. None of them had ever contemplated such a thing before, but a light seemed to go on. They each answered that they wouldn't like it, except one boy who shrugged his shoulders and muttered under his breath.

Much of my focus went to the young lady and the three friends sitting with her. She was sweet, very mild-mannered, and was so shy she could barely get a word out. I could tell she felt things deeply and made the effort to be nice to others. I explained to her that it was her body, and no one could touch it unless she gave them permission. The word *no* was the most important word in her vocabulary, and she had the right to use it anytime. However, giggling when the boys began to pester her communicated something other than *no*. It was important not to worry about hurting anyone's feelings by saying clearly, "No. Do not do that." Her friends seemed to be glad we were having this conversation, not only for their friend but for themselves.

The second young lady, I suspected, had already been sexualized. She was a beautiful nine-year-old girl wearing a pair of jeans and a mid-drift top. It wasn't what she was wearing so much as how she was wearing it. She intended to be sexy to receive the attention of the boys. She spent quite a bit of time on that bus ride brushing her hair and looking at her image in the mirror while putting on lip gloss and then flirting and playing with the boys.

The aspect that was powerful to witness was that she did not seem to be the child she was; she was deeply rooted in her sexual power and appeared to have some consciousness of it. Unlike the other young lady, she was pursuing the attention of the boys and getting frustrated with the attention she got. Unaware of the energetic boundaries she was setting for herself, the boys were acting much more aggressively. Again, I had similar conversations with all of them, as I did with the first group. It wasn't the bus ride that was potent for me with the second young lady, it was the news that she'd given birth to twins just a little over a year and a half later.

Personal authority

It is your ability to own every bit of space you take up in the world. Speak loudly and clearly when you have something to say; own every choice you make, being accountable for their consequences. Of course, it can take years to cultivate this type of personal power, but it doesn't have to.

It is through people challenging our personal authority that we learn to champion ourselves and communicate effectively. However, it is our spiritual patterns that set up the kind of challenges we receive and by whom. For example, let's look at someone who has lived a past lifetime being trafficked for sex. The spiritual pattern ingrained in their soul in future incarnations—until the patterns are resolved—is one of attracting sexual power and conflict in order to claim respect, own personal space, grieve past trauma, and learn independence in all ways (including personal and environmental awareness and safety).

Boundaries

Boundaries are set energetically, emotionally, verbally, and physically. A pedophile will groom their victim over a period of time by making small bids for attention and invading personal space to see what kind of reaction they will receive; it is the same for the victims of sexual assault—only it is through the landscape of their entire life. Instead of being perpetrated by one person, they have a victimized relationship dynamic to many people, known or unknown to them. Every time they are disrespected and it goes unaddressed, every time their personal space is invaded and they laugh it off or say nothing, and finally, when they are sexually violated and they just want to *put it behind them* without confrontation or grief—these are the steps to a slow descent into victimization from the victim's point of view.

Expectation of violation

It is possible for people to carry with them the karmic burden of expecting to be emotionally overrun, abused, or violated in some way. This presents as feelings of self-pity and powerlessness in regard to one's ability to manage their life without help—and even sometimes with help. This spiritual imprint often supports addiction as well. Often, the imprints for abuse and sexual abuse can be passed down from family member to family member.

Bad Uncle

I counseled a woman who was victimized by her uncle; neither parent fully acknowledged the abuse nor championed the young lady while the uncle was still living. When the knowledge of the abuse came forward, the uncle was no longer welcomed into the family home, but nothing more was said. Both parents had been abused, and in turn, unwittingly allowed the abuse of their daughter.

It wasn't until the birth of the next generation of daughters, that the time for grieving became imminent. Because there hadn't been any intellectual or emotional support for the woman to move through her trauma, the energy of the trauma passed down to her most sensitive daughter. That girl began to have terrifying dreams of the great-uncle she'd never met and of whom they rarely spoke. In these dreams he would attempt to attack her—chastising her until she awoke in panic. At this point, she'd not been told of her mother's abuse.

The mother had quietly sought to put the trauma behind her without dealing with the devastation of the abuse, and her resentment of the parents and family dynamic that allowed it. She'd put all her time and energy into a wildly successful business, and several failed relationships, but she hadn't yet done the work of grieving. Now, she had no choice. Her daughter was emotionally, spiritually, and psychically suffering from the dynamic of ancestral abuse that had been placed on the girl to resolve.

The night terrors that were triggered allowed for many positive things to occur. Such as, the entire family could talk about what really happened and unearth the repressed feelings that had imprisoned them. The young lady could learn spiritual boundaries by enacting them in her dreams with her great-uncle. She could speak to the great-uncle once and for all, telling him to leave them alone and assisting her family in finding a way to forgiveness. Setting boundaries in the spiritual world translates into vocalizing them in the physical world as well. At last, the entire family could find a way to grieve and move forward with the new level of safety that setting boundaries creates.

The Karma of Abortion: The Dynamic of Power

People who take away the power of others will inevitably experience the same thing. So the debate around reproductive rights and a woman's right to make choices for her health is amazing to me. This fight exists, in part, because of the systemic misogyny that prevails, but also—in part—because of a lack of focus on the true karmic impact to those who are systematically disempowered. It may sound counterintuitive to some, but the issue around abortion is not really about the unborn child. It is about the power structure set up for women based on the options they have at the time an abortion is considered.

Often, those seeking to impose a pro-life doctrine do not consider that many of the women seeking an abortion do not have the resources to provide for the child, putting that responsibility on others—mainly county and state care providers that are not funded to do so. They have been raped and have had their power stricken from them—once, during the crime and twice, being forced to bear the child of a rapist. They are women whose vulnerabilities, such as addictions and other diseases, preclude them from taking care of the children that outsiders fight so hard for them to bring into the world—placing those children in an already overwhelmed foster system.

This topic has not been delved into on deeper spiritual levels, beyond the illusions of life and death, as our society has sought to create shame for those women who want or who have had abortions, making it safer for them to keep quiet. This derivative of slut-shaming has been an effective tool in keeping misogyny afloat and the discussion down. So, I'd like to talk about the spiritual repercussions of keeping women subjugated in society, the spiritual reality for the soul whose body is aborted, and the cost to a community when an unwanted child is brought into the world.

The circumstances around my own decision to abort were emotionally and spiritually profound. Being a 25-year-old rape survivor and still suffering from PTSD, I hadn't had a period in several months before I conceived;

consequently, I was already a few months pregnant when I learned of my pregnancy. Unbeknownst to me, I'd been targeted by a reproductive abuser. (I tell the full story in *Heal Your Soul History: Activate the True Power of Your Shadow, Volume 2 of DSHS*.)

I'd not heard the term *reproductive coercion* until a few years ago. This type of predator seeks to impregnate women, often by bullying them or sabotaging the birth control (the technique often used by female coercionists). The latter is what happened in my case. The man I'd been seeing sabotaged the condom we used in our first sexual experience, and a child was conceived. As it turned out, I'd found out about the pregnancy the night before leaving for an extended stay in Pheonix, Arizona.

I am a spiritualist. So, recognizing that life is eternal, I've always been pro-choice. However, when this happened to me, the decision was deeply painful. I loved and wanted my baby so much, but my spirit wouldn't allow it. I grieved for days in hopes of fully understanding the spiritual reason I could not bring this child into the world. Although I'd had enormous anxiety and dread the night my baby was conceived, at the time I chalked it up to residual PTSD that I still often experienced regarding any sexual encounter.

I hadn't made the decision to abort until I spoke with the father (we'd broken up two weeks after that first night, when I found out he'd lied about being married with two children). During the call, he wanted me to know what he'd done, and went on to tell me how he'd put a hole in the condom before our meeting. He said he'd been following me for weeks and knew I was pregnant; he'd seen it in a dream. He was so proud of himself. His reasoning? He thought we both had spiritual gifts and we'd have a gifted child. He gave no consideration to the environment he'd be bringing the child into, nor did it occur to him we should both have choice in the matter. I was devastated.

My grief became more intense as the days passed. I called to the spirit of my child asking him to come into the world another way. It was only then that an enormous sense of peace came over me. Neither this child nor I wanted anything to do with a father who'd taken away my choice. Once the child was at peace, I was at peace.

Perpetuating the disempowerment of women in any society is diminishing for everyone. The consciousness of the divine feminine inhabits all of us. It is the energy that brings awakening through all who honor it. To repress or oppress, in any form, the gentle flow of this wisdom, education, love, and compassion, creates confusion, self-hatred, and rage in all who bind it. This is the sickness from which our culture of fear and power-mongering suffers.

When any woman makes such a powerful decision, the world doesn't see the real considerations of such a choice: all the people involved, the environment, the availability of resources to provide for the child, the spiritual contract made with the child, and, no matter what it looks like from the outside, the suffering that comes to that woman until her contract or relationship to that child is fulfilled (whatever it may be). My karma was to make this choice consciously and to consider everyone before making it. But what of the karma for those who force their beliefs onto others?

From the outside, the stigma of abortion comes from an absence of understanding about the spirituality of birth, death, and eternal life. Within the understanding of eternity is a compassionate creator and a universe that thrives on forgiveness. Here's the thing: if these aren't your beliefs, then you must make the choices that follow your ideology as it pertains to your life. If you must, find a way to forgive yourself for being powerless against controlling others. Everyone grieves in this situation, but the choice to bring a child into the world is between the parents and the child.

Every situation is so unique to the individuals involved, it's not logical that an outside party could have a voice, or a choice, based upon what is righteous for them. In any situation, there is only one decision that fulfills the karmic contract between the parents and child. The relationship of a woman's right to choose versus a society's desire to control is about power. The karmic response to this power struggle occurs in the spiritual imprints that ultimately form in the souls of those who disempower others. Often those seeking to express righteousness already feel powerless in some facet of their lives. I made the choice that needed to be made, giving more respect to the father than he'd shown me, and giving the child a voice in our world.

I've not ever felt an ounce of regret. I am grateful to have met the incarnation of the boy who eventually made it to this planet and had exactly the parents and love he needed. Don't get me wrong, I grieved the loss from my life on every level, and it was deeply painful. But I think of him from time to time and only feel love. When you eliminate fear by facing what you're afraid of, there is only Truth.

Death, Hauntings, and Karma

Apart from our physical world, there are multiple dimensions that function in a spectrum of vibratory rates which contain entities (angels, spirit guides, extra-terrestrials, demons), energy constructs (running thoughts, beliefs, curses), and imprints (spiritual memory, ghosts, residual energy from traumatic events, and unprocessed emotional energy in a space). As we grieve, we change our relationship, or lose access to all of these different spiritual dimensions.

Death is inevitable for all of us, and resistance to the process is futile. It is this experience of resistance around death that keeps us in the dark about the process of dying. Hauntings exist on a plane of resistance or fear. Often, when someone dies abruptly, their soul cannot transition to a higher state of consciousness because they were unaware of the process that led them to their demise. The soul stays around or is stuck in this dimension in order to gain their bearings in this new existence, to access further understanding around their demise, and, sometimes, to continue comforting those they left behind. Hauntings aren't good or bad, they exist for a purpose.

Death and Grief: Heart-Breaking is Heart-Opening

When someone dies, there is a process of grieving and mourning that takes place. Grief is the energy and emotional release that helps to transition how you emotionally relate to the physical loss. Mourning is the physical conversion of your past daily life with the person who died to now experiencing it without them, including all the changes it requires. Everyone will experience grief and mourning in different ways, based on many factors regarding the death.

- Was there a long-term or short-term illness?
- Was it a suicide?
- Was homicide involved?
- What was your current or pre-existing relationship?
- Was it an accidental or unexpected death?
- Was there pre-grief involved (the grieving that happens while a person is still living about their impending death)?

Grief is the way our body and mind heal. Crying for ten minutes at a time actually changes the neurons in the brain and allows for the healing of unwanted feelings and behaviors while transforming outdated spiritual patterns. Crying and grieving is not weakness.

Every person grieves in their own way. Some people will deny their feelings in front of others and become extra busy, while others will cry continuously and experience many triggers. Here is a list of some other possibilities:

- Crying several times a day
- Experiencing vivid visions and dreams
- Interrupted sleep
- Angry, controlling, and hypervigilant behavior
- Extra sleep
- Over-indulgence in food, alcohol, or drugs

- Careless or reckless behavior
- Deep and thoughtful reflection

Your karma around death pertains to every innate feeling and belief you have around grief, life after death, and the experience of freeing yourself from fear. If we've lived a life guided by fear, then most likely we will experience it in our death process as well. But even if someone fears death, it doesn't mean they won't have an easy spiritual transition. It is a part of the death process to investigate the concept of where we go next—the acknowledgment and distinction of seeing yourself as a spirit that resides in a body. While that body may be losing its energy, the spirit becomes stronger, freer, and more in tune with the environment and other spiritual dimensions.

The Karma of Death

The most potent spiritual imprints we carry in our soul pertain to death. If we've caused someone's death, died abruptly, been murdered, or caused our own death in some way, either in a past life or the current one, the spiritual trauma can take lifetimes to overcome because it takes specific work. The presence of guilt points to the grief-work that needs to be done.

It is common to experience a past-life recall and sometimes briefly relive your own death from other lifetimes. Personally, I've experienced several different past-life death events, reliving them as if they were yesterday. They were a spear to the heart, taking my own life and the life of my unborn child by drowning, a gunshot to the gut, a lynching, a public hanging, and a stabbing to name a few. Each one of these past-life recollections came at very different parts of my process and in different ways: through spontaneous visions that made me relive the trauma, or through dreams and meditative visions. All of these experiences were life changing and allowed me to grieve and integrate each of these lost parts of my soul.

Reliving a death experience, whether it's traumatic or peaceful, has a purpose: it reveals the impact of that life and death to everyone involved. The karma is in knowing how and why a death occurred and the events that led up to the death in question on a spiritual, mental, emotional, or physical level. When one relives the experience, they open themselves to the psychic energy of that event so that they may grieve it—and find forgiveness for themselves and all others connected.

What happens to people who create, promote, or provoke mass killing? Remember, karma isn't meant to be punitive: it is about understanding the conditions present that led to the traumatic event. A person who participates in mass killing in any way will eventually experience psychic guilt and the spiritual weight of those they killed, either in the same lifetime as the traumatic event or another. But it is the process of this spiritual grief that clears the way to forgiveness and the understanding necessary for redemption. Spiritual grief can be ignited through feeling or being victimized in some way; anything that causes empathy will create the space for deeper levels of clarity and self-mastery.

Culture and Death

The cultures that embrace the process of death—and welcome and teach the witnessing of the death process of loved ones and community members—have less fear, less guilt, and a better quality and perspective of life because of it. When you do not fear death, you are able to focus on and enjoy life.

Death is a spiritual concept that many religions disagree on. Without getting into a religious conversation regarding the different approaches, I'd like to address what we each need to embrace as individuals: death is beautiful and sacred. It's more important to spend our time and resources with our loved ones during their death process and their final days, enjoying them and loving them out of this dimension, rather than the thousands of dollars we spend on separate hospice facilities, caskets, funeral processions, and burials.

It is the nature of modern western habits to send away the dying, possibly making a visit or two, then waiting for a phone call with the final news of the end. In relationships that are conflicted, it is important to use the final days to have honest conversations with the person dying about them and their impact on you—it allows them to *leave it all on the stage*, as they say.

Suicide and Karma

I've had spiritual experiences with dark energies since I was a baby; the story I want to tell now is about the suicide demons. Previously, I'd never once considered suicide despite enduring enormous suffering for years. I think because I was spiritually minded, had a relationship with many benevolent beings, and came into this life knowing to ask for help.

However, this one day I was the lowest I'd been: broke, sad, tired, rejected, and existing with no inspiration whatsoever. I'd run into a friend I hadn't seen in a while, and we chatted, making a date for later to go to a movie. When I arrived at his apartment, he opened the door a crack and looked at me with one eye, not really saying anything. I said, "We had a plan tonight. Did you forget?" Still he said nothing.

"Are you okay?" I asked.

He responded by opening the door and walking away from it—back to the video game he was playing (something about the different levels of hell). He was wearing nothing but a sarong (which I found surprising as it wasn't traditional moviewear). I could see that there was something very wrong. I walked into his studio apartment, and though it was still light outside, his home was completely dark. I sat on the bed, which was about five feet away from where he was sitting, and said, "Hey John, what's going on?"

"Nothing, just playing this game," he responded.

"Do you not remember that we made plans a few hours ago?"

His demeanor was slow and lethargic, and the energy in the room was heavy and stifling; though, I knew he didn't use drugs or drink. Finally, he responded: "Oh, I can't go."

Normally, I would have been pissed, but whatever was going on here was beyond his control. I'd only been there for five minutes and began to feel tired. Asking to use the bathroom, I walked out of the room. I sat in the bathroom for a few minutes but began to experience such exhaustion that my head bowed. When suddenly, my phone rang. It was my sister.

"Hey, what are you doing?" she said.

"I'm at John's. Something's wrong here. I'm so tired."

"What is he doing?"

"He's in the living room," I said, "playing some video game about the demons of hell. He's wearing a sarong, and the house is completely dark."

"Tracee, you are mumbling your words. You need to leave right now. Just leave."

"Lynne, I'm confused. ...I feel woozy. What should I tell him?" I asked.

"You don't have to tell him anything. Just leave. Call him later," she said.

Leaving was exactly what needed to happen. I told John that I had to go, and I'd call him later. He didn't look up from the game.

Once outside, I began to get my energy back immediately. Later that night, I wasn't feeling well as I went to bed. Things seemed darker than usual, and as I closed my eyes I heard, *You might as well do it; it doesn't matter anymore.* I thought, *What are you talking about?* It said, *Life, it doesn't matter. It won't get any better. You should kill yourself.*

And for the first time in my life, killing myself seemed rational, and that made no sense. Luckily, something inside of me got angry, mad enough to recognize that I was under spiritual attack. I had been feeling so low and apathetic about hope that when the calm, rational, voice told me to kill myself, it seemed normal.

That night, and for the next several weeks, I had to chant myself to sleep. I couldn't think straight, so I chanted, "Christ, Christ, Christ," over and over again until I fell asleep. During the days, I got out of the house or found someone to stay with me. I didn't trust myself to be alone. I knew that whatever this was I would overcome it, but it was powerful.

A few weeks later, I again ran into my friend whom I'd seen the day it started. I was still deeply distraught, and he could see my vulnerability. I asked if I could join him in whatever he was doing that day. As it turned out, he was running errands, getting a haircut and going to the grocery store—now with me in tow. It was in that meeting that again the demon transferred from me to him. I left him, feeling better than I had in weeks.

It appeared he'd been battling this demon for some time, and had been free of it for a while, but now I had returned it to him. After seeing him that day, I understood what had happened. A few months earlier, I'd had a dream showing me my past-life with this man who was John today.

In the dream, he was carrying me up a flight of stairs into his apartment; I was unconscious and strung out on heroin. At the time, the dream didn't make sense to me, but now I understood that my friend saved me in that life, taking away the entity that had a hold on me. It was the return of it to me, and the ensuing spiritual attack from it, that let me know what was happening.

In reflection of my day with John, I realized he'd taken the entity back, as I was feeling normal again. I performed a remote deliverance, and the next day John was relieved. It was necessary I help deliver it from him, as he'd been the one who'd taken it from me in my most vulnerable time.

I was profoundly grateful for the experience. The darkness was all-pervasive, and I felt many things that were unfamiliar to me: confusion, apathy, futility, and the idea that suicide was rational. Despite how I felt, I'd had enough practice making choices based on what was right for me rather than from my feelings. I also had a relationship with my Creator and understood that I was divinely protected, which I believe we all are.

One of the most powerful conversations you can have with anyone is about suicide. One of the biggest misnomers is that suicide is like a virus you can catch. The truth is we are spiritual beings in a physical world, and our human karmic directive is to find ways of anchoring spiritual light into our physical body without leaving our physical body. We can do that in a thousand different ways, but in order to do it, we must create links between the light and the dark—transforming the darkness every step of the way.

It's important to talk about suicide. Speak about it all the time and make it a regular household discussion. Discussing it at the dinner table, when everyone is sated and relaxed, allows for a deeper receptivity and sense of safety. Or, talk about it in any casual scenario—versus starting the conversation when you're in a crisis.

In many cultures, thoughts of suicide, mental illness, ultra-sensitivity, or interacting with the spirit world are looked upon as a weakness, which perpetuates the shame and embarrassment already often felt by those who have these experiences. The only way to truly overcome that shame is to talk about it. The truth is, almost everyone at one time or another feels like they don't want to be here anymore, which is the beginning of suicidal ideation (thoughts of suicide, imagining what it would be like, how you'd do it, or making a plan to do it).

Max and Margay's Story

I have a longtime friend, Margay, whose son Max died of suicide. Although he'd struggled with emotional highs and lows his whole life, things had finally begun to turn around for him. Max was twenty-seven years old, a DJ, and holding down another job as well. He had parents and a sibling who loved him, a girlfriend who adored him, and friends and fans who loved his music. One summer morning in a fit of panic and rage, he ended it all.

Although Max had spoken of suicide before, he hadn't made a plan. Max was diagnosed as a child with ADHD (attention-deficit/hyperactivity disorder) and medicated from around the age of eight through his high school years. At that point, the medication wasn't working, and Max was finding activities he loved to put his energy into, namely music. As a young adult, he struggled, but his family kept him close as he forged his way into relationships and the world on his own.

I was called when it happened, and made plans to visit my hometown of Albuquerque, New Mexico. Upon my arrival, I immediately felt Max's presence. He was angry at himself and so sorry. He hadn't meant to kill himself. He knew it the minute his body hit the floor and his spirit was still standing. The one most important irrevocable moment of his life.

It's important to know that life goes on in different ways for everyone. The person transitioning their life through suicide, continues that life in a similar spiritual dimension without a body, and the folks left behind continue on, often with questions, confusion, and regret. Everyone will do the work of finding peace and resolution for the unanswered questions. Throughout the next few pages: Margay's journey, in her own words.

> "So many have said to me 'There are no words...' and it's true, but please know that the words are not so important to me. It's the love behind them that I feel. Just when I think I can't possibly make it to the next moment, someone reaches out to me, hugs me, cries with me, shares their sweet memories of Max with me and there I am...in the next moment. So that is how I will do this. One breath at a time."
>
> – Margay Erne

How to start the discussion

Sometimes, we are afraid to speak to our friends for fear they'll feel judged, they won't like us, or we'll hurt their feelings. When you want to speak to someone about their most inner secrets, your only goal is to listen, not give advice. Do your best to open your heart and feel what they are feeling. Often, those who have died from suicide didn't feel acknowledged or heard in their life or the time preceding the suicide. When taking on this topic, it's important to:

- Be direct
- Be compassionate
- Don't judge
- Let go of fear
- Be patient

Don't be afraid to hear the words, *I want to kill myself*—but always take them seriously. Acknowledge them by saying, *I am so sorry you feel that way. That feeling must be such a burden for you. Do you know why you want to kill yourself?*

If someone says, *I just don't want to be here anymore*, respond with, *I'm sorry you feel that way. Do you want to kill yourself?* If yes, *How often do you think about it? Do you have a plan to kill yourself? Have you ever known anyone who died of suicide?* Listening and not reacting to someone's plea for suicide isn't giving them permission to kill themselves.

In my experience, suicide isn't limited to only those with mental illness or chemical imbalance. Suicide is a reaction to a deep-seated need to control what feels uncontrollable, desperate, and devastating. Often people who attempt suicide are experiencing the illusion that the only way to overcome the pain they're in is to end it through death. And, many times, it is a spur-of-the-moment decision.

In the last 10 years there has been a huge uptick of suicides related to conditions or circumstances where impulse control is a factor: traumatic brain injury, PTSD, teen-suicides, bi-polar disorder, and schizophrenia (to name a few). Many people who've died of suicide have had some sort of mental condition at the time of their death, with depression remaining the most important risk factor.

We can never know, absolutely, what someone will do when their emotional, mental, and physical state reaches the perfect storm of angst, depression, rage, apathy, pressure, and volatility. This uncertainty is the best reason to speak often about suicide and the aforementioned feelings of intense emotion.

Some tell-tale signs someone is considering suicide are:

- They speak about it.
- They make a plan.
- They withdraw from social situations.
- They are rageful and erratic.
- They overindulge in substance use, food intake, and risky behavior.
- They experience intense apathy and depression (nothing really matters anymore).
- They sleep too much or too little.
- They experience intense grief, humiliation, or guilt.

Never be afraid to ask questions! Expect it to be awkward and uncomfortable. Know that once the discussion begins, it gets easier. Here are some questions you can ask:

- Are you thinking about suicide?
- Tell me about the thoughts you're having?
- Do you have a plan to kill yourself?
- If you have a plan, can you tell me about it?
- How long have you been thinking about suicide?
- What is the first thing that you think of when you consider what is causing these feelings?

Healthcare and wellness providers lead the conversation about suicide in our culture, and they are the most obvious interface when it comes to speaking about it. They are also a demographic at high risk for compassion fatigue and suicide themselves. So let's not put it all on their shoulders. If every person reading this took responsibility for starting ten conversations a month about suicide, we could eliminate the shame, ignorance and stigma attached to it.

> "After Max died, the first time someone asked me if I had kids, I panicked like a deer in the headlights. I knew the question would come but I was totally unprepared for it. I answered, 'We have a son, Jake.' WTF!?! I immediately regretted it. It was a betrayal of Max to spare myself and others and I felt guilty about it for a long time. I swore I would never do that again and I haven't. I usually just stumble my way through a vague, awkward reply that includes Max. Today, someone asked if I have children and how old they are and I answered calmly, without hesitation, 'I have 2 sons, Max and Jake. Jake is 25. Max passed away in 2015. He would be 30 now.' Then they asked the dreaded question: 'How did he die?' (Yes, people actually ask this a lot.) I answered simply and truthfully, 'He died by suicide from depression.' It rolled right off my lips like I'd said it a thousand times. It felt so good to say it just like that. The truth. I know it makes some people uncomfortable, but I owe it to Max. He lived and he was deeply loved. As I write this, I feel proud of myself. I have a smile on my face and peace in my heart."
>
> – Margay Erne

Understanding Depression: Forgiveness is the Key

Spiritually speaking, depression is the way we turn inward and self-reflect. Often, when we are confronted with seeing things about ourselves we don't like or reflect on things we've done or that have happened to us (for which we carry pain, guilt, or shame), we tend to shut down our emotional channels.

Doing this puts extra pressure on our minds to metabolize the intensity of the emotional energy through our thoughts. It can create loops of the same thought over and over, or many thoughts that are related but may not express our truthful specific feelings. There is no better, more efficient way to process the enormity of certain emotions than to feel them. Finding a safe place and way to allow the emotions to move through you will keep you from letting them build and turn into erratic irrevocable choices.

To help someone who experiences depression, listen to them with an open heart and without judgment. Encourage them to feel what they feel without shame. Offer them the idea that the cause of their depression wants to be healed through confronting it directly. Ask about it, talk about it, feel it, and forgive it.

Forgiving yourself and others for the traumatic events in your life doesn't make them okay. It says, *I will no longer allow it to run me or my choices; I am willing to start fresh without the attachment to this burden.*

Times on the planet, right now, are difficult to say the least. It's easy to feel depressed and hopeless just from watching the news. All the wars, natural disasters, and crime can make life feel uncontrollable. If you or someone you know is feeling threatened by the state of world affairs, admit it, communicate it, and find a way to do something nice for someone else. Get involved. In my darkest times, being of service to someone else kept me going.

Why People Attempt or Complete Suicide

A person who tries to kill oneself, successfully or not, has an underlying mental, emotional, physical, or spiritual condition. We've addressed mental and emotional conditions but as a spiritualist, for me, everything begins on an energy level. Mental, emotional, and physical conditions all exist because of spiritual patterns. These are most often soul memories or hauntings: people feel them but have no rational justification for their presence.

That experience can make a person feel isolated, tired, apathetic, out of control, burdened, confused, unwanted, depressed, and angry. When someone is sensitive in this way, they can also attract energies from their environment that amplify the burden they feel. Getting caught up in this experience can make it appear there is no way out—leading them to take an irrevocable action.

The one thing I've learned by working with people over the years through the deepest burdens they would ever face is that every spiritual obligation we carry comes in a complete package (the burden and the resolution). Facing the malady head on reveals the way to its healing.

Suicide Stats

The highest rate of suicide today occurs in the LGTBQ, Native, and Military Veteran communities: 23 a day! Men committing suicide is four times higher than women. It is highest in the 65+ age group. Children between the ages of 10–14 is the fastest growing demographic.[13]

Spirituality vs. Religion

While learning about and understanding the symptoms of mental illness is positive, I believe the underlying cause of them is the lack of spiritual understanding—even if there is no religious confusion. Our culture is suffering deeply from an imbalanced spiritual ideology. In this case, religion is not spirituality. Religion is the ritual that helps to cultivate spiritual understanding.

This means spiritual understanding includes everyone. I love religion and believe they all tell a variation on the human story. But it cannot be ignored that the ways we relate to religion today have been compromised by human ignorance and greed.

It is our birthright:

- To acknowledge a higher power, no matter what you call it.
- To trust that every person was born perfect and is deeply loved by their Creator.
- To understand that being yourself is your life-purpose, no matter what.
- To know you were born at this time because the planet needs who you are—as you are.

"I've always hated the wind, but tonight I felt drawn to it and found myself standing alone in the middle of our land, in the dark, arms outstretched, hair flying, tears falling, imagining all my cares scattering away on it. Dorky and wondrous…"

– Margay Erne

Suicide and Telepathy

You can never be responsible for another person taking their life, but you can have a very strong influence on another's choices. Human beings are telepathic, whether they have awareness of it or not. What you say to a person in your mind and heart can impact them as much as your spoken words.

If someone you know is in crisis, acting erratically, and are saying they are going to hurt themselves or someone else (and they have access to the means to do it, or you think they do), this is the time to let go of betraying their confidence or how they feel about you. Call 911.

Telepathy can bring strong results: it's a form of prayer. If a person's suicidal ideation or behavior hasn't reached crisis level, and your loved one is not allowing you access to them, or if they are unwilling to speak with you honestly about what they are going through, take the opportunity to speak with them telepathically. Speak to them as if they were in front of you, or write down these thoughts while thinking about them:

- I love you.
- You are amazing and valuable exactly as you are.
- You may not be able to see your purpose now, but you have one.
- You are stronger than you feel.
- Taking your life won't make the pain go away.
- Please let me help you.
- The burden you feel will be lifted.
- Darkness always gives way to light.

> **Some other things to consider:**
> - Write down any other personal positive affirmative thoughts you may have because of your relationship with them.
> - Call on your Higher Power. For those of you who are religious, religion neutral, or just willing to call on an angelic power in time of crisis, doing this activates and calls on your powerful higher self.
> - St. Michael (who appears in the Bible, the Torah, and the Koran) is an archangel—a spiritual being and the patron saint of warriors. All cultures have an equivalent being who specializes in transforming darkness and slaying or transmuting demons, which are often a spiritual factor for those who kill themselves.
> - Call on St. Michael in your own words, asking for a complete and total intervention of light over darkness and for the strength and vision to overcome all pain, apathy, and confusion on behalf of the person who is suffering.

You can do this for anyone, even if you don't know them. Darkness is a perspective, and although it is an all-pervasive viewpoint at times, it will always give way to the light. We have all the power if we will take it. Let your loved one know they are valued, and what they are feeling is more normal than they realize. Talk to them. Like any grieving person, they need structure and reliability. This is not the time to not follow through with your word. Most of all—be honest.

> "Every day is Suicide Awareness Day for me. People who complete a suicide are neither weak nor selfish. They don't want to end their life. They want to end their pain. I'm deeply saddened and forever changed by the loss of Max, but I'm not ashamed and I will never stop talking about him. I've been awed and humbled by how many people have reached out to me in the last year to share deeply personal stories of loss, despair, anxiety, depression, suicidal thoughts and even suicide attempts. You often speak of suffering quietly, alone and too afraid or ashamed to tell those closest to you. Maybe there is a sense of safety in our shared experience. Maybe my spirit searches you out, like seeking like. I honestly don't know, but I am certain of this: You are unbelievably strong and courageous. Keep holding on."
>
> – Margay Erne

Suicide and Addiction

Addiction is being caught in a loop. Doing the same thing over and over hoping for a different result. The loop often feels safer than what we are trying to cover up with its presence. The type of substance or activity you are addicted to can give you an indication of the energy of the entities that are connected to you. For example, methamphetamine is a completely different vibration than alcohol.

Of course, it goes without saying, getting sober allows you to better see and understand what you are covering up with your addiction; ultimately, you must face off with the entity and reclaim your space (mind, body, and heart). You have everything you need, right now, to take authority over yourself and your circumstances.

Make the battle about reclaiming yourself and acknowledging what is causing you pain—forgiving all involved. In this situation you cannot be passive or think it will change with time. Things will change when you change them. It's a paradox: once you've discovered and healed the underlying cause of the loop, the addiction will be easier to address. And vice versa, once you've addressed your addiction, the underlying causes will begin to heal.

I knew a woman once who lived next door to me. She was afflicted by this huge octopus-looking entity that got my attention when it flicked me in the face with its tentacle one day as she passed by. (It was as strange to experience as I'm sure it is to hear about it.) It's really funny, as I look back on it, being smacked in the face by something no one else can see!

That night, my neighbor came to me in a dream and began to pick a fight with me. I found myself fighting with her, until I realized it was the entity on her. She wanted to be delivered from it. So, I proceeded to call on St. Michael to do that.

During the next couple of weeks, I didn't see her around. What I didn't know was that she was an alcoholic, and the day after my dream, she checked herself into rehab. Allow for a miracle and one will happen.

> "I wonder why it's so hard to admit to ourselves that we're not okay. Why we spend years, even lifetimes pretending we are. I've spent every single day since Max died trying to convince myself that I'm okay. It literally became my mantra. 'You're okay, you're okay, you're okay.' I would say it to myself over and over, sometimes out loud when I was alone, rocking back and forth like a baby, or just in my head if people were around. Every day I would wake up thinking 'Today is the day you will be okay' and it scared the hell out of me that it wasn't that day, or the next, or the next. I was so consumed with being okay that I cheated myself out of grieving. A wise woman recently said to me, 'That shit will not be denied.' Shazam! It's taken 2 ½ years, but I'm finally learning to be okay with not being okay. Feels like I'm onto something."
>
> – Margay Erne

Discussing Hard Topics

The most important thing you can do is speak about it (whatever *it* is) every day, in non-crisis settings. Often, we only speak about difficult topics when we're launched into a crisis. The more we get comfortable talking about it without judgment, the more members of the communities at risk will feel safe to be honest about the depth of the anguish they feel. Consider this, if everyone sat down with a psychologist, everyone would very likely walk away with a diagnosis. We need to allow for the possibility that our mental balance is conditional and changes often; we can all be vulnerable to self-harm given the right circumstances.

When I was under spiritual attack and was deeply apathetic and hopeless, suicide seemed like a reasonable option. I told someone at the time, and they laughed. They made a joke about it and moved on with the conversation. The futility of living in a world where people are unwilling, don't know how, or cannot comprehend such levels of distress is an unnecessary reality in our culture. The time of waiting for someone else to do the hard work and have the hard conversations is over.

Ice Breakers:

- What upsets you the most?
- How many times a day do you cry or feel like crying?
- Do you ever feel homicidal or suicidal?
- In your family, how do they respond to grief?
- Do you think that grief is weakness?
- What do you do with your anger?
- What enrages you?

Spiritual and Mental Suicide

I was asked one time, about committing spiritual and mental suicide. These were terms being floated around social media and the person wanted to understand the validity of them and what they meant.

Ultimately, suicide is physical. Depending on your religious affiliation, or relationship to the Universe around you, some people consider being non-religious as committing spiritual suicide. The truth is, spiritual suicide isn't a possibility. There is a resolution for every spiritual malady, no matter the amount of time it takes to find balance in the eternal spiritual construct. One may traverse every religion over many lifetimes in order to find out, in the end, that they had a relationship to the Creator the whole time.

Every relationship to the Creator, including *non-belief*, contains valuable lessons and wisdom. When you expand your world and begin to acknowledge the larger cosmic picture beyond your personal and familial survival, it inevitably becomes safer to include others rather than to exclude them.

The term *mental suicide* is an urban term expressing the stress created from not being able to process emotions with thoughts. In other words, *thinking too much*. So, not really a thing. Suicide is physical. The heart processes emotion, and the mind creates strategies to move forward—two different functions. It's common for people needing to grieve a transition in their life to avoid the emotional process. But make no mistake about it, there is no other way to process emotion than to allow it to flow through your heart.

Again, crying for 10 minutes or more changes the neurons and ultimately the chemicals in the body that help us to feel emotion and to express ourselves. It helps create clarity, concise thoughts, and a strategy to move forward. Once you've processed old beliefs or experiences emotionally, the heart can receive a resolution from the higher self. Or the brain will interpret a way forward, sending signals of what action to take. Every level of us—mental, emotional, and spiritual—is interactive and designed to help with a portion of the job of living. Mental and emotional balance happens when the heart and mind do their own jobs.

When there is a union between spirituality and science, the need for shame and stigma attached to the process of self-awareness and spiritual integration (what people call the treatment of mental illness) will cease. We can do that by telling our honest stories.

"Earlier this week I read a beautiful essay by a woman whose grown son recently died. Before he was buried, she asked the funeral home for a lock of his hair which she placed in a locket and now wears 'over her heart' every day. When I read that, I felt sick. Literally. Like someone had punched me in the stomach. Why didn't I think to do that? Why didn't I have such foresight? What the hell was wrong with me?! Even though it never once occurred to me since he died, I suddenly, desperately wanted a lock of Max's hair to wear over my heart and I was so damn angry that I didn't have one. Angry as in furious. Enraged. Cursing. Screaming. Throwing-things mad. Questioning: 'Why?' 'Why him?' 'Why me?' 'Why our family?' I know it wasn't about the hair but I don't think I've ever been as pissed as I was in that moment.

"Flash forward to yesterday. While sorting and throwing out some old stuff, I came upon the boys' baby books which I hadn't seen in years. As I sat on the floor leafing through Max's and reading the highlights of his first year, I was finally able, for the first time in many years, to really remember the sweet, high-spirited baby and young boy he was before his long struggle with mental illness overtook him. At the end of his baby book, I found a little sealed envelope with the words 'Max's 1st Haircut' scrawled on it and inside were several locks of his white, baby-soft hair.

"I know there are no answers to my questions but I am grateful for things found and things remembered. As Max used say, 'Let it be enough.'"

– Margay Erne

How Do You Know if Someone is Homicidal or Suicidal?

The truth is, I've heard many accounts of people who've reached out to a hotline and have been put on a lengthy hold, or who reached an operator not equipped to deal with the weight of what they are experiencing. This is no one's fault. The problem of suicide and mass violence is of epidemic proportions, and we must all get involved. A hotline is an opportunity to create an intervention, but sometimes it's just too late to really intervene.

All of us need to practice speaking about these issues without shame or judgment. Create the space for your friends and relations to feel honored and included no matter their circumstances. Another truth: all of us have some form of a mental, emotional, or spiritual issue. All. Of. Us.

Most often, these are left undiagnosed. Whether they are diagnosed by a professional or not, they need to be acknowledged by us—each individual, for ourselves. Western medicine and pharmaceuticals intended to help balance one's behavior or outlook are created without the benefit of the entire spiritual picture. They won't ever be the cure as they don't often address the origins of the imbalance. Unfortunately, some of these therapies can sometimes cause side effects that exacerbate or promote suicidal ideation. However, on the other hand, when someone is at risk to harm themselves or others, pharmaceuticals can help to alleviate the crisis.

When someone you know is speaking, listen for these key words to identify possible suicidal or homicidal ideation.

Listen for these key words:

- Hopeless
- Trapped
- No reason to live
- Humiliated or ashamed
- Unbearable
- Bullied
- Devastated
- Burden
- Obsessed with firearms
- Feeling isolated
- Intense reaction to minor things
- Change in work or school productivity

If you hear any of these key words or see any of the listed behaviors, make the effort to dig deeper into the conversation—or to start one. Your goal is to keep yourself and others safe. There is no shame in asking for help for yourself or someone else by calling 911 when your situation has escalated to a crisis—or even if you're not sure. If you don't feel equipped to handle the situation you've found yourself in, ask for help.

"They say what you resist persists. This summer the darkness came for me and I finally understood what Max tried to tell me for so long. It's unforgiving and unrelenting. You can't wish it away or pray it away or drink it away or write it away or travel it away or hike it away. It always comes back and demands to be acknowledged. You can hide out and cut yourself off from the people who love you (I have) and bury yourself in work and other 'important' things pretending you're fine (I do it all the time) but you can't fool your heart. It always knows the truth. You just have to face that shit no matter how painful. Every day you must get up and try again.

"I had an amazing epiphany today. I've always had a fear of stinging insects, especially bees and wasps, to the point of literally knocking people down (including small children and animals and food and drinks and chairs and plants) trying to get away from them. I've been stung before. You can't grow up in NM without a few ant bites and I was once stung by a clover bee while walking shoeless in the park and another time I leaned onto a wasp when I was washing windows. Totally my fault. It's embarrassing and irrational, but I could never seem to overcome it.

"Until today. Sitting on my back deck, a wasp began buzzing around me and I just sat there watching it thinking 'Why am I not freaking out?' It landed on my arm and still I sat there, almost outside myself. For whatever reason, I thought of when Stuart told me Max had taken his life. I haven't shared this with many people because I felt ashamed for a long time, but in the moment I learned he was gone, one of my first feelings was near euphoria—because he wouldn't be able to do it again. My biggest fear had been realized and I knew nothing in my life would ever hurt more. I realized today there's really nothing left to fear."

– Margay Erne

It's been a few years now since Max died. I've had the honor of acting as a medium in this world between him and Margay and her family. Helping them cross the bridge to their own communications, dreams, and visions with Max. Letting them know that within time, all people heal, and Max was doing that work; as were they. Grief has a special way of requiring us to confront our guilt, shame, and fear—dissipating it into thin air when the grief is complete. And, finally, diminishing the illusion that death exists.

Death and Reincarnation

Death is inevitable and reincarnation is a matter for another time—if you need it to be. Whether or not you relate to your spiritual imprints as past-life memories, relating to death and spirit are everyday occurrences for everyone; the more you understand what that means and begin to cultivate your awareness of it, the better for you. Both, death and our spiritual imprints, govern the way we engage, participate, and embrace life.

Spiritual Healing

Spiritual healing is the idea of shifting the origin of, and circumstances around, an imbalance so completely that it can no longer exist. People are motivated with the desire to feel good. But when demon-battling, people must face and process their deeply painful and devastating pasts—which does not initially make them feel better.

I've had clients immediately get frustrated with the process because of the difficult honesty and shattering catharsis it requires. Ultimately, if they stay with the work, they will be more balanced, self-aware, compassionate, loving, and present human beings—and they won't be in pain any longer. With every breakthrough (spiritual and emotional transformation) a person feels less burdened, until one day they wake up and their entire life looks and feels different. Doing spiritual work means connecting the dots to how all their experiences impact them. Here are some of the processes:

- Soul Retrieval
- Spirit Releasement Therapy
- Past-Life Exploration
- Transition Strategy
- Altar Building and Sacred Spaces
- Grief and Emotional Processing or Counseling
- Mediumship
- Spirit Guide Work

When a person is experiencing intense futility and darkness, elements of it have been occurring for a long time. A common feeling is being weary and tired of it all, apathetic and unable to see how to change it, or that the change just doesn't come soon enough. Often, there just aren't words to counter what the person is feeling in those moments.

However, countless times I've spoken to the spirits of people who died by suicide, and every time they see that killing themselves was not the answer.

Many were in a confused and futile frenzy, sometimes being encouraged by demons or other spiritual entities. These people carried the expectation that dying would help the pain go away—until they died, and saw that their pain was still very much intact.

After death, a person lives in the same condition they were in when they died. It is every soul's journey to complete and heal what they bring into life; destiny will happen with or without a body.

Many years ago, I was called to a home being renovated. It was haunted, and it was my job to clear it. Once there, I found—among many things—a boy who had shot himself in the head. After communicating with him for a bit, it became evident that something else was present. He had been demonically influenced over a long period of time and the demon was still with him. Once I helped him release and transform the demon, his spirit was free for the first time since the 1970s when he died. He was then able to crossover into the light.

No matter how futile things seem, there is always an answer; it must be searched for, and you can be the bridge a person needs to find it. I use soul-retrieval and past-life work to connect with the origin of a conflict or spiritual pattern. Once something is healed and transformed in the space where it began, that energy shift creates a healing process that expands out to every other level of energy: from spirit to emotions (grieving); from spirit to mentality (ideals and thoughts); and finally, from spirit to the physical (where any habits that are in play because of the pattern can be changed with little effort).

Soul Retrieval

Life is eternal, so nothing can be lost forever. A person's soul, if they've died in trauma, does not ascend to what is called the *over-soul* (a dimension of the spiritual collective). It stays, discarnate, in the dimension where it died in order to find peace. In fact, any trauma a person experiences creates an exchange of energy or spirit with all the people involved in the traumatic event. It is the build-up of that energy we call karma. It requires us to remember the events until we can heal. And no matter how long it takes, we will heal.

The trauma can be spiritual, mental, emotional, etheric, or physical, and the healing can happen in a single moment. Which is relevant when dealing with someone who may be one impulsive action away from suicide. And, I'll say it here again: dying never creates peace. It can produce space from the issues at hand, but never resolution of them. You must be at peace before you die.

Soul retrieval is the spiritual journey to consciously remember and travel back in time to the origins of the trauma (via meditation or visualization). This can be a past memory or past life that is reviewed and understood from an objective spiritual perspective. It's an opportunity to witness, once again, all the circumstances around an event—to grieve, and forgive, all those involved. This directs the part of your soul that has been stuck in the trauma, back to the collective over-soul, and clears the place in your physical and etheric body where the energy of the trauma has been stored.

How Past-Life Death Sequences Create Trauma in Future Lives

It has been my experience in the regressions I've done with clients who've had consistent suicidal ideation, that they've often killed themselves in previous lifetimes, or carry a spirit with them who has. Revealing and healing it has released them from the need to resolve their anguish in the same way in this life experience.

Anytime the spirit leads us to a specific lifetime in a person's history, it's because seeing it from a perspective of power or objectivity allows them to be released from the pattern through finding forgiveness for themselves and all others involved—ultimately, grieving the experience. Many times, people die and don't have the opportunity to grieve their circumstances. Grieving in the next life integrates the soul, and it anchors the focus of their spiritual power in their current reality.

I facilitated a past-life regression for a woman who had been experiencing night terrors since childhood. We regressed her back to a violent death scenario where she was able to reconcile the loss and grief of that time. She never had a night terror again.

Spiritual Battle

There are many signs someone is in a spiritual battle. Although every culture has their version of describing malevolent entities, when we refer to demons it is commonly a biblical reference. So if it's a demon, it makes some sort of comment regarding or relating to Catholicism and the beliefs therein.

There are many other spirits that can be troublesome as well, but know this: all disruptive spirits have a story to tell, are in pain, and want to be heard. You slay them by hearing their story and encouraging them to forgive themselves through grieving their own loss and trauma. Ultimately, this changes their form—even demons.

The density of a demon's presence is often intense and scary, so if you are experiencing spiritual attack, feel free to call in any higher angelic or ascended master you feel comfortable with for support. Most of all, know you have all the power. The entity needs your permission to be in your reality; sometimes your fear is that permission. Here are a few of the signs to look for:

- Where demons are concerned, they make some form of Christian reference, quote scripture or demean God or Jesus. It's a telltale sign.
- Erratic, unexpected behavior, or language that's out of character
- Vulgarity
- A demon's purpose is to cause chaos, and they capitalize on your insecurities.
- Every demon's nature is related to the seven deadly sins (envy, wrath, sloth, lust, pride, gluttony, and greed).
- A person may experience the loss of time, saying and doing things they don't remember.
- Being asked or commanded to do something bad or normalizing inappropriate actions.

Demons and other malevolent entities target people in flux, often those on the spiritual path and seeking to find and create peace. A demon's purpose is to create chaos—so the most important thing to know about demons is they were created by us at some point in time and space. They couldn't exist without us, and they are personal to us. Once we identify the energetic connection, we can shift it and eliminate their access on every level. They gain access to us and our dimension through manipulating our emotions and beliefs about ourselves or our circumstances: anything in our world for which we experience insecurity or feel shame are easy targets.

Ultimately, demons and other spirits can be passed down from incarnation to incarnation or from family member to family member (spiritual or biological family), waiting for the opportunity to be delivered and transmuted into another frequency of energy. This type of healing happens when the soul in question can understand what energy connects them to the entity and can resolve the dynamic or event through forgiveness.

Cultural Karma and Genocide

It's important to consider what becomes of the groups of souls that die in genocide or the souls of the people responsible for their killing. No matter how one justifies it, killing others will always carry the karma of learning to progress or accomplish one's goals without killing. The lesson beneath the idea of taking a life is not about ending life—it's about obtaining power, identity, and superiority.

Each individual in humanity experiences a personal impact when we are taught to ignore, diminish, or repress any aspect of ourselves. Repression of this energy amasses internally when we have confusion about the elements of true power, identity, or superiority.

- **Power** is the idea of being and feeling self-sufficient.
- **Identity** is knowing who you are and embracing all of it without shame.
- **Superiority** is actively being all we can be—recognizing our power by supporting others to acknowledge and cultivate their own power.

These truths are individual, not cultural, and they become active the more each human includes all other life in their construct of society—creating space for all forms of life to live simultaneously and peacefully. It is up to the individual to create a life that teaches these truths. And clearly—on a societal level—there is a lot of trial and error on the path.

The Slayer's Altar and Ritual: Face or Challenge the Things You Fear

Nothing is an energy stealer or happiness killer more than the habit of avoidance. The truth is: the more you know, the better able you are to think clearly, process your emotions, and make positive decisions. All of which allow you to lock onto the flow of beauty that is yours to claim every day.

There are a lot of things you cannot have control of in this life. What you can have is the confidence, commitment, spirituality and self-awareness to decide what you will receive from the world around you. This is a powerful spiritual concept that offers joy, safety, and the opportunity to cultivate happiness.

Feeling safe in an uncertain world happens when you connect to the larger construct around you: your God, the Universe, or the compassion that connects all sentient beings. To reveal your personal truth, first to yourself then to others, gives you power and freedom from which the experience of happiness can be chosen.

What You'll Need for this Ritual:
- Two seven-day jar candles, the color of your choice
- A metal burning-pot or fireplace
- Cleaned and cleared sacred space for your altar
- A dish with dried corn, tobacco, or glass of water for an offering
- A journal
- Loose paper and pen

Release What no Longer Serves You

At the heart of any transition is grief; everything must be grieved. No matter if you liked it, loved it, or hated it, grief allows for the emotional, mental, and physical transition of replacing one energy with another.

Many years ago, I had this car. It was a fine ride, but as it was getting on in years, I felt safer having a newer vehicle. I still had a 150-dollar-a-month payment, but the harder I tried to find a buyer for it, I couldn't get anyone to purchase it for what I owed. Finally, I decided to keep it and purchase the new one, hoping it was just a matter of timing. Flash forward two years later, and I was still paying for both vehicles.

It occurred to me that I'd spent all this money on paying off the loan and was in the same position. So, I found and accepted a buyer. On pick-up day, as they drove away with the vehicle, I doubled over in tears.

As I cried, a whole world of emotion opened up to me. I realized that it wasn't the car I was sad about losing, it was recognizing all I had accomplished while in its ownership that came to mind.

It was the first car I'd bought completely on my own—with no help, in any way, from anyone. It was paid for with money from a job it took so long to find. Plus, I'd traded in the vehicle I lived in for the first six months I was in Los Angeles, for it. As I stood there, becoming smaller and smaller in its rear-view mirror, it was the first sign I was safe in this new city where I resided.

As that phenomenal world was moving out of view, and I was deposited back to my reality, I was just a girl on her knees crying in the parking lot of the apartment complex where she lived. Things are always much more layered than they seem.

What Do You Need to Release?

In order to gain self-mastery, you must first cultivate self-honesty. The ritual for you today is to write your story, twice. The first story is written in first person, present tense—who you are and how you got to the place or condition you are in (begin with: my name is…). Be honest, descriptive, and unashamed. No matter your circumstance, you are alive and have worked hard to get here. Claim forgiveness for all that has happened in your life, and all the people that have impacted you—creating space for newness.

The second story is to be written in first person, present tense as well. But imagine how you'd like things to be and write about them as if they are that way today. Allow your imagination to fill you with the emotion of what it feels like to live in a new way—in a new relationship or peace in an existing one. Living without fear or lack. You are successfully running that business or position you've always wanted. And, finally, what does it feel like to have all that you need? Again, be descriptive and unashamed of your desires.

Take the time you need to write these stories; grammar and punctuation aren't important here. Once you've written the first one, fold up the paper it's written on and place it under the candle on your altar, burning the candle for a few hours every night. All the while, writing the second story. Once the first candle burns down to the socket, take the paper from underneath and set it aside. Always keep a journal with you during this ritual. You'll want to pay attention to your dreams and experiences, night and day—writing any thoughts or images that come to mind.

Now that you've completed the second story, repeat the same process. Once the second candle has burned to the socket, sit and read the first story and the second story in succession, answering these questions:

- How do these two stories make you feel?
- What events have taken place during this ritual?
- Do you feel the same way as the person in the first story (you)?
- Are there any changes in how you see yourself and your circumstances?
- What changes does it inspire you to make right now?

Once you feel complete with the entire ritual, take all the stories and your notes and burn them in a metal burning pot or fireplace, dousing the fire with the glass of water when the burn is complete.

PART FIVE

INFINITY

Your Karmic Relationship to Sexuality, Creativity, Spirituality, and the Divine

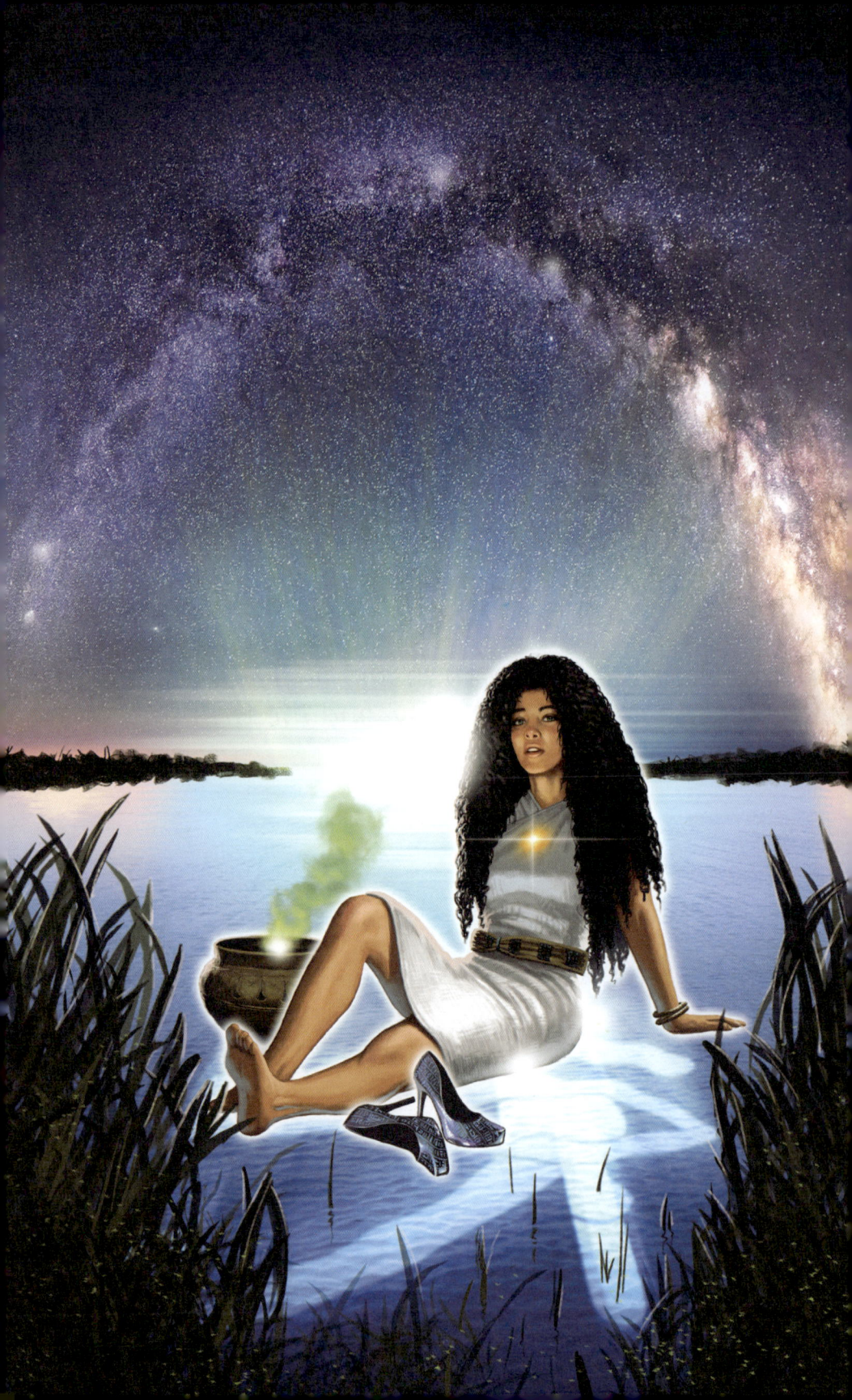

Karmic Relationships are Meant to Create Freedom—They aren't Forever, but They are Eternal

The Slayer's Weapons:

Steadiness, Conviction, Commitment, Vision, Courage, Forgiveness, Magic, Transcendence, Faith

The Karmic Story:
The African Queen No One Remembered

Every moment became consumed with the destruction of what was, the bitterness of what is, and the fear of what would be...

Ahtiaahmas' heart was pounding right out of her chest as she was helped into the priest's quarters. Many throughout the royal court knew about the troubles of the monarchy and their wavering fruitfulness. After the queen's first child didn't survive birth, she was luckily able to assuage the king's anger by quickly conceiving him another opportunity for a first born; although still, it was not without his berating her for her loss of the first child with cruel words and spitefulness. He began to despise their marriage, and he took up with his sister Meritites— as was the plan before he had married Ahtiaahmas.

In the beginning young Khnum Khufu and his second cousin Ahtiaahmas were in love. They shared such a deep connection that Khufu was jealous at the thought of her going to anyone else but him. Although their relationship wasn't forbidden, his mother had strong leanings towards a possible marriage between he and Meritites. But Khufu would have no part of it: he was the king and aimed to forge the world with his decisions—and he was infatuated with Ahtiaahmas.

Tall and shapely, she was the most beautiful girl in the land. The rich dark brown tones of her skin strikingly offset the green of her eyes and highlighted the billowing black hair that surrounded her face and fell down her back. Even though she wore her hair braided most often, Khufu always thought of her with her beautiful locks framing her gorgeous face. He'd often told her that if he couldn't have her, no one could.

Ahtiaahmas could barely walk as she was escorted into the priest's room, and she knew from the cramping that the baby wouldn't make it to term. The priest, who was personally close to her, helped her to his chambers for what the king believed to be her weekly oracle session. Khufu needed for this child to be born, and he was now well versed in what he called his wife's deficiencies; he would likely fly into a rage if he knew. Once again, another miscarried child! She was approximately four months along and it could only be kept from the king for so long. After his vindictive and unforgiving response at what he called his humiliation eleven months ago, Ahtiaahmas was certain she would not be allowed to survive this, and the priest knew it. He'd been teaching Ahtiaahmas the ways of Heka (magic), and she was becoming quite skilled. She needed to have a way to protect herself from the king's rage.

Devastated from what she considered the two deaths of her first child (he died once being still-born, and twice: not yet having received a name before his death), the gods would not recognize his soul or remember him in eternity. Ahtiaahmas had mourned him twice, and she was not about to let that happen again. This child she'd carried in her belly for four months, she knew he was a boy and gave him the name of Seti—he of the god Seth, who was the god of war, chaos and storms. Surely the gods would remember him now. It wasn't long after she arrived in the priest's quarters, that she lost him.

In pain and afraid, Ahtiaahmas needed to figure out what to do. Whatever it was, it would take some planning. The priest called for Ahtiaahmas' loyal servant to come, and at nightfall they would get her back to her quarters. The priest would tell Khufu that Ahtiaahmas must take her rest without disturbance. This would buy them some time to devise a plan.

After some rest, Ahtiaahmas burned some herbs and special plants, to call on the spirit of her son Seti. She knew he would be the one to lead her away from the tyranny of her husband. The stars were consulted, and in five days' time, the cosmos would be right for her safe passage up the Nile and away from the compound. The priest would make sure that a boat would be waiting. And although it would be certain death for Ahtiaahmas' trusted servant, she would make sure no one would enter Altiaahmas' quarters for at least three days upon her departure. They placed a powerful spell of protection over the door to ensure no one entered.

The time in question arrived and the moon was full and ready to receive Ahtiaahmas into the night. The further away the boat carried her, the stronger she became. She'd been with Khufu since she was twelve and had been removed from her family and all she had known. Now, with every mile, her senses were on fire and her rage was igniting, revealing the hold the king had on her and all she'd given up for the him. The priest had prepared the boat with some simple tools for building and catching food, supplies, and an iron pot for her spells and burnings. As terrifying as this new future was, even as the anger began to surface, Ahtiaahmas was also exhilarated and relieved.

She'd lost track of the time she'd been traveling upriver, when finally she arrived near a Ta-Seti stronghold,* where she felt she would be safe for a while. Ahtiaahmas could feel Khufu's fury—she felt him the minute he realized she was gone—and knew he would send a search party for her, but she was tired of being under his tyranny. She found a safe place to pull her boat ashore; it would feel good to sleep on dry land.

---

* Nubia

For the next three years, she was embraced by a family of cowherders in Ta-Seti; they were willing and able to keep her secret based on the remote nature of their village. She would need to stay in hiding, as those who protected her would be in jeopardy as well. Ahtiaahmas stayed out of sight during the day and practiced Heka at night. She'd been working with the god Sobek: he was the god of the Nile, and he promised her success for the bounty of the village and protection from the waters.

Mostly she spent her time claiming revenge against Khnum Khufu and his years of abuse, and she used the spirit of her son Seti to do it. Seti was strong and not the spirit of the young infant he would have become. Every night she focused on bringing humiliation to Khufu, strengthening Seti to visit upon his father and bring him the fear he so continually placed upon others. She held no ill will towards anyone else.

Each night, Ahtiaahmas felt Khufu's frustration increase for his inability to control her, and she loved it. She was certain by now Khufu had divorced her and, in fact, had removed any trace of her presence—as was his way when he felt betrayed by someone. But in all her vengeance, she missed the nuances and signs that heralded the presence of the team of assassins whom Khufu had sent.

One morning, just before dawn, she snuck down to the river to bathe and wash some cloth. She was making her way back through the tall reeds when the assassins attacked. One grabbed her and slammed her to the ground, another rolled her on her back, while a third plunged the spear through her heart into the hard ground beneath. Ahtiaahmas was now united with her son Seti—for the first time at peace, and loved.

Death Reawakened

All my relationships in this life have been discovered, thrived, and ended because of the past-life patterns and soulmates through whom I've received insight and healing for my personal spiritual history. The dynamic embodied in this story reawakened in me the rage of rejection and oppression, and a need for vindication: an opportunity to grieve what was, in order to create space for compassion, love, and peace, now.

Many years ago, in the middle of the night on Redondo beach, I sat witnessing a dear friend's grief from the unexpected death of her mother. She was intoxicated and crying, running and throwing herself at the dunes of sand—summersaulting in every direction. A man ambled out of one of the pier's eateries and noticed my friend. He came over, asking if she was all right. I explained the situation; he asked if he could keep me company. We sat together for almost another two hours chatting away as my friend began to tire out.

His name was Dan, and there was something in his green eyes that was familiar to me; of course, I had an affinity with someone who could witness this form of grief and not judge it or fear it. Finally, when my friend was sufficiently plastered in sand, worn out, and the tears were at bay, I said goodbye to my new friend, and we drove home.

Dan and I went out a few times after that—he was gentle and easy to be around—but he lived almost two hours from me, and a relationship of commuting is not something he could do. All of this he explained as we spoke over the phone. I was sitting on the terracotta-colored velour couch in my living room, nestled in its over-sized pillows; I wasn't surprised or sad. I thanked him for his honesty, and we hung up the phone.

Without a moment's warning, I was transported back in time: I felt the spear press through my chest to the desert below. Safe in my living room, I sucked in some air—gasping for breath. In my mind's eye I saw my dark golden-brown body and black, curly, unbraided hair—my green eyes frozen in time.

I began to cry uncontrollably. I was completely confused about everything, except that I had just witnessed my own murder in another time and place. I cried for weeks. The mourning was revolutionary. It was all I could do to get up and function, but somehow I was able to compartmentalize it on days that I worked. I didn't understand the connection between my vision and Dan, and the few times I reached out, he was unable to speak. It was almost as if it had nothing to do with him; his goodness made him available to the spirit who was trying to communicate with me.

Over the years, this spirit would make efforts to let me know they were there by connecting with me, sometimes through the men that I dated. Eventually, all my questions would be answered.

The Slayer's Path:
The Practice of Forgiveness

I'm sure you've heard that forgiving others is something you offer yourself, and it's true. But spiritually speaking: the most important person to forgive is you. This kind of forgiveness underscores the idea that everything occurring in your world is purposeful and deliberate—even if it is generated from a subliminal level and unwanted. If it happened, it was meant to happen. While it's not always clear to us when, how, and why we choose certain experiences, they are resolute, and our response is divine. Through understanding this, we can change what happens in the future.

This spiritual vantage is valuable in helping us to experience radical acceptance and unvarnished honesty in all aspects of our lives. The pivotal relationship that changed the longstanding dynamic of personal hauntings, grief, and spiritual attack I'd been plagued with my whole life was with the reincarnation of the man who was the spirit of my (Ahtiaahmas') son Seti. He incarnated in this life as a man I'll call David. I met him just shortly after my mother died. He was authentic and unable to don the masks of illusion most of us learn to wear early in life.

He had a good heart, in spite of a childhood that required autonomy from an early age. This self-preservation lead to dealing drugs and then incarceration for the majority of his adult life. Unbeknownst to me, I met him only a few months after his release, but I recognized something familiar in his green eyes. Although we had many interactions and stayed in touch, it would be five years before we would come together in any real way. There was an intense and enduring love between us that my life had allowed me the luxury of feeling and expressing in every way, while his life had not.

From the moment he crossed the threshold of my front door, the spiritual attack I'd experience for decades stopped. Completely. I was strangely in awe of the feeling of freedom, space, and clarity that began to emerge in my life. For the first time I could begin to focus on other things rather than the hypervigilance that had pervaded each day before. The relationship with David lasted a few years and ended with the same love with which it had begun.

It wasn't until one night—I hadn't seen him in a couple of years—but had gone to sleep thinking of him; I was awakened around midnight from something crashing to the floor in the other room. I got up in the darkness, rounded the corner of the living room doorway and as I walked into the room, I reeled back at the shock of seeing a man standing there. He was a very tall, thin, regal looking man wearing ancient Egyptian garb with a stern look on his face. He was a spirit, but looked as vivid and real as you and I. I stepped back from him and he disappeared just as my phone rang in the other room—it was David.

For the first time, everything began to make sense—the Divine was answering all my questions. David and I shared some truths that night that reignited our karmic love and allowed both of us to find peace in the imperfection of our lives, the relationship between us, and the spiritual history we shared. The energy he brought with him ushered in a new channel of love and courage that cleared the way to the redemption and forgiveness I was seeking. The spirit in the room that night was the king from my previous life, and as David (the incarnated Seti) and I were expressing forgiveness to one another, so too was the king. Now we were all free.

So many of our human foibles have occurred to initiate and maintain an illusion of perfection—when the real magic happens from all that remains a little rough around the edges. We need to learn to be honest with ourselves about ourselves, to be confident in what exists and change what doesn't serve us. So, forgiveness means to accept who you are, or what has happened in your life, by saying: *I'm sorry, forgive me, thank you, and I love you*—to yourself.

Ho'oponopono

The Huna of Hawaii have a practice of forgiveness, it is the phrase Ho'oponopono. It is used as a mantra in any situation, especially those that invoke intense emotions. Using this mantra helps you to develop calmness. Its literal translation is "to make right, establish harmony, correct what is wrong, and restore things to order,"[1] or: *I'm sorry, forgive me, thank you, and I love you*. So, when you're facing down those things that befall you, don't overthink it—Ho'oponopono.

When in need of forgiveness or quelling anxiety, recite the phrases: *I'm sorry*, *Forgive me*, *Thank you*, *I love you*, or *Ho'oponopono*, until you feel your energy shift (remember, you are speaking to yourself). This notion of healing allows you to recognize that everything outside you is a reflection of your inner self (your shadow and subconscious mind). Finding forgiveness for that part of yourself transmutes the energy in your life altogether.

This level of spiritual accountability is a powerful challenge to sustain in the face of all the personal and world tragedy we experience today. Your goal is to consciously reconnect yourself with the universal flow of energy that reminds you of the limitless support you have at your beck and call. Connecting yourself to the flow of forgiveness helps you detach from the effects of that which you seek to forgive, allowing you to consciously find your path to the Divine.

Three Rivers that Lead to the Ocean: Understanding Your Connection to Divinity

In this vast, multi-dimensional changing world, understanding all the ways energy flows through our body, heart, and spirit to the Divine helps us to receive, manage, and create all the experiences we have in life. The path then, of our relationship to the highest and best we can be, begins with our sexuality and expresses itself through our creativity; it cultivates our spiritual understanding, and finally, defines the way we comprehend the vastness of our concept of Oneness.

Each of those aspects to our humanity have their own natural vibrational flow that is adjusted based on our experiences. If we've been nurtured and supported well, our flow is steady and continuous. If we've been rejected or abused, our flow will be choppy and sidetracked. Both are positive paths to Oneness, and neither requires that we expand our knowledge or personal awareness—this is still an individual choice regardless of our circumstances.

The River of Sexuality

Human sexuality inspires the path of life-force energy in the physical body that leads us to the awareness of our relationship to the Creator. The understanding of one's sexuality is paramount to comprehending Divinity. A place we go wrong is believing sexuality is ungodly and unimportant. Our sexuality takes us on a journey of the multi-leveled creative path, opening us to the many dimensions of our spirit—paving the way to our understanding of the Divine. Should it be diminished, oppressed, or repressed in any way, a person's perspective of creativity, spirituality, and ultimately their relationship to the vast world beyond their knowledge will be skewed.

Sexuality is not just the physical manipulation of the body to open to orgasm, it is the slow seduction of intimacy that opens us to other spiritual dimensions of thought and emotion—allowing partners to know each other or one to know themselves. Intimacy is connection, presence, and reflection—all are part of the sexual journey and path of the kundalini in the body. Essentially, our sexuality is our channel to awareness of ourselves, others, and our environment.

Unfortunately, this aspect of sexuality isn't taught in schools, and yet it is this expression that provides the basic awareness that keeps us safe, present to learning, and conscientious of our own behavior and that of others. These subtle psychic channels are governed by the sexual organs and our relationship to emotion—oftentimes commandeering our ability to communicate.

So, when you consider your sexuality, consider the whole picture and purpose; it is the path to enlightenment.

Romance with Spirit

For almost the entire decade that I lived in New York City, I experienced many profound psychic, and telepathic sexual encounters with the men I dated and the spirit that followed me. Consider this: I was in my twenties—suffering from PTSD, anxiety, and depression—and having spiritual and psychic experiences I couldn't communicate about to anyone. When it comes to sex, people can be judgmental, cruel, and lack a magnitude of understanding. I'm not sure I could have spoken of the experiences I was having, as my comprehension was based on intuition and faith. I knew I was safe and there was purpose in all that was happening with me. I somehow had a sense of familiarity and peace.

Everything for me in NYC was transient. I moved eight times and had many deeply psychic-sexual relationships. Basically, that meant I could have a telepathic sexual relationship with a man who wasn't physically present in the room; I masturbated often. Although I had many sexual partners, many of the encounters with them were spiritual in nature. It was difficult to get physical with the people I dated as I would experience post-traumatic stress symptoms from the rape. This manifested itself in meeting emotionally and spiritually open love interests.

I met Harmony (that was his name) on the subway platform. I'd had a long day working at Bloomingdale's as a make-up artist; I yawned and stretched, oblivious to anyone around me. Evidently, that caught his eye, and from that moment on, we were connected. We remained lovers for several months. For some reason I didn't experience the post-traumatic stress with him, as I did with others. Harmony was a gentle soul. He was smart, funny, spiritually aware and a jewelry designer of the most magnificent wearable art pieces—but he suffered on levels I could only sense from him.

One night, I awoke to see him sitting at the side of my bed. He was wearing a red bandana around his head I'd seen him with earlier in the day. In a flash, he was gone. I was so confused. It wasn't a vision—his body seemed real—but it wasn't of this world. The next day he called to ask if I'd seen him the night before. He'd astral traveled (sent a spiritual body) to me. Harmony told me that I had been visiting him frequently. Who knew I was a spirit-stalker and had no idea? I knew he was right as I dreamed of him frequently. My mind couldn't quite accept my spiritual ability until this experience with Harmony. And I was grateful: if I'm going to stalk someone—I should know about it.

Our sexuality isn't only a physical experience. Often when we have a sexual connection with someone it precedes having sex with them. It is this energetic channel through which we begin to relate to the multiple dimensions of feeling, thought, and perception. This sexual connection creates spiritual cords from one to another that keeps the partners in intuitive and emotional contact. The sexual channel brings far more to our lives than pleasure and children; it is our road access leading to information on the spiritual superhighway that allows for healing and expansion on all levels.

The River of Creativity

No matter who you are or what you do in life, creativity is an integral part of your world and paramount to your self-expression. Creativity isn't only fulfilled through arts and crafts, it is your ability to innovate regarding your thinking, feeling, and energy, on all levels. Creativity can be expressed in limitless ways: numerically, mechanically, biologically, and structurally. These are but a few of the languages of creativity we all speak. It's your charge in life to transform what doesn't work into another workable form using your creative and innovative ability.

I've had hundreds of clients, over the years, who walk in with the idea they don't have a creative bone in their body. I always receive this as a challenge. A person's creativity is often predicated on their confidence and entitlement, however, neither are necessary nor an accurate assessment of ability. One must have courage to use their creative expression. Creativity is cultivated through a need or desire for change. Some of us have had a lot of change, and some of us haven't had much at all. Every time we must innovate our thinking, we are using our creativity; our courage becomes stronger.

It is through our creative energy center (third chakra) and our emotional center (second chakra) that we assert and define ourselves in the world. Our creative flow is paramount to helping us express ourselves and our divinity in the world through all that we do. Being engaged creatively is what connects us to the higher vibrational flow of the Universe, and it connects our being to Divinity itself.

Romancing Creativity

One sunny afternoon in NYC, I sat for a Viennese coffee at the Hungarian Pastry Shop, a favorite of all the locals. I was sitting next to a young man who was there alone, frantically turning the pages of a newspaper. I could see his anxiety buzzing around him like a swarm of bees. He looked so confused. I reached over and gently held the corner of his newspaper to briefly keep him from turning the page, and said, "Are you okay?"

He looked at me with wide eyes but couldn't speak.

I said, "It looks like you're feeling a lot of anxiety."

He shook his head in discomfort.

"May I make a suggestion?" I asked, regardless.

He nodded yes.

"Close your paper. Place your hands on top of it, flat on the table, and close your eyes. Take four deep breaths." He did as I suggested.

Once he resumed his balance, we began to chat about what was bothering him and then, about life. Thus began a many year friendship. Daryl was a college student, a brilliant artist, and deeply intuitive. One afternoon, he and I were talking: I was pregnant at the time but did not know it, and therefore, I was worried about my health. I was experiencing bouts of anxiety and trips to otherworldly dimensions; I didn't understand what was bringing it on. Daryl understood this aspect of life well. He pulled out his sketch pad and began to draw. Within minutes, he'd created a picture of the man I'd recently broken up with (the man who impregnated me) wearing a huge tribal headdress. He'd never met him, and it was startling. I explained to him it was Ron, and we were both perplexed.

It hasn't been until the last several years that I discovered my past-life as Higuemota[2] and recognized the spiritual connection I'd had with Ron—as well as Daryl's ability to channel that incarnation into life on paper. Our creativity is a channel of vibration we lock on to, receiving it's information by opening our heart and releasing the control of our mind. My experience with Daryl was evidence for me that we are all connected—our creativity links us to our Divinity.

The River of Spirituality

Our spirituality is our connection to our inner selves and the formation of our outer world. Remember this deep truth (something for which the opposite is also true): *the clarity you hold inside defines the clarity you witness outside.* It is the connection to our soul that focuses the lens through which we witness our lives and ultimately the Creator.

If we see ourselves as lowly sinners just trying to get through the day, then our Creator will certainly be critical and ready for judgment at any time.

Our personal divinity is connected to the Divine: the aspect of ourselves that transcends earthly attachment, expanding our awareness and possibilities in ways our minds cannot readily comprehend but can connect to at any time. Spirituality is the matrix of our soul and all its many connections, leading us to the consciousness of the Divine.

The reason we connect spirituality and religion? Religion and ritual are two of the many bridges we use to experience and express our soul's spiritual imprints. These spiritual contracts we have with ourselves and others are the impetus for us to find the understanding, forgiveness, healing, and release from old patterns of experience and behavior that no longer serve us. The choices we make are the key to spiritual transformation, and they keep us aware of our flow in the river of consciousness.

Michelle Obama's Shoes

Many years ago, I awoke from a dream that gave me a part of my spiritual integrity back, eternally freeing me. In the dream, I was getting ready to do a big presentation of some sort; although, after riding multiple long escalators to get there, it was more like a fashion show. Everyone participating had to walk a long runway, which was magnificently lit with a multi-colored light show as a backdrop.

I was in the dressing room getting ready, when I realized I didn't have any shoes. I was worried and began to panic. I'm not exactly sure where I was going, but I started to make my way back to the escalators. Just as I reached the entrance, Michelle Obama was waiting for me with a shoe box. She handed me the box and said, "These are for you."

In the box was a pair of Michelle Obama's unworn shoes. I was filled with relief and gratitude.

"Oh, my goodness, thank you!" I responded.

"Don't forget who you are," she insisted.

Her words reverberated in my head and heart as I looked in the box. The shoes were iridescent rainbow-colored stilettos with Egyptian hieroglyphs imprinted on them. I was enamored with and slightly frightened of wearing such powerful shoes. Frightened of the path they were acknowledging in me, let alone of breaking an ankle (I'd never worn shoes like this). I ran back to the runway, put on my new shoes, got ready to go on stage—and woke up.

The Divine Feminine is the aspect in us that communicates to all our other levels of energy. It is creative, sensual, magical, intuitive, and inspiring. It is the connection we have that expands our options, releasing our fears and opening us to possibilities beyond our current beliefs. The Divine Feminine as it presented itself in my dream was letting me know I was guided and supported on all levels. Consciously connecting with the universal flow by walking the new path (what the shoes represent) on the world stage (the fashion show), I could use my magical powers to support myself and others for higher pursuits than exacting revenge or expressing agony (what Michelle Obama represents). Magic is the connecting force that brings all the pieces of our intention together, manifesting it into the physical world. And it was now time to find a creative, positive way to help many.

The Warrior's Hidden Motto: I am Unworthy

When a warrior feels unworthy, they are becoming aware of the inventory of knowledge their soul contains. This concept of unworthiness is your personal roadmap to what you will need to fulfill your destiny: the completion of all your karma requires. Feeling unworthy is more accurately interpreted as being unprepared. We are worthy of all that comes our way, whether we know it or not.

It is this illusion of unworthiness that opens our heart and requires a deeper look at the thoughts, feelings, and words that infuse our world—what we say to ourselves and others, and the feelings we harbor without complete expression. Expressing sadness or anger is different than harboring it. Unexpressed emotion attracts to you the same emotional vibration from your outside world.

So, naturally, the insecurity or confused esteem we experience, which makes us feel vulnerable, is the evidence that our self-understanding is on the move. We are learning, changing, and expanding, and it feels awkward. Unfortunately, what do many of us do with that? We get stuck on the feelings of unworthiness and attached to the phase of confusion. We somehow perceive them as permanent conditions, rather than the passing transits of life they are.

Many years ago, I had a friend who became my lover for a brief period; his name was John. We'd known each other from the neighborhood for years and had this intense ability to be telepathic with one another. For months I had a crush on him, and by happenstance, we would meet at the oddest times and places. We didn't exchange phone numbers for two years but somehow managed to run into one another at least twice a week for a chat or spontaneous coffee. He brought me enormous calm, which was a welcome departure from the chronic anxiety I experienced daily.

But it became more and more frustrating that he was keeping me at arm's length. I knew he liked me too, but the push and pull was getting ridiculous. Finally, after two and a half years, we spontaneously ended up at my apartment. I remember sitting on the couch, looking at him standing in front of me. I felt awkward and unsure of what would happen next: this man never did anything I expected. When out of the blue he said, "Are you sure you want this?"

I laughed on the inside but was a little stunned on the outside. *Was this a romantic ploy?* (I was deeply connected and attracted to him.)

I responded with, "I think so? I'm not sure what you mean."

"I didn't think so," he retorted. "Let me know when you do." He kissed me and left.

The man I am talking about is John (from Part Four), and it was the night I had the dream of our past life together when he saved me from myself and a heroin overdose. Before I had any conscious idea of what it meant, he was asking me if I was ready to face the demon. He was then carrying it for me, until I was able to reconcile it, by helping him.

The demon in this situation was an entity created from a past-life coping strategy of heroin. I used it to help tolerate the continual abuse I was subjected to in that lifetime; however, my body and spirit became unable to continue carrying it. John, in that lifetime, gave me relief, until I was able to process and become accountable for myself by healing the entity that was on this plane because of me.

Remember, everything you experience is temporal and will eventually pass away to something else entirely, so learning to breathe deeply during confusion helps to easily transition into times of acceleration. Ultimately, being prepared for both opens you up to the many options that lie in-between.

The Slayer's Dilemma: Building Spiritual Integrity

What is spiritual integrity? It means your fitness to flow with the course of change you've been handed by your life. Do not judge yourself by how other people handle things, or compare your life to others, but radically accept every aspect of your own experiences, whether you like them or not. It is only when you completely accept the reality of your physical world that you can change it—and all the mental, emotional, and spiritual links to it.

The more flow you have in your body, the more you must be prepared for movement. Did you know most people subtly hold their breath when they are confused or are experiencing other understated emotions? When this happens in children, it can make them pass out. We naturally tend to hold our breath when we feel unsure (and we learn this from an early age). The movement of the breath leads to the movement of other emotions that may be lurking such as sadness, grief, anger, humiliation, embarrassment or self-pity, even the general movement of life itself (i.e., taking action). We hold our breath in hopes of getting grounded and prepared for what comes next.

The kicker is: what grounds us, calms our experience, and brings understanding is deep, long breaths. They connect us to our lower body, chakra system, and the stability of energetic flow. The more slowly you breath, a deepening of awareness takes place connecting you to your divine knowledge and your energy link to the planet through your root chakra.

Kundalini Movement in the Body

Kundalini is life-force energy in the physical body. It begins its journey from a repository at the base of the spine near the coccyx. This life force is the opener, or instigator, of our mental, emotional, and spiritual development. As it moves in the body, it activates the glands of our endocrine system and essentially releases our next level of higher knowledge, which is energetically contained in the glands. The chakras and our energy system in the body manages the flow of energy, information, and some parts of the physical body. The body's energy system, or aura, is extensive, and it connects to or can access any other dimension of energy through our awareness.

When these activations take place, the energy movement can be startling, sometimes painful, and can result in a healing crisis (some form of temporal malady) or an emotional release. All these things are perfectly normal, but sometimes frightening if you've not had the experience before. The first big one I remember happened when a friend of mine was standing in front of me. Right before my eyes, his image replicated three times in my vision—as if I were going to lose consciousness (but I didn't). This in turn scared me, and I began to cry. I was opening to my clairvoyance. I sat there crying and confused for at least an hour before things resumed to a somewhat normal state. From that point on I began to see other dimensional beings and light in a different way: clearer and more concise.

Quantum Spiritual Shifts

A quantum spiritual shift is similar to your kundalini life force being activated but much more powerful. It can feel momentarily debilitating—at times accompanied by a multi-hour or day-long emotional release. Quantum shifts are recognizable by the experience of seeing light—a light that connects to any of your chakra points. The third eye in the center of your forehead is the most common.

These spiritual shifts can be triggered by recurring spiritual patterns in the area of your life they are connected to. We experience a quantum light shift when we have transcended a pattern and must release it through the transformative quality of the spiritual shift. I once worked with a client who had deep-seated pain regarding feeling rejected by her father. As an adult, she began to challenge the things she would repeatedly tell herself: *My father doesn't love me*, *My father doesn't help me*, and *My father disapproves of me*. She began to question those statements' validity and power over her, and her thoughts and behaviors began to change. Suddenly—and for a period of about three weeks—after her bi-weekly yoga class, she began experiencing intense emotional jags that felt uncontrollable.

Every week she'd go to class and inevitably, as the breathwork and movement began to connect, she would experience a flash of light in her mind; immediately, the tears would begin to flow. She recognized that the more she experienced relaxation through her yoga practice, the more her mind would begin to think about her father. That's when the flash of light would come, and then the tears on the drive home would start. Many times, she would have to pull over to the side of the road until she calmed herself. The first time she had this experience, it was so traumatic and alarming to her, she pulled to the side of the road and called me so that I could talk her through it.

These kinds of experiences aren't uncommon for someone beginning to challenge the thoughts, ideas, and emotions that no longer serve them. Although they can accompany exercise, they need not be triggered by physical activity, or specifically yoga. They can also be ignited by some form of emotional upheaval or conversation. They can even be brought about by a sexual experience: the shifts of all the chakras can be activated by orgasm.

Healing Crises

A healing crisis follows a spiritual shift. The physical body is an echo of your spiritual, mental, and emotional makeup; when there are changes on any of those levels, the body must change as well. Healing crises can be many things: anything from an illness, like a flu or cold that includes a fever, to something more intense if you are already physically out of balance.

The spiritual shift isn't the cause of the physical response, but it often activates the immune system to eradicate certain viral or bacterial strains that vibrate at the same frequency as the spiritual, mental, and emotional energy leaving the body. In addition, I've had multiple clients become aware of cancers and other maladies that previously existed but only became obvious as healing on other levels was imminent. Once you upgrade on one level you must adapt on all the other energy levels as well.

While I have rarely needed or desired to be under a doctor's care during a healing crisis, I've always used supplements, massages, acupuncture treatments, and other integrative healthcare to help me complete a spiritual shift. Trust your intuitive leanings, and get any additional assistance you need to get through the healing crisis at hand. Don't be afraid to reach out to others for help.

> When we lie, spiritually we are living in two places—the lie and the truth—and over time it's impossible to keep them straight.

Building Spiritual Integrity through Honesty: Everyone Lies

Everybody lies. Seriously. And I'm not being cynical. Studies show that only approximately one third of us can identify our emotions as we feel them, which means there are two thirds of us who are lacking in self-awareness.[3] That's an important thing to take into consideration. Furthermore, between half and three quarters of the approximately 590 million online-dating participants have fibbed, embellished, and flat out lied on their profiles.[4] In non-online interactions, studies show that people lie almost two times a day about topics like true feelings, income, accomplishments, sex life, and age.[5] All the while, teens lie about money, alcohol and drugs, friends, dating, parties, and sex.[6]

I wanted to give you an idea of the facts, a scope of the panorama of human behavior that you're sure to run into out there. My own research shows that of approximately 150 conversations with men on dating apps and during about 50 meetings, I experienced that upwards of 90% of the men lied directly in some way, withheld valuable information, or admitted to lying during their dating experiences. (Some studies say that women lie more than men.)

I once met a man online whose profile said he was 40. He was very good-looking, showing off his washboard abs in a Jacuzzi photo, complete with him wearing a cowboy hat. He and I really hit it off, and we chatted online and by phone for about two weeks before we set up our lunch date. At the time, it was customary for me to do a bit of a background check, and at least verify the age and other vital information of my dates prior to meeting them, but I didn't this time. Wouldn't you know, upon my arrival, I found out the sixty-year-old at the bar was my date. Honestly, he didn't look anything like the photo, and my first impression was that he didn't look well. I think it was his sickly appearance that kept me in a place of compassion as I said, "Hi, are you Dave?"

The minute he saw the look on my face, I saw guilt come over his. I didn't address it directly; for some reason, I didn't feel the need. He was the same charming intelligent man I'd been communicating with, and we ended up sitting and chatting at the bar of the restaurant. Luckily for me, they'd already closed the kitchen. I had a glass of wine while he downed four beers in our forty-five-minute visit. We talked about the state of the world and previous relationships until I finished my beverage and politely thanked him. To his credit, he made no attempt at seeking further communication.

> **Trust but Verify: Things to Do When Meeting Someone New**
> - Do an online search and maybe a short background check to make sure the person you're going to meet exists: their name, birthdate, and home need to match. If you can find them on social media that's a good sign.
> - If there are huge discrepancies, ask about them before you meet.
> - If the information you find is accurate, move forward with an open heart and mind.
> - Know that everyone has insecurities and be willing to deal with them head on with compassion. Doing this will weed out the folks you need not have any business with.
> - Be honest, and remember humor makes everything easier.

Most of all, consider that we live in a society that is rife with judgments about who we are, what we like, and what we look like, so much so, that it sets us up to lie in the face of judgment—every time. Of course, we must all strive for truthfulness and honesty—but the truth is, we need the love, compassion, and humor of others to support us in achieving it. So, *if you see something say something.* Give people the chance to be honest, and give yourself the opportunity to be gracious and compassionate. There is always a future in that.

Karma's Impact: Why People Lie

People lie for three different reasons: survival, self-deception, and to deliberately deceive others. It's only a person's incredible courage to see and accept themselves as they are that will get you the whole and true story. The honesty you need to start with is your own. Consider that every person you meet, every relationship you have will have some omissions or embellishments. Men lie about their height, job, and financial standing; women lie about their weight, job, and financial status—just for starters. But, most importantly, why?

The answer to this question is found in the soul. Each of us has a profound constellation of attributes that contribute to our desire to be honest and truthful in all situations. Humans naturally seek to avoid pain at all costs (at least most of us do). Because of this, we are likely to take into consideration the response we expect to get before we share the information we have. If we've been bullied, abused, chastised, criticized, or deceived, we may just forget or opt out of the complete truth—especially if we don't feel safe.

People feel unsafe for many reasons: they are avoiding physical harm or lie to themselves to prolong the avoidance of feeling grief, which the truth brings. Even more so with con-artists and criminals: they have lifetimes of spiritual memory that leave them feeling unsafe and seeking power over others (regardless of the image they project). When you consider that there is much more to someone than can be seen, you open your intuitive channels to a person's spiritual truth. Trust your own feelings and be willing to talk about them.

Ultimately, when it comes to lying, our most important obligation is to ourselves and our well-being. However, when we lie, we are spiritually living in two places—the lie and the truth—and over time it's impossible to keep them straight. It is the natural flow of the spirit to integrate and release the things that no longer serve us; inevitably, those two places will become one, and the truth will prevail. Not only does telling the truth feel better, but others are able—consciously or unconsciously—to see or feel the disparity of your energy when you lie. Others are more likely to trust you when they feel your energy as integrated.

Sexuality and Intimacy: The Birth of Creativity

When we consider sexuality from a spiritual perspective, the focus moves to the idea of seduction and intimacy: all the energetic connections and communications that have taken place long before actual intercourse happens. We are speaking of the spiritual information in our soul that determines our initial attractions before the physical body's physiology takes a hold of our desire.

It is within seduction and intimacy that we can easily get lost, especially our pre-teen and teenage society members. But, it is also in these dynamics that we forge our ability to set boundaries and self-soothe—the two most important lessons in anyone's personal development.

My Human Story

I was sexualized very early in life, not by other people, but by the memory of my spiritual history and the damage that was caused in those lives from sex trafficking and abuse. I had an awareness of my sexuality by the time I was three. The burden for me was the sexual attention I've always received. From a distance I must have appeared like a pedophiles dream: open and apparently naive. In my grade-school years, predators would seek me out: on the street, in the park, at the mall, and as I grew into high school, they'd seek me out at the night clubs and bars where I'd go with my fake ID. But once they found me, they'd quickly realize I was a force to be reckoned with, and I was never hurt or molested in any way until being raped at eighteen. I attribute this to the many vicious spirits I carried with me at the time—they protected and haunted me at the same time.

My earliest memory of sexual attention was in kindergarten, by one of the boys in my class. I mentioned him earlier, his name was Daniel. He was a karmic love of mine in this life, and although we only shared a few moments of affection together in our early years, we lost track of one another once we entered high school, and he died young. Daniel and I still have a relationship in spirit, and the love has never diminished.

My sexuality is an arena of life where the lack of parental influence really supported my need to make my own decisions and learn to be confident in setting boundaries. Sexuality wasn't defined in my house, though there was never any slut-shaming or identity bashing. My folks were friends to all, and everyone was accepted in our home. What I learned came from other articulate open-minded adults and from the spiritual history I carried with me. I learned to communicate early about setting physical boundaries and had planned to be a virgin when I got married. No doubt, this was a Christian mindset I opted for as it suited my need to remain grounded.

My unconscious reticence to become sexually active was the only thing protecting me from the onslaught of my spiritual history and emotional grief that was waiting to break through into my waking world. Spiritually speaking, our karma is present in our energy and dream world until we hit certain developmental milestones or other spontaneous events occur, such as puberty, pregnancy, or sudden losses and accidents that cause quantum spiritual shifts. When these things take place, our life-force energy moves throughout the body activating the spiritual imprints of our karmic stories. It moves them into our waking world via our emotional responses, thoughts, and visions—all as we relate to our physical world and to the subtle clues that reveal the hidden chronicles of our soul.

Sexual Orientation, Gender, and Karma

Karma is created by actions, behavior, traditions, or customs that create a mark on the incarnated or collective soul's patterning. Gender karma is not only the relationship to the physical attributes of each gender but the emotional makeup, thought patterns, and the traditional roles we have attributed to each gender. Our world and our consciousness are moving beyond the need for a patriarchal society and the illusion of pedigree; in fact, we have more than enough humans on the planet as it is. Our human identity is shifting to a purpose and worth beyond just having children.

Consistently, over the last two decades in my practice, I have met many multi-spirited people whose gender and sexual identity (and any confusion therein) has come from the subtle awareness of spiritual beings that are non-binary. The presence of female and male focused personality-imprints, past-life memories, or other spiritual entities (including discarnate humans) creates internal conflict. When you have a spiritual entourage living inside of you or a strong spiritual memory of being male when you are in a female body (or vice versa), it is a unique experience and often one you'd like to ignore as long as possible—until the need to embrace and discover those parts of yourself becomes tantamount to living itself.

We all have masculine and feminine aspects—it is a part of being human and the larger construct of life. Within this construct each human has their specific spiritual goals and the goals of the DNA evolution of the body they were born into. Our relationship to ourselves and one another is forever evolving, growing into a common understanding of value, health, and spirituality—all requiring self-sufficiency, accountability, and connection.

Gender Identity and Fluidity

Our gender identity is a way of owning our karma and accepting all that we are by requiring us to choose our gender. This choice must be made by the person living the experience and not by the society outside them. Although I share the concerns of others about the unknown impact to the physical body taking synthetic hormones will have over long periods of time during gender reassignment, I understand the commitment and sacrifice those who have this choice are making.

My experience of being multi-spirited, left me in a position to recognize the multiple men and women I carried in spiritual form. In addition, I understood their male and female gender roles, but had no inclination to follow them: I was clear that I was female with a deep understanding of what it felt like to be the male spirits I carried. My sexual identity was heterosexual (while understanding bi-sexuality). My sexual karma is with men.

The path of understanding and self-identification can be frustrating and confusing; being able to reconcile the hormonal commands with the requirements of one's spiritual makeup are challenges in and of themselves. Make no mistake about it: the quicker you accept your leanings and find truthful ways to communicate about it, the better.

Personal Sexual Identity

Our sexual identity is not only our orientation but our ability to be intimate and with whom we choose to share our energy. As an empath, I am vastly receptive to feeling and understanding all that others experience. This is often interpreted as sexual attraction and openness by others, as my ability to share intimate details and compassion isn't average.

It has been a topic of conversation and confusion on many occasions as I meet new people. My experience of spiritual and emotional openness connects to others on emotional/sexual/heart levels, making the connection feel like sexual attraction to some. I'm often approached sexually by men and women—people from all cultures— and thought of as promiscuous, prudish, or as everybody's surrogate mother. The only way I've managed such a diverse sexual identity is with patience, compassion, and boundaries.

My spiritual patterns dictate that my perception of my sexual identity is very feminine, that I only seek to be with men, that I am open to all who are truly open to me, and that I'm a serial monogamist. While sex is important to me, the relationship is always much more important than the sex. Having abstained from varied sexual experiences, I've not ever felt I was missing anything; my feelings haven't changed since I was a toddler and first remember having them.

So, when you are considering your personal sexual identity or dealing with someone who is managing this process, here are some questions to ask:

- List five people you're attracted to.
- Who do you feel comfortable sharing secrets with?
- List five people who generate sexual feelings for you.
- What do gender roles mean to you?
- What type of people express attraction to you?
- Who do you experience telepathy with?

- Are there any commonalities in the people who make you feel the best about yourself?
- Are there any commonalities in the people in whose company you feel bad about yourself?

Sexuality and Trauma

There are many ways to become sexually traumatized in our global culture today, anything from physical sexual violation and disrespected boundaries to spiritually and emotionally being inundated with unprovoked or unwanted sexual information and attention from people and in media of all kinds. The most insidious type of sexual or intimate trauma is the violation of trust on any level. When our trust is violated it can take lifetimes to overcome completely, based on our willingness, or ability, to do the spiritual work necessary to inspire healing and the spiritual and emotional condition we were in when the violation took place.

If someone violates our trust when we've allowed ourselves to be vulnerable and open with them, the pain is penetrating. How one processes that pain is up to the individual.

Pedophilia, Incest and Abuse

I've worked with several clients who've experienced sexual abuse from a person whom with they've had a trusted relationship: a parent, family member, teacher, coach, or close friend. The presence of sexual abuse where a relationship is present can be an indication of a past-life history between them. The spiritual familiarity of a karmic connection can often be disguised as sexual attraction and feelings. Leaving a person sexually connected to their perpetrator long before it is legal, or they are ready.

This bears mentioning not because it changes the circumstances of the life they are in now and it's relationship restrictions, either legally or otherwise, but because when the victim is doing the work of recovery and healing, the spiritual link they have with their attacker can inspire feelings of attachment and intimacy that are deeply familiar and not rational—for which they carry guilt. Many sexual abuse survivors experience these deep emotionally intimate connections and struggle with their presence. These connections are often the excuse an abuser gives for grooming and violating someone with whom they've built trust.

If you find yourself on either side of this equation, getting to the karmic root of the attraction to or the abuse from an inappropriate partner can help release the need or desire of the perpetrator to engage—and the victim to find forgiveness, grieve, and move on. On the other hand, I'm not referring to serial rapists or pedophiles. While the existence of past life karma exists for these serial predators, they are dealing with patterns of control, dominance, and lack of empathy, which may or may not be the case with a person who is unconsciously reliving a past-life dynamic.

Healing must occur for all of us to live in peace, and we must be willing to go back in time and space as far as it takes us, to find healing and forgiveness so that criminal patterns do not continue.

Sexual Attraction and Karma

In general, sexual attraction can be generated in several ways: by the DNA compatibility that produces pheromones; by spiritual familiarity and karmic connection; and similarly, by vibrating emotional patterns interpreted as sexual openness. The spiritual purpose of all these pathways are not necessarily to lead you into a sexual experience but to encourage further investigation of the object of your attraction. Intense sexual connection doesn't guarantee a good relationship, and often, it is an indication of negative relationship patterns seeking to be brought into balance.

Your sexuality and attraction for others is a guidepost for you to look more deeply into yourself and the awareness of the world around you. Your sexual connection is the root of your creativity beginning to attract, process, and innovate your thoughts and feelings regarding the object of your attraction or yourself. Paying attention to this subtle flow of energy before sexually engaging with someone is a very powerful habit to create. It opens you more efficiently to the information your spirit is receiving.

Sexual Attraction: Breaking karmic patterns

People are sexually attracted to one another for many reasons: their DNA is compatible (chemistry), they are emotionally open, they perceive power and seek dominance, or maybe they just like each other. Whatever the case may be, if you've found someone you like but need to break out of past sexual patterns, there's hope if you're willing to do the work.

As an empath, I experience a lot of emotion—emotions of my own and those of others. When a person is in an emotional space, it means they are open for giving and receiving energy. This energy flow is centered in the second chakra which governs the sexual organs and where chi (Universal Life Force) enters the body. Although it appears that a person may be sexually attracted to you, they may be merely emotionally open. Conversely, if a person appears interested but not sexually attracted, it could be because they are emotionally shut down.

There are several components to sexual attraction, and throughout the life of a relationship they will all be tested, cultivated, expanded, and contracted as is the way of one's life force. Below are a few things to think about when you are looking to connect sexually with your partner and break old sexual patterns of thought, feelings, and behavior.

Trust: The number one factor in a balanced loving sexual relationship is trust. There are two kinds of trust: emotional and physical. Emotionally trusting another relies on your ability to trust yourself. In the face of your own vulnerability, above all things, know you are safe, whole, and loveable. You must know and love yourself first so that your response to what is causing the disconnection—trauma, immaturity, misunderstanding, or misdeed—is compassion, which is reestablishing boundaries.

In addition, you must be viewed as emotionally trustworthy. This means when your friend or lover reveals something precious to them, you receive it without judgment and with kindness, sensitivity, and compassion. Whatever you do, don't use it against them later.

Of course, physical trust is self-explanatory. It means that boundaries must be respected in order to have all the other components you'll see below.

Relaxation: Many folks experience daily stressors and anxieties and while for some, sex may be a stress reliever, for many it is not. The biggest aphrodisiac in a relationship is kindness and care. Pay attention to your partner's needs and desires. Listen to them while creating eye contact when they speak. Respond to their subtle bids for attention. Help them get or resolve what they need in order to relax. Understand that sexual interaction happens as a result of many subtle emotional connections over a period of time.

Patience: For the average person, sex won't happen without patience. I clarify, the *average* person, as it deems mentioning that there are a lot of extraordinary people out there with sexual proclivities too numerous to mention. Guaranteed, all of them have their sexual habits rooted in their emotional balance and openness: the way they have been treated and their personal experiences in relationship. Everyone comes with a past, and having success transforming sexual patterns and cultivating sexual attraction rely on your ability to be patient, open, and understanding of what someone has gone through before you met them.

Intimacy: Intimacy requires a bit of everything mentioned above, in addition to a little love added in. While love doesn't need to be present for sex to happen, it is a major component of true intimacy. A person who is good to themselves will have the capacity to be good to you and vice versa. Intimacy is connection, comfort, trust, closeness, joy, understanding, and acknowledgement. You cultivate intimacy by doing all those things.

I'd like to share a story of what not to do when meeting a prospective lover. These are the types of sexual beliefs and feelings one might desire to change. I met a man on a dating app. He was good looking and appeared smart, funny, successful, and charming. As the instant message conversation continued, he disclosed he'd used a fake name for his profile. Continuing our conversation, he told me he was nontraditional in dating. He expected the women he dated to pay their way, otherwise he considered them weak and selfish. If for some reason he decided to pay the check, he would have sex with them (not the term he used) "like the prostitutes they were." At this point, I suggested he had more on his heart than paying the check and wished him luck.

I don't need to point out to you his lack of fitness for dating or cultivation of a rewarding sexual connection. However, should you run into a person like this, and not allow their demeanor to change you, it's an opportunity to cultivate compassion for yourself and embrace your own worth.

Finding Balance in Your Sexual Relationship

Getting on the same page as your partner in your sexual relationship can be easy and harmonious, or precarious at times—due to busy schedules, stress, mixed messages or other unwanted karmic patterns as a part of the relationship dynamic. Sex is many things to many people: sometimes it's a definition, an esteem booster, a nemesis, a drug, a sacred expression of love, or a varying combination of all of them. So, how do you keep that connection going?

It depends on different factors: like how long you've been with your partner and how you relate to sex. While there may be differences for men and women regarding sexual patterning, at our core we share essential needs. Here are some things for you to consider.

Respect

Respecting yourself and your partner in a relationship means leaving sex out of the power struggle. Although it's easy to withhold or dole out your sexual favor with purpose (within a relationship), it's not kind and doesn't build on everyone's need for trust, openness, and relaxation within the sexual experience. Power struggles are a natural part of getting to know someone, but if you don't feel safe or find you need to be in control of your partner or the sexual experience—maybe you're not quite ready to respect yourself or your partner in the way that a loving sexual connection requires.

If you find yourself having resistance to being kind to yourself or your partner, reevaluate your motivation for intimacy; you may need to cultivate other ways to self-soothe when things don't go your way or you feel rejected. These are two dynamics often found underneath the inability to be respectful.

Accept

Body image is a big deal in your sexual relationship but no matter what you feel or look like, there is only one amazing you. Feeling sexy is different than looking good, and it comes from how you feel about yourself and how much personal power you experience. Everyone has thoughts of comparison to others or changes they'd like to make. At a time you are not engaging in sexual expression, strategize about one change and make it, or accept yourself for the hottie you are today. So when it's go-time, you're not self-conscious. It's amazing how much our inner thoughts inspire reactions from the people witnessing us.

Try this exercise:

Starting on a Monday, repeat this affirmation 30 times a day, and see how it makes you feel by Friday.

> I am the sexiest, most loving person on the planet.

Be Authentic

Many aspects of our sexual expression are negotiated. It's a belief for some that in a marriage or monogamous relationship, it's your partner's responsibility to make sure your needs are met. This is magical thinking. Being able to connect with your partner and reach climax are the two elements of your sexuality that only you control. Your partner will contribute to your feelings, but they are your feelings. It's not anyone else's responsibility to ensure your sexual happiness, only you.

When you are upfront about your needs to your partner, your partner can address these things outside of the sexual experience, for example: if you need monogamy to feel comfortable sexually, whether you're into bondage and discipline, if you like oral or anal sex, or you feel most aroused in the morning. Talking about sex early in the relationship is important. When you tell a partner early on about your needs and desires, you will either have the love and support you need from your lover or plenty of free time to find the right one.

Be Kind

Everyone is tired and stressed, let's just start there. My go to remedies are *be kind* and *lower your expectations* when it comes to having any form of sex. Sexual activity creates and releases endorphins that ignite warm and positive feelings that carry you throughout the day or can help you sleep better at night; they go a long way to reducing your stress and fatigue. Rejection, however, creates the opposite effect.

Kindness is an aphrodisiac to a frazzled partner. Considering your current mood and that of your partner before making a bid for attention is a powerful step. Then lowering your sexual expectations to adapt to the situation allows time for you to show some form of kindness to your partner. If they need to talk, let them talk. You're not going to have the energy for earth shattering sex all the time: consider initiating sex with your partner in some form and then finishing it yourself, if need be. The more this dynamic is a part of your sexual history with your lover the more energy you'll have.

Communicate

Communication, understanding, and compassion are the three biggest generators of a lasting love connection. As early as possible and as often as necessary, have a sit down with your partner and write out what you like and don't like regarding sex. What, if any, are your changing experiences in your mood or your body regarding sex? If your partner doesn't know, they can't adjust to your changing needs. If you want to have sex more frequently, find ways of staying connected daily: little kindnesses, sweet text messages, notes left in pockets or purses, or simply picking up after yourself.

Talk about heavy topics in a room other than the bedroom, and preferably fully clothed: it's usually easier for everyone when you're stripping down emotionally. My philosophy is the more you share your sexuality, the more you share love—no matter the phase of your relationship. You may not always have those *in love* feelings, but you can always be loving, which leaves you openhearted. So, decide what you want, be where you're at, love yourself first, and all the love in the Universe will flow your way.

Understanding Intimacy

One time, I asked a boyfriend: what makes a good lover? I was about nineteen and had very little experience. His response surprised me. He said I should want to have sex. Being with someone who wants sex, changes the mental and emotional connection. I expected there was some sort of action or secret to be a good lover, but just the simple idea of wanting to be doing what you were doing? Did people have sex when they didn't want to? As I've discovered over the years, people have sex for all sorts of reasons that don't include actual desire for their partner.

Love and compassion create the space for someone to want to connect with another, mentally and emotionally. For many folks, sex is about power and control and intimacy is resisted or feared. The less you connect with a person, the easier it will be to move on should the need arise. It is in these subtle mental, emotional, and spiritual connections, beliefs, and memories that the foundation of our relationships can be found. Our personal history in relationship to our body, heart, rejection, and comfort level with honesty are the building blocks to the fabric of intimacy woven in all our relationships—sexual or platonic.

Many people have an irrational perception of their physical body, the clinical form is called body dysmorphic disorder. It is the negative perception of our bodies (feeling too thin or too fat, disgusting, deformed, or ugly) based on varying circumstances, hormonal cycles, and can often be found with a karmic root. The most loving thing you can do for your sexual partner is to be willing to work through any obstacles you have about the way you feel about yourself. Being comfortable with exactly how you are in this moment gives you a freedom in your loving sexual expression.

For some, being openhearted in our society is akin with being vulnerable to manipulation, but in fact, we're only vulnerable to the information we don't have or don't want to have. At the least, openheartedness is trusting yourself. At the most, openheartedness brings the experience of unconditionality into your sexual experience. It is a complete openness to your partner and their needs, in addition to the ability to know and express your own needs.

Loving your sexual partner doesn't necessarily mean to be *in love* with them. It means accepting them and being willing to be generous with your truth, honesty, kindness, and to negotiate a relationship that works for both of you. From a fully accountable position, we let people treat us how they do. Setting a boundary the first time a partner expresses a behavior that we're not interested in, is the key. Rarely, does bad behavior just present itself all at once. Unloving behavior happens in increments over time.

For example, it's easy to allow yourself to be called a name in anger because your partner had a bad day, and it wasn't personal to you. Over time, you are teaching your partner that there are times when it's okay to treat you badly. Just saying, "Hey, I know you've had a bad day, but don't call me names. That's unacceptable," can change the course of your entire relationship. Expressing a deliberate boundary in a peaceful voice is enough to change the direction positively, especially when you're just getting to know someone.

Being present in your sexual relationship requires courage. When you're present, you're connected and open to receiving loving energy. As you know, a natural response to being uncomfortable is contraction: to pull back emotionally or withhold sexual expression. Opening to someone's loving energy expands and moves you on every level: spiritually, mentally, emotionally, and physically. Letting yourself receive your partner on all levels creates an unforgettable experience. When you love yourself and meet your own needs, it allows you to show authentic interest in your partner.

Why People Resist Intimacy

I think it bares mentioning here that the openness that intimacy requires also leaves you vulnerable to receiving energy and feelings of anger, grief, frustration, hatred, disappointment and humiliation—and any other form of self-loathing one can muster. Remember, you cannot receive energy that you do not possess on some level, yourself. We take on energy from others to bring its presence into our conscious awareness so that we may reconcile it in some way.

This means acknowledging its presence. Searching your life experiences to discover the origins of the discordant energy—grieving any and all people and events related to them—finally finding a path to forgiveness. You cannot process what you do not know is there.

Hook-ups and Other Sexual Encounters

I dated a guy, on and off, for about five years in my twenties. During that time, he lied to me about everything. This guy lived with his *cousin* (girlfriend), was having sex with my good friend, and even being fellated by our co-worker (40 years his senior) in the parking lot of the mall where we both worked. Of course, I didn't know about any of this at the time; although, I intuitively suspected he was being untruthful about something. But when I confronted him directly, he'd reassure me of his honesty every time. Our relationship was a series of dangled carrots, until finally I discovered the root of what was going on was much deeper.

One night, at a small dinner party, a friend and her husband had created for us, my date asked me, "So, have you slept with him?"

"Who?" I asked.

"Your friend's husband? You seem to get along really well."

"No," I replied.

"Why not?" he said.

"For starters, because he's my friend's husband!?"

I was surprised. All in one brilliant *Maury Povitch* moment, it occurred to me that if this was his expectation of relationships, how was he conducting himself out in the world?

From that moment on, I began to pull my energy away from my relationship to him, and soon, all the truths came flooding out. The truth rocked and devastated me at the time, but I was given an immense opportunity to channel my rage at this betrayal into something productive, rather than annihilating him or myself. In that, I was successful.

Slut Shaming and Other Disparaging Illusions

Today, in hindsight, I feel sad for both of us. The sexual culture we live in sets us up for failure. Doing one thing but saying another always leads to conflict, and the hook-up culture is about being honest. Let's all take a deep monogamous breath and face it: it's the dating culture and the illusion of monogamy (before two parties are ready) that creates the problem. Society sets it up: the consensus is when a woman wants to sleep with multiple people, she's a slut; when men do it, they're impressive. Of course, that's ridiculous, and all it does is set folks up to be untruthful about their desires and choices with one another.

I'd like to define two things: dating and hook-ups. Dating is the process of getting to know someone, ultimately to move towards an enduring union. Hook-ups, on the other hand, are getting together for the purposes of sexual interest or companionship. And, no matter how well you negotiate it, feelings will get hurt on either path. That's life: embrace it. Now before we go on, I'd like to offer a defense as to the purpose of such a long running moral notion as monogamy.

Spiritually speaking, when two people share in a sexual connection, they transfer energy back and forth to one another—possibly unbeknownst to one partner or the other. Some people are better than others when it comes to the ability to transform or metabolize the energy they've taken on. So, the fewer connections you have, the clearer you're able to experience your spiritual truth.

Physically speaking, our DNA requires that we are continually given the message to procreate our species. Rightfully so, for at other times in history there were fewer people and multiple cultures that supported polygamy (one man impregnating several women) for the purposes of childbearing. Today, however, is not that time or circumstance. In fact, I am certain we will never have the need to populate en masse on this planet again.

Having said that, I'd like to make a few suggestions on how to hook-up or date with honesty:

- Be who you are from the beginning. There will always be someone who likes exactly who you are.

- Take time out to be honest with yourself about your desires. Write them out and practice saying them out loud. There will always be someone who wants exactly what you want.

- Don't deny the discomfort you feel from going against the monogamous or free-spirited grain of your particular society. It's not their life and they don't matter. The more you embrace the discomfort of being different, the stronger you are in every aspect of your life.

- Strive to achieve love in any relationship in which you participate. Love yourself completely and love will flow from you and to you.

- Don't fear rejection. Of course, everyone you meet won't want what you want, but if they don't want what you have–it's for certain you won't find happiness there.

Bondage, Discipline, and Other Creative Forms of Connection

Sexual fetishes, at their core, are ways of building trust of yourself and others. Because there are far too many fetishes to name here, I chose B&D as a representative of all fetishes. Anytime you have a proclivity (especially in your sexuality) that goes far outside the cultural norm, and strays beyond the need to procreate, you are beginning to cultivate self-esteem by acting in a way that brings conflict or criticism from others. Facing rejection in any form is a spiritual integrity builder. In life, we will all face rejection in one form or another. When you face it head-on or call on it, as in bondage and discipline, you learn to love yourself, be vulnerable, and authentic in spite of what others say or do.

If you're not sure what B&D is, it is the practice of sexual roleplay (not necessarily sex) between a dominant and submissive partner; it enacts the natural power struggle all partners go through usually at the beginning of the relationship. However, in bondage and discipline, the dynamic between the dominant and submissive is pronounced and deliberate, whereas in many other relationships it remains hidden or dismissed. In B&D the submissive is in control of the situation, while the dominant is the apparent leader—until the submissive pulls the proverbially rug out from under the dominant.

In my tenure of managing a Los Angeles apartment complex for about a decade, over the years we had four tenants who created *dungeons* in their apartments for use in their bondage and discipline sessions. We're talking several *mistresses* and *submissives,* with their clients coming and going at all times of the day and night. It was common to see professional athletes and CEO's rolling through an hour at a time. Occasionally, there'd be a submissive in his underwear gardening in the back of the building or doing some housecleaning for one of the tenants as a part of his session.

The dominant and submissive power structure is a part of the human progression of developing confidence, learning to be authentic, and accepting responsibility for all your behavior and leanings on all levels. People who express themselves sexually, through fetishes, are doing this deliberately and honestly for themselves.

> Anxiety in a relationship is a note from your lover saying that they're in your house but not necessarily home.

Monogamy and Karma

Monogamy is another option for your sexual expression, but it's important to be clear: it is a choice not an obligation. I understand this may differ from many cultural points of view, but it's true. The Universe would rather have you happy, honest, kind, and loving—than monogamous. However, going against the cultural norm and negotiating a plural relationship has the potential to be unnerving.

The truth is, dating isn't just a lead-in to marriage and family anymore. Many people date for many reasons: some for companionship, connection, loneliness, networking, and sexual interest. However, the most palpable unspoken reason to date is for self-realization.

People who are engaging with multiple people are often looking to find their own hidden truths mirrored in another. Making efforts to shut down that process for someone, before they're ready, doesn't work. Commitment is cultivated in your relationship to yourself, not in a relationship to a partner. Those who are ready to commit to a monogamous relationship, do. Those who aren't, won't. So, it's best to allow you and your companion the opportunity to be completely honest without emotional consequences. Otherwise, they will certainly rear their ugly heads down the line in the relationship. Take this opportunity to reset your viewpoint and your purpose for dating with the following tidbits of perspective.

Truth #1: Nobody wants to get hurt. It's common for a person who's been hurt before to easily attach to a partner in a dating relationship. But hoping you're on the same page with your partner doesn't make it true. If you're in an emotional space where it's difficult for you to date someone who is dating others, that's okay. Don't date them. Be honest with yourself and truthful with them, and if they're valuable enough to you, you'll find a way to cultivate a friendship that can grow into a stronger romantic connection at a time where you both can get your needs met in the relationship.

Truth #2: The real power struggle is within you. Fear of rejection is what's at play here. Don't buy into it. A wise friend said to me when posed with the question, "Why is it, dating can be so difficult?" Her response made me chuckle a bit: "Because people change their mind." Folks can be fickle, superficial, self-centered, self-serving, and flat out fair-weathered. When and if they are, it's not about you. They aren't rejecting you, they just have no need for your value. It doesn't mean that you don't have value. The more quickly that you move on from someone who doesn't need, appreciate, or want your value, the better for you.

Truth #3: Tell the truth and negotiate from there. I've seen, many times in the relationships of couples whom I've counseled, that the less willing a partner is to know the truth, the easier it becomes for the other partner to lie. Many people aren't self-governed, they rely on the boundaries set for them. When you set a boundary for things to be a specific way, and they are not that way for your partner, it makes it easier for them to lie—especially if they like you and don't know you well.

I had a friend who was so stringent with her companion in the first three months about everything from only dating Leos to not dating men who've been married or have children. And yes, you guessed it: they were living together for four years before it all came crashing down. She found out he was really a Sagittarius, had an ex-wife and three children (with whom he would visit daily from nine to five after he'd lost his job in the first year they lived together), and those are just the highlights I remember. His lies were not her fault—clearly, he had much deeper psychological issues at play—but when some people get forced into a corner they feel ill-equipped to handle, they also are ill-equipped to be honest.

Truth #4: Love yourself unconditionally and accept your needs. When you enter a new connection with someone, it's okay to let yourself explore who they are rather than vet for who you want them to be. If you are attracted to someone, trust that. Allow the relationship to move at a pace that makes you comfortable. When you learn something about someone that isn't agreeable to you, take some time on your own to process what and why it is. Don't make a rash decision about inclusion or exclusion from your life. If you'll allow yourself time and exposure to other people, everything will eventually be put in the needed prospective for you to make a solid informed choice for your highest good.

Truth #5: The grass is always greener, until winter comes. Life transforms through cycles and every relationship has them. You won't ever be in a relationship with someone you like all the time. Unless, of course, you like yourself all the time, and if that's your case, I'm certain you don't need relationship advice. So, please disregard the following: the way through an enduring relationship is to always choose your own goodness—your love, your compassion, your integrity, your truth, and your honesty. If you will cultivate those five things you will attract and promote them in others. They will be the green lens you'll need in colder, leaner times.

All in all, despite our immediate-gratification social structure, our one true goal is to learn to satisfy ourselves: first by what we give ourselves, second from what we receive from others, and ultimately, what we give to others. Relationships and the process of self-reflection that we experience in communing, can give us enormous clarity on how we're doing.

The rejection, jealousy, conditional love, conflict, and frustration we feel in the face of engaging with someone who has many love interests, is certainly a path to an open heart and more generous spirit. Eventually, when you do find a partner that you connect with on many levels, you're going to be prepared to do what it takes to endure in that relationship no matter the season.

Love is something we are and do, so why does it seem that people fall in and out of love so quickly? This is a phenomenon that participating in a karmic relationship brings—feeling in love one day and feeling nothing the next. But is it possible to start or stop loving that quickly? What does it mean about you?

Falling in and Out of Love

What we are talking about here is the vulnerability we feel when we fall in and out of attachment—not love. A karmic connection is like a lock and key coming together to open the door to a specific experience between two people. Often, the markers of this liason are intense emotion, sexual attraction, and an undeniable, overwhelming, conditional or unconditional love.

Attachment, Vulnerability, and Receptivity

The best way to address anything is to investigate it directly. Find a way to break it down into smaller digestible pieces and eventually understand it. That's why so many of us get overwhelmed in relationships when we're in the process of getting to know someone. Sometimes the emotional doors fly open and we feel intensely close to someone in a very short period of time, or conversely, we spend an inordinate amount of time and energy trying to keep those doors closed.

I thought it might be helpful to look at attachment as a skill and from the prospective of personal responsibility. After all, it's your door and you can open it if you want. It takes more work to keep the door shut, and if you keep inviting someone to knock at your door but never open it for them, they'll get bored and leave. Nobody wants to sit and stare at a closed door; unless of course, they have open doors in other houses.

The most important thing to understand is that attachment and openness in a relationship are the same thing. The only difference is your perception and level of self-trust. Our sense of self comes from many factors like our spiritual patterns and what we think, see, and experience. You can only change what you know to change. Here are the three main levels to take note of:

Attachment: Feeling attached to someone is experiencing an immense, and at times, abrupt spiritual-emotional connection. It's most difficult to manage this when you've just met someone and aren't quite sure of the content of their character. When this happens, try your best not to sweat the small stuff, be too pushy, emotionally overbearing, or give ultimatums.

This is the time to communicate freely and deliberately about who you are, what you like, and your circumstances. Often, when people feel overly attached, they focus on what they want and don't want in a relationship, which can be a good thing; however, in this instance, it can be generated by a fear of not getting what you need.

Instead, focus on what you like. Be willing to set gentle boundaries and respect the boundaries of others. If you're in a long-term relationship: strong or untenable feelings of attachment often stem from dishonesty, minimal communication, or a crisis within the relationship. In this case, communication is king. It's natural to feel insecure when you're not getting all the information or when your emotional and mental bodies are being taxed because of trauma. Stop, breathe, speak, and listen. Know that this, too, shall pass.

Vulnerability: Attachment can mean being vulnerable to someone. When you open your heart in an authentic way, or are emotionally or sexually connected, you intermingle spiritually and energetically with your partner. Anxiety, intense emotion, or thinking about someone all the time lets you know that their energy has entered your spirit. Anxiety in a relationship is a note from your lover saying that they're in your *house* but not necessarily *home*. Attachment doesn't mean you are in love: it means you are connected and there is an openness and opportunity to love.

Being vulnerable to someone means that you are in a natural place of openness. It requires three things of you: maturity, patience, and kindness. Those are the first three trust-building skills we must master in order to find peace and authenticity in our vulnerability.

Being vulnerable to someone means the power they have over us is directly related to the value we give to them. How you value someone is in your control alone. Have patience to allow the natural unfolding of getting to know someone. No need to push the river—maturity allows you to know when and how to set personal boundaries, and kindness is the key to persevering through confusion and enduring in the relationship.

Receptivity: When we accept who we are, we become aware of the constant communication with ourselves. She knows the things that trigger her and is willing to talk herself through them. He knows that a deep level of connection with someone ebbs and flows all the time, and when you're in a deep state of receptivity with another person, you feel when they are present in the relationship and when they are not. If your lover has pulled their energy back, they've not necessarily left the situation, they've only connected to other things of value in their lives.

This pulling back of energy can be unnerving to you if you're the least bit unclear about the reason. That's why your willingness and ability to speak openly with candor and grace is so important. The subtle way you phrase things will be the difference between peace or conflict.

Staying in the first-person present tense, with a focus on personal responsibility, is your friend.

Say things like I am, I will, I feel—all for the purpose of expressing yourself and then promoting the expression of your lover. When you're receptive to another, they in no way are the cause of your feelings, experiences, or troubles. You are. How you feel is an indication of your possible need to express yourself, to grieve, or to set boundaries—all things you control.

You don't need to know how, or do it well, but you must be open to work through difficulties in communication. Believe me, it's a skill with a huge learning curve and takes daily practice. It is frequently our romantic relationships that bring out our most submerged wounds to be healed, for they connect with us the most deeply—at least for a time.

As a spiritual empath I am in a deep connection with a few people, always: understanding that my attachment is the way I telepathically communicate with them at any given time. It's been quite a journey to understand that things weren't necessarily the way I felt them to be but rather an expression of my connection and perception. Knowing myself first is the way to recognize what I'm feeling—versus what I may be empathetically or intuitively aware of in another.

Knowing and trusting yourself has its own learning curve that is cultivated over time and through self-awareness. Surrendering yourself to attachment, vulnerability, and receptivity is the shortest path to get there. Our media focuses on being pretty, young, talented, virile, happy, successful, or smart, and the list goes on. The reality is we are all unique individuals with varying elements of these things that make us the amazing vulnerable humans we are.

Whether or not you believe there is a person out there who wants you, and will love and cherish exactly what you have, is the question. And by the way, it's also your combination of beliefs and ideals that make you the terrific individual that you are.

No matter how you look at it, relationships are work and sometimes hard work. People can be lazy or unskilled at communicating what they want and negotiating a compromise that works for both partners. Yes, compromise, understanding, patience, and kindness are the four self-mastery keys necessary for a loving enduring relationship. Any relationship will help you build on self-mastery and the four keys—helping you transform any spiritual pattern you may have outgrown.

Adjusting your relationship lens to look at and engage with specific partners through what your true desire is, allows you to communicate truthfully—taking the illusion of rejection out of the equation. When your partner knows what your goals are, they can make an honest and open assessment about how they want to move forward with you—not because of your worth and value but for your aligned relationship goals. Any relationship is an investment of time, emotion, and energy on multiple levels that will absolutely take away from other things that you're doing.

What I've found is there are people you think aren't interested, but they are fearful or unable to express themselves and negotiate the relationship they want. Then, there are potential partners who say and do all the right things and are talented at doing what's necessary as a means to an end—without actually communicating what that end is. The reality is, we all want to be loved, acknowledged, respected, and appreciated. When any of those elements don't manifest, or begin to wane at the start of a relationship, we begin the exodus (at least in our minds). You can't endure in a relationship when you've already ended it in your head.

Relationships reduce to the way we negotiate them and whether we are willing to go with the flow of the partnership we enter rather than trying to fit our partner into the mold of our agenda. People need love, kindness, nurturing, and patience but are at varying levels of ability to say and know exactly what they want; many times, they give up on the relationship before they achieve success.

Affirmations for The Four Keys:

- **Compromise**: I am willing to embrace a relationship that meets the needs of me and my partner; I am willing to compromise.
- **Understanding**: I am willing to accept the truth about myself and my partner; I embrace understanding.
- **Patience**: I have all I need and receive everything I truly want; I am patient and embrace the time things take to manifest.
- **Kindness**: Being kind makes me feel good; I embrace giving and receiving kindness.

The Slayer's Motto: I Am at Peace with Myself and My History

Peace is not the absence of conflict; it is the commitment to work through any inconsistency that should arise. When you make that agreement with yourself: acceptance, empowerment, and peace become the new lenses through which you experience life; life becomes fluid. You are then empowered to embrace all your soul contains: your spiritual history and physical experiences. Complete with the thoughts and feelings you have about that history and experience, you are free to transmute, transform, and heal all of it.

Your Personal Cultural Identity: Finding Your Tribe

A part of getting to know yourself more deeply is discovering all that you are, spiritually. Your personal cultural identity will include all that has been nurtured in you, all you believe about yourself, all you have been, and all you will become. Consider that you are not only the DNA your ethnicity would suggest, but that your spirit has imprints with leanings and knowledge of other cultures and traditions and the experiences those imprints draw to you.

It is this spiritual element of ourselves that has given rise to many people identifying as ethnicities, and with cultures, other than those in which they were born. We are spiritually and emotionally complex beings and will always gravitate to those people and communities that fulfill, on some level, our image of ourselves: spoken or unspoken. This gravitational pull is the way we begin to recognize the inner images we carry.

Finding your tribe doesn't eliminate the experience of feeling alone or isolated, as those are a part of your spiritual development. You may align with many tribes in your life and connect with people in all walks of life: this is a community in and of itself. The common denominator to all your connections: your willingness to let go of defining yourself and opening your heart to becoming a witness to your own life.

Magic and Healing

Magic is the link between your sexual energy (life force) and creativity. It is used in traditions all over the world to create innovative, protective, and fertile relationships to all life has to offer. It is governed by the etheric body of energy, which manages your habitual behaviors and manifests the condition of your physical body.

The energy of magic has the power to integrate the spirit through truth, justice, balance, order, compassion, harmony, and reciprocity. These energies are the new foundation from which you will perceive all other dimensions of life. The increased focus shifts your awareness to mindfulness—the experience of self-awareness without judgment.

- **Truth:** practicing magic will always bring truth to the foreground in any situation.
- **Justice:** focusing your energy and intent on another person cannot take away their power; nor can yours be taken.
- **Balance:** there is only one true balance and it is that of the Universe; we will all find our place within it.
- **Order:** practicing magic connects you to a natural progression of energy flow; your intent advises the vibrational frequency of your connection.
- **Compassion:** magic requires you to see all that you are, before you see the nature of others.
- **Harmony:** magic reveals the concise configuration of the intricate design of our spiritual lives.
- **Reciprocity:** the natural ebbs and flows of the Universe are inevitable; magic helps you to define yourself within them.

Being at peace with your history means that you accept everything about you, who you've been and what you've done. There is no room for shame, embarrassment, criticism or judgment. Your history embodies all that is contained in your lower self, unconscious mind, or shadow (all names for this part of ourselves). Your historical judgment of yourself, your actions, or others is no longer relevant, you do not need to experience shame in order to cause self-awareness. Now, you are free to acknowledge all you've done, and what you are drawn to do without mistake; your self-awareness allows you to recognize and appreciate the purpose in all your choices. Most certainly, you will come upon actions taken that need not be repeated, but it is especially in the reflection of those that we solidify the foundation from which to create our lives.

Fascia: The Magical Connection to the Physical Body

Fascia is the incredibly powerful yet, mostly uncelebrated, densely woven sheet of connective tissue beneath your skin that attaches, separates, stabilizes, and encloses the muscles and other internal organs; it is primarily made of collagen. Fascia is your friend and determines many things in the body, including flexibility, strength, cellulite management, and body symmetry (to name a few).

Energetically, your fascia is directly related to your habitual behavior and etheric energy body (or body double); it can influence how you respond to movement on all levels. It will hold you in place or be the impetus to make change. Its quality is impacted by the body's level of water and inflammation. In its natural healthy state, it is smooth and protective to the entire body. When unhealthy, it can be bunchy and uneven: restricting the bodies blood flow to the muscles and other parts of the physique.

If you're feeling stuck in life or lacking flexibility in any way, fascial massage is a great way to support spiritual and emotional movement. Your fascia can harbor old feelings and emotions and be sensitive to the psychic environment in which you find yourself. There's a good chance that if you're feeling at a standstill, so is your fascia.

Working with your fascia once a week (giving yourself a massage at the pressure you can tolerate), beginning with the feet and moving up the physique, will help the blood and energy flow to your body and ultimately to the areas on other energetic levels that are reticent to flow at a healing pace. And just so you know, doing fascial work can sometimes be painful because you are breaking down what has become hard and lumpy just below the skin. Make sure to prepare by doing a short cardio warm up, or even work on your arms and legs in the bath. When you take deep breaths and intuitively tune in to your fascial layer, it will tell you everything you need to know about how to get moving again, and possibly what slowed you down in the first place.

The Magical Use of Breath and Words

Speaking words to, about, or over someone can be one of the most impactful things you can do. It's important to be clear about your intention and the influence it will have. Speaking words over someone creates affirmative or unfavorable karma. Spiritual essence is carried through our breath out into the world, solidifying the intent of our words, causing them to stick where we and others are receptive.

Many cultures focus on the magical use of words and breath as our ability to effect change on the outer world and cultivate control of our inner world. The function of spells, prayers, healing incantations, and affirmations is the same no matter your cultural or spiritual leanings: they use your life-force energy to claim an outcome and connection in all the dimensions of matter and spirit.

When you take deep breaths—completely filling the lungs and using the muscles of the diaphragm—you not only oxygenate the blood bringing energy into the body, but you also release tension and life-force essence as you exhale, naturally bringing your awareness to the center of the body. When you release your breath consciously with intention, you are breathing life into the outer world to effect change. This healing technique is found in many spiritual traditions.

> **Here are six affirmations to get you started in creating your own:**
> - I am love and loved on all levels of my mind, body, and spirit.
> - I am safe to embrace my sexuality without judgment.
> - I am creative beyond my belief: ideas flow naturally, and I effortlessly act upon the ones that bring me joy.
> - Money comes to me from sources known and unknown all the time; I always have more than enough.
> - I am free to be successful and generous on all levels.
> - The Universe is conspiring to give me all the goodness I desire.

Speaking Your Way to Health

We can talk our way to health, not only from the unburdening that comes from expressing all you know and feel, but from literally speaking to each cell in the body. Our physical body is in the same condition as our spirit. If we find our body in a place of *dis-ease*, regardless of the condition, try telling your body: *I'm sorry*, *Forgive me*, *Thank you*, and *I love you*.

Then, speak to the part of your body that is out-of-balance, directly. Tell your heart, liver, kidneys, bones, or blood what you need from them, and what you're willing to do for them to encourage their repair. Speak to them often, asking questions about *what they need from you?* Or, *how they got into the condition you find them in now?* Understand that you are creating a pattern of body awareness that you can relate to other aspects of yourself and your life.

If this idea works for you, take it to the next level and create a 15–30-minute mindful meditation every day: sit with a paper and pen and write out your questions and your body's response to them. If you are experiencing cancer or some other chronic malady, ask it what it needs to tell you? Your body loves to talk to you, if you'll listen.

Illusion of Time and Space: The Hermetic philosophy

Hermeticism is a name given to a variety of ancient spiritual ideas going back to the first century C.E. (Common Era), originating from writings by the master Hermes Trismegistus. They stem from the idea that we as individuals are equipped to address the Divine and our Universe individually; essentially, these laws of the Universe govern us all. They are principals from which we can conceptualize the way our world works and our relationship to it.

Throughout the centuries, and especially the last few decades, these laws have been brought to mainstream philosophy in many ways: from religious ideology to traditional magical practices. It is through these understandings that we can comprehend our accountability to ourselves and our Creator on all levels of our relationship to the outside world.

The Principle of Mentalism: *All things are mental and a part of the One Universal Mind.*

We are all interconnected and a part of Divinity. At a fundamental level the Universe is mental and a part of the infinite, living mind. The material world manifests from our thoughts, and it is through the illusion of separation from the Creator that we can bear witness to ourselves and others, and know we are never alone.

The Principle of Correspondence: *As above, so below; as below, so above. As within, so without; as without, so within.*

Our outer world is a manifestation of our inner world. You can begin to change one by making changes to the other. In relationship we often attract partners that express aspects to our hidden self and inner life.

The Principle of Vibration: *Nothing rests; everything moves. Everything vibrates.*

The world, you, and your world are inherently moving and changing all the time. This means that all things are temporal and that which appears permanent is moving at a pace set forth by you and that you control with your perspective. In relationships, emotions and dynamics aren't permanent, they are consistently reevaluated and chosen again.

The Principle of Polarity: *Everything is dual. Everything has poles. Everything has its pair of opposites. Like and unlike are the same. Opposites are* identical in nature but different in degree—extremes meet. All truths are but half-truths. All paradoxes may be reconciled.

This concept lets us know that everything exists in duality, and to varying degrees. Nothing is absolute; therefore, everything is predicated on your perception of those varying degrees and how you relate to them. Who's to say at what degree hot becomes cold or love becomes hate?

The Principle of Rhythm: *Everything flows, out and in. Everything has its tides. All things rise and fall. The pendulum swing manifests in everything. The measure of the swing to the right is the measure of the swing to the left—rhythm compensates.*

Rhythm allows for the flows of transition to happen incrementally. In relationships, the rhythm of the flow of new information and experiences creates space for both individuals to have expression within the new current, dictated by the coming together of the two individuals.

The Principle of Cause and Effect: *Every cause has its effect; every effect has its cause. Everything happens according to law; chance is but a name for law not recognized. There are many planes of causation, but nothing escapes the law.*

This truth posits that nothing happens without explanation, and the law here is the eventual result that comes from all actions. In a relationship, every thought, word, and deed has an impact on your partner and therefore determines the natural flow and expression of the relationship and its outcome.

The Principle of Gender: *Gender is in everything; everything has its masculine and feminine principles. Gender manifests on all planes.*

Everything expresses itself through nuance and action, especially in relationships. There is what a partner thinks, speaks, and does—all with specific consequences in different spiritual dimensions.

Contemplating these Universal Truths and applying them to your relationships, to yourself and to others, allows for all challenges to be resolved, all love to be returned, and all individuals to be whole just as they are.

Falling in Love with Love

I love love. There is no other way to say it. I love the giddy stomach churning, heart palpitating joy of a loving connection. I even enjoy the heart wrenching struggle of overcoming the inevitable disappointment that comes with it. You know, the cosmic turn of events that require you to champion the fun love, which seems to have briefly disappeared, so you can get it back? Yes, I even love the work that love, at times, requires.

There are many phases to a relationship, but there are only two intertwining phases to love. The first is the initial connecting of the body, mind, heart, and spirit. The second is the succession of choices made continually that contribute to the varying degrees of the living love that two people end up with in their relationship.

Make no mistake about it, love is a lot of work: working to overcome your fears of intimacy, trust, and even a dawning happiness. (Being happy can be a daunting task.) I'd like to take a moment to simplify love.

The Experience of Love

People connect on many levels: mentally, emotionally, physically, and spiritually. You can fall in love with anyone when you connect on any of these levels. The idea of *falling* in love is the experience of being receptive to the connection and allowing it to move you.

However, people falling in love with each other first fall in love with themselves as they see who they are or who they wish to be in their partner. We experience the *falling* feeling of love as each of the following elements open (see below), but when they inevitably close again, as is the way of the Universe, the feelings of love are temporal. We are then left with the opportunity to choose love based on our relationship to each element, individually.

More specifically we connect with another person through our sense of security, power, openheartedness, communication, values, and ideals. We fall in love as we connect on each level. The more we acclimate to the new experience, the newness of it leaves us. So, too, might the love, with only a choice left behind to champion what once was.

The experience of security in a relationship comes when a person feels stronger because of the connection to their partner and the relationship itself. They may feel taken care of or safe, with their most basic needs met. True security, however, is a product of our self-acceptance and acceptance of our partner as they are.

The experience of power in a relationship is present when at least one of the partners has confidence and the other partner benefits, leaving them both feeling powerful for a time. Real power, however, is a product of the partners working together in unison.

The experience of openheartedness in a relationship comes when two hearts connect for any reason: compassion, sympathy, empathy, joy, grief, or love.

The experience of communication happens when there is an easy flow of expression or the support, education, and permission that someone needs to do so.

The experience of shared values with another comes from common knowledge and experiences, whether they be: geographic, cultural, racial, experiential, spiritual, or emotional.

The experience of shared ideals with another comes from either a deeper belief in humanity or the shared recognition in a higher power or, at the very least, a focus on anything outside the self, like family or community.

The Process of Love:

Loving somebody is a series of choices we make daily for the opportunity to experience the original rush of love. As we fall more deeply in love with ourselves, we can cultivate the most powerful tools required for an enduring loving relationship to another: trust, kindness, patience, motivation, inspiration, and joy.

- **Trust** is your ability to know that you can recover from anything.
- **Kindness** is your ability to choose a firm graceful boundary where necessary and forgoing the need to be right all the time.
- **Patience** is the willingness to let things happen in their divine timing rather than the timing that you hope for or expect.
- **Motivation** is the underlying set of beliefs that support a person's reasons for being in a relationship.
- **Inspiration** is the set of cosmic ideals that perpetuate going outside of traditional beliefs in order to keep the loving flow in a relationship.
- **Joy** is the mutual experience of power combined with happiness that creates confidence in a relationship.

Everyone can fall in love, but having and sustaining the opportunity to love someone is a privilege.

The Slayer's Pact: I am Free to Thrive

What does it mean to thrive? It means taking comfort in small things until the big things come. It means feeling grateful for all things, not just some of them. It means having more than enough and sharing what you have. And it means finding peace, patience, grounding, and joy in your successes and recessions—preparing for both.

The most important element of thriving is your understanding of where you are in the cycle. You must be willing to accept and embrace all that prospers you, and to acknowledge and respect what holds you in place until you are free to prosper again. It may seem counter intuitive, but many people unconsciously hold themselves back out of habit or unfamiliarity, and they fear flow in their lives. If you've not cultivated spiritual integrity, creativity, and emotional intelligence—thriving can be quite uncomfortable and detrimental to some. There's a reason why many folks who become millionaires through the Lotto are broke in a few years. Learning the subtle nuances of receiving and having are a skillset to be practiced.

The concept of religion is an example. Any religion is a bountiful set of understandings about life that can help us cultivate a relationship to the highest and best we will become on any level. When we use that religion out of fear or to exclude others, it can only reduce our lives, not prosper them. Whether or not you feel spiritual, you are spiritual, and you are spiritual despite religion.

When you use religion to prove your value, or disprove another's, you focus your energy on a universal untruth, and you cannot prosper continuously until you can sustain your attention on the oneness of all things: that means everyone's prosperity. To be clear, being selfish or fearful will not keep you from being rich, but it will never actually prosper you. For whatever is built on a faulty foundation will eventually fall to be built again.

A slayer finds ways to use all their beliefs to strengthen their connection to the vibration of themselves that is linked to all things. Make efforts to look for the common ground that is inevitable to find: you and those you don't know or understand are both standing on it. When you thrive, you recognize the inherent movement in all things, including your attitudes, beliefs, hopes, and means. Know that when you embrace the successes of others, the Universe promotes you.

Creativity: Your Connection Between Your Higher and Lower Selves

Everything between your higher and lower selves is a part of your creative energy. It is the energy you use to innovate, create, sustain, propel, embellish and promote. However, this creative energy is influenced by the subtle thoughts and feelings of your lower self (unconscious self) and all it contains.

While living in NYC, I was privileged to do a cabaret show with a good friend and profoundly talented partner named Julie. Julie was smart, funny as hell, and deeply empathic. She and I had amazing comic chemistry together and the same brutal sense of humor. We took on parodies about the music industry, misogyny, addiction, and cultural isolation to name a few. Our show was called *The Deadly Medley: Songs by Dead People with the Mangler Sisters* and was as successful as it could have been, as it offended some.

In my young and immature ambition to propel the show to higher heights, I was consistently more and more frustrated when Julie didn't do the things I thought she should to move us forward. I didn't feel she wanted the same things I did because she wasn't working towards them in the same way I was. So, I opted for a very hurtful response to my frustration: I demoted her. I told her if she didn't want to have the same level of success that I did then she should take a lesser role. I would become the headliner; essentially, it would become my show.

Now, all things considered, I didn't really have the right to do that, but as Julie was a little older and a lot wiser, she allowed me to have my way. We reworked the show to be a parody on what an asshole I had been; it was now called *Patty Mangler: On the Road Solo*. For the first time, we added a few additional characters to do walk-ons in the show, including Julie's character, J.J. Mangler.

This left me in a position to rewrite the entire show by myself, and I struggled. It had been weeks since I'd come up with an idea, and the show was coming up in less than seven days. Plus, it was the largest venue we'd ever played. Finally, after seeing Steve Martin talk about what helped him get through a creative block, I decided to take his advice which was to place some bologna in my shoe and walk around with it. I walked the entire East Village on a Saturday night with a quarter pound of cold-cuts in my ladies' official-issue combat boots (they were my standard at the time).

It was the antidote I needed to get my creative flow back—the flow that undoubtably had been generated by Julie and her laser focus. The show went well, it was the largest audience we'd had, but the glaring truth: I wasn't really prepared to go to the next level myself. Something inside of me (I didn't know what at the time) struggled with all the things we made fun of in the show: the sexual attention, the misogyny of male controllers in the industry, the environment of drugs and addiction, and the feeling of being isolated and alone.

Julie and all her brilliance had been the salve for me in those dynamics. *Patty Mangler: On the Road Solo* was the last show we ever did. Looking back, I'm certain I could have moved forward in attaining my epiphany without being so self-centered and hurtful. I did follow my heart, and I learned many valuable things about myself in the process. I dug a little deeper into my spiritual matrix to connect to another layer of the karmic relationships that I related to music, show business, and addiction. I learned an enormous amount about forgiveness, wisdom, and compassion from the dignity Julie portrayed throughout our entire relationship, but especially in the face of my hurtful rejection of her ways. I am grateful she still considers me a friend and has given me the opportunity to rebuild what I tore down.

The path of creativity takes us on a road to the unexpected, where all things can be made even, and our many worlds collide if our hearts are open to it—all we need is a little courage.

"FORGIVE YOURSELF FOR NOT BEING AT PEACE. THE MOMENT YOU COMPLETELY ACCEPT YOUR NON-PEACE, YOUR NON-PEACE IS TRANSMUTED INTO PEACE."[7]

– ECKHART TOLLE

The Art of Saying No

No is a one-word sentence. It's not rude, obstinate or selfish. It claims a boundary that is desired and must be respected—without explanation. Learning to use the word no is an artform that grows as we do. One of the lesser known commandments? Thou shalt not fear the use of no. Learning to say no can be the most loving thing you do for your friends, lovers, and soulmates.

It may seem counter intuitive, but saying no is productive. When you set up a clear structure for people to connect or communicate with you, it creates a space for everyone to feel safe and be comfortable; nothing is worse than feeling like you consented to compromising yourself. But what if you are being threatened or intimidated?

The #MeToo movement addresses the dynamic of receiving consequences within an unequal power structure, when a subordinate is threatened or intimidated into unwanted sexual attention or activity. Sexual manipulation leaves you feeling that you gave your power away, which is why so many have gotten away with it for so long. The entire game for a manipulative abuser is to do just that: get you in a position to give them what they want so they can justify their actions by making you accountable as well. However, at the end of the recovery process from any sexual assault, you are left in the position to deconstruct the order of events and reclaim your power. Here are some things to consider:

It is your body and your life. There is no threat for which the Great Spirit cannot help you overcome, if you will take the first step by saying no and walking away from the situation.

My experience of the music business: almost every male musician, producer, or club owner I worked with made some sort of sexual advance. Saying no, often meant the end of the collaboration. Although I became more comfortable saying no, it grew tiresome and was the reason I let go of the music industry. I met a lot of amazing musicians and was elated at the opportunity to connect with them, and then devastated at their integrity and the burden it placed on me to deal with the constant sexual attention.

What I eventually came to understand about my experience, was that the burden I carried was karmic: an internal spiritual conflict with a music industry and addiction dynamic that was still living in me. All the spiritual partners I encountered had come forward to assist me in exorcising the pattern by creating an opportunity for me to make another response, repeatedly, to the dynamic at work.

Saying no early and often sets a precedent of respect in any power structure.

As a waitress in my twenties, I had a boss who was a predator and eventually arrested for sexual assault. It began for him with making sexual innuendo and remarks to all the girls; it angered and unnerved me to witness it. The first time he made one of his sexual comments to me, standing at the desert case, I was enraged and prepared.

I said, "Don't even think you can speak to me that way because it really pisses me off." And he never did again.

Saying no takes preparation and practice.

Your assertive response in any situation doesn't just happen overnight. By the time I arrived in that situation I had already been sexually assaulted and was deep in my process of rage about it. I was prepared and had thought through what I would say to this restaurant manager when he approached me (because I had witnessed his treatment of others and knew what to expect).

On some level, I already knew about the process of grooming and devious influence a manipulative abuser exerts over their target. If you find it even slightly uncomfortable to be direct in saying no, practice. Sit with a friend and roleplay until you feel confident, playing both sides of the equation. It's important to understand both sides of the dynamic, as it solidifies your power in the choice you make.

Remember: people don't respect others when they don't respect themselves, and they judge others as they are judging themselves.

The only thing that makes a person's behavior personal to you is when you allow it. Consider that the behavior in any dynamic may be set forth by a karmic pattern and look to address it.

Often, people who have big personalities are deemed selfish and disrespectful. They could, however, just be capitalizing on the glitch in someone's inability to be firm in their communication. I am one of those people. One of my most memorable conversations with someone was offering them some chocolate: I asked the friend if she wanted half the bar, stating that I couldn't eat any more.

Her response was, "That's okay, you go ahead. More for you."

I was perplexed. I had just said I couldn't eat anymore. I received it as she wanted some but was uncomfortable taking it.

I responded, "I don't want it. Do you want it?" It took about three go arounds to get her to say directly, "No, I don't want it."

I know it may seem that the onus was on me to recognize she was saying no, but at the time, I didn't. As silly as this exchange was, I remember it to this day because I learned what I needed from others: directness. I didn't want to spend my time figuring out the subtleties of someone's communication. My brain did not comprehend *no* unless it was clearly stated.

I am a self-motivated person who started out early in life working (age 13) and taking care of myself—being assertive and not taking no for an answer from the Universe was a part of the dynamic for me. I learned early to ask for what I wanted, and if I didn't get a *no*, it was a possible *yes*. I would keep on with my pitch until it was shut down. Not knowing that about myself led to much conflict, bad feelings, and disappointments in relationships. Now I'm able to recognize when someone has difficulty in saying no, and I can address it accordingly; everyone has the right to be who they are.

Setting boundaries isn't about power, it is about values and standing up for them.

This is a difficult one when it comes to men, women, and sex—so many confusing dynamics at work in sexual foreplay: emotional desire versus sexual desire, unspoken emotional and spiritual receptivity, difficulty in knowing what you want and being able to communicate it, and most importantly, trust. That is, having enough experience with someone to have cultivated trust. The energy and spirituality of our sexuality can confuse one about their own desire versus their values. A person can want sex but be unwilling to have it. It is paramount for all parties who desire sexual encounters to exhibit enough self-mastery to say no and hear no.

In a karmic relationship, where two people are coming together with deep spiritual patterning, influence, and often an exaggerated sense of familiarity, they must learn to recognize these markers and compensate for them by taking time and being patient in new relationships. If you are willing to set a boundary in your relationship the first time it is necessary, the response you receive helps you discern how to move forward.

The truth is, we are all interconnected and surrounded by people who mirror us in some way, so your ability to set boundaries will be evident in your environment: how clear you are in making the choices you do and being accountable to yourself for them. In addition, your feelings of safety, security, and clarity in the people you attract, or the relational dynamic you consistently come upon, can illustrate any karmic patterns and partners you may be engaging.

A good habit to get in: taking some time at the end of every day to reflect on what happened during the day, such as who you saw, what you spoke about, and thoughts and feelings you had. Doing this allows you to become aware of the spiritual patterns you are unconsciously complicit in and how to change your response and relationship with them, effortlessly saying no, if it is required of you.

The Art of Saying Yes

The art of saying yes is for those of you who are already experts at saying no and use it often. For some, saying yes can be as difficult as saying no; saying yes is about letting yourself receive from the Universe. Many times, consenting to something requires effort or change on our part, which, in our mind, can be prohibitive to the experience we're looking for. We can even say no so often that the offers we're seeking stop coming. However, one affirmative utterance when you are feeling immobile, helps to shift the energy of being stuck and allows for new and exciting adventures to come.

Here is the magnificent upside of saying yes: it pulls you out of the orbit you're in and launches you into a new vibration of positive expression between you, the receiver of your yes, and the Universe. It helps you to become confident in every aspect of yourself by connecting to the faster pace inherent in yes. Of course, it goes without saying, that as you practice the affirmative expression, you'll not say it out of obligation or fear but embrace the joy of consenting to your heart's desires. This lets the wings of yes carry you on into your successful future.

The Art of Apologies

Apologizing is a bridge to reestablish a connection with someone. It can help you move through guilt and shame because it's for the giver and not the receiver. You can't guarantee that the person receiving the apology will want to accept it, but at least they'll have a deeper understanding of how you feel, and you'll be able to be accountable by acknowledging your impact on another—and the self-reflection that brings.

Showing and feeling remorse is different than saying you're sorry. Apologizing isn't necessarily about being sorry: it's a path to understanding what happened, how it made everyone in the situation feel, and a way for behavior to become clearer in everyone's perspective of the situation. You may not be able to take back what you said or did, but making a heartfelt apology brings you one step closer to the respect, compassion, and connection you're seeking with others.

The Art of Prayer

The use of prayer, affirmations, and mindfulness is a way for your focused mental energy to connect your humanity to your divinity. When you speak your prayers, mantras, or affirmations, you send your spiritual essence out into the world with commitment and intention to effect change. That essence gains momentum as it is nurtured in all the spiritual dimensions to which it travels. People often consider praying when the purpose for the prayer is clear and they're looking for a desired result. In my experience, prayer can influence all aspects of life—those that we witness and call a sign of the Creator's love or mercy, and those whose impact we may never see directly.

All prayer, affirmations, and mindfulness offer the opportunity to heal. When we pray for others, the healing vibration begins its work with us. Prayer is a form of internal conversation we have with all the aspects of ourselves. It's like a spiritual council meeting where everyone involved shows up to reconcile, innovate, and expand you, on every level. Mindful self-awareness becomes engaged in the process. You begin to address directly every thought you have and why. Being able to ask yourself *Why are you saying this?* creates the beginning of a discussion with you and your higher or lower selves. You'll be surprised how easy it is to have an entire conversation with yourself.

Mental and Emotional Healing: Often, when we carry guilt, shame, anger, or humiliation about experiences we've had, we must find a path to forgiveness. All our thoughts are messages to us on some level. Negative thoughts pierce our consciousness to ensure the higher-minded message gets through. Don't be afraid of them, master them. Our negative thoughts are generated to help us become self-aware, mirror our unconscious patterns, and strengthen our integrity. They are not there to hurt us or diminish us in any way.

Inevitably, we will all need to find peace in the routes we and others choose for ourselves. We must embrace their teachings, recognizing that our prayer, affirmations, and mindfulness exist to help cultivate a conscious awareness of our relationship to our connection to the Divine. This constant communication raises the vibration to our expectations and creates opportunities to grieve and release what no longer serves us. When we pray for others, we help them on all the levels they are energetically open to, strengthening their integrity for the path they are on.

Many years ago, a client brought her 16-year-old grandson to me for a session. She was fearful that he would meet with an early demise, and rightfully so. He was in a gang and spent almost all his time running the streets.

Sitting with him was an amazing experience. He generated such power in his presence. I spoke honestly to him, about details I don't remember, but within those few minutes spent—his destiny was clear. He had a *live by the sword, die by the sword* philosophy, and nothing would move him from it. He saw himself as indestructible, and I could see he was not. In fact, I felt that moving in the direction he was going, there was not much time left.

Being an empath, I can usually connect with everyone, but with this young man, I could not. I couldn't persuade him to change his path in exchange for a longer life, and I knew it. The impenetrable wall I was up against in him, I could only express through the tears I cried all the way home—I've never forgotten. I think this is a dilemma we all face—accepting the purpose and value in another's path. When you pray for others, you will first be healed of your desire to change what their Divinity requires of them—then you will lend additional focus and light in support of their process.

Spiritual Healing: Prayers, affirmations, and mindfulness help one focus and discern between themselves and their soul generated imprints—or otherworldly entities. If an entity such as a guide, extraterrestrial, or angelic being is charged with supporting you on all levels of your process in life, they will always respect your boundaries and offer loving, gentle support and consolation. Other lower-vibrational entities will connect with you on a frequency for which the both of you must heal, even demons and other malevolent spirits—there is always a common ground. All these entities will communicate with you through your thoughts, feelings, and sometimes your surroundings.

And as a reminder: if you are having thoughts of hurting yourself or someone else, respond back directly with, *No, I won't*. Repeat it until the voice subsides. Sometimes these types of thoughts are generated by negative beings who seek to feed on your anguish and create additional chaos. Do not let them. You hold all the power. Under no circumstance can hurting yourself or someone else bring you peace, retribution, or make pain go away.

Finally, don't ignore any being. What you resist persists. Address them with firmness and compassion, find out why they are connecting to you, and take authority over them, or receive the loving help they are there to offer. If you need angelic or ascended master help, ask for it. You can call on St. Micheal, Quan Yin, Buddha, Jesus, Mother Mary, Sanat Kumara, St. Germain, and Kuthumi, to mention a few.

Prayers/Affirmations

- I am the master of my mind on all levels. No one can speak for me or through me.
- I choose goodness. I see goodness. I am goodness.
- Good things come to me from sources known and unknown, on all levels, all the time. I am grateful.
- I am at peace with myself and others as we are, and I am free to say no to anything I choose.

The Lord's Prayer is always helpful.

> Our Father, who art in heaven, hallowed be thy name. Thy kingdom come. Thy will be done, on earth as it is in heaven. Give us this day our daily bread, and forgive us our debts, as we forgive our debtors. Lead us not into temptation, but deliver us from evil. For thine is the kingdom, the power, and the glory for ever. Amen

Prayerful Art

Give yourself permission and opportunity to draw, paint, garden, or perform any other mindless or mindful craft. We all need to doodle, fantasize, and wander our way to freedom without expectation of a productive result. Being unproductive or producing without expectation can be the most valuable time you give yourself and can open your spiritual channels through which higher-minded wisdom can flow to and through you.

In these experiences, allow yourself to open your heart to whatever feeling is present, and let it move through you, using the art or craft you've chosen to express it. As we spoke about earlier in this chapter, we all access the creative.

The Spiritual Matrix of Multiple Dimensions

The best description I've ever received explaining the spirit world was this: a great map of infinite horizontal lines and infinite vertical lines crossing one another; every intersection a spiritual dimension of essence, thought, or emotion of the individual soul that expands into the matrix of the One Mind. It finally put everything into perspective. Every thought, feeling, dream, or uttered word creates its own spiritual dimension of energy to be nurtured and expanded, or used and transformed into a new facet of one's life. Each of us is born into this plane with our own cosmic map with plot points that connect with all others, somewhere in the great beyond.

I had just moved to Los Angeles and was battling a fierce depression. Because of this, I rarely left the house. One Saturday morning, spirit awakened me with the notion of going to my favorite Chinese restaurant—for breakfast. It was a small family owned place on Broadway and 7th Street, in Santa Monica; they opened at 8 a.m. I arrived as they were opening the doors. The place looked like an American diner with red vinyl seating, and it had a traditional Buddhist altar, which was dressed first thing in the morning: incense burned before the customers arrived. The woman who owned the place always made me feel at home, which soothed me and my depression.

Existence was a ridiculous struggle at the time; I was living out of my truck on the couches of friends, and at this point, a job had been evading me for months; somehow, this day felt different: prosperous. I paid the check with my last ten dollars and left with three bucks to spare, just as the bookstore down the way was opening. I stopped to browse the table of discounted books when a book cover with a big beautiful flame got my attention. It was only two dollars, so I bought it and headed back to my truck. That book changed my life, giving me the words to express the spiritual mysteries in ways that transformed my outlook and chronic depression. The book—long since given away and title forgotten but whose cover and contents are imprinted on my brain—ignited a fire from a barely burning flame.

Healing the Rift of Illusion

The grand illusion is that we are separate from one another and the Creator. Our broken heart is the cause of our suffering, and death is real. Each of these illusions causes a rift in our understanding on every level. This gap in our recognition of the infinite spiritual universe causes confusion, pain, hatred, and strife. But worst of all, it causes the most common illusion: we can get or be *stuck*, or our lives are static. The truth is, energy is always moving.

The Illusion of Separation: What would it mean to you and how would you see the many facets of your life if you knew there was no separation between you and your Creator? How would you handle your money, relationships, time, and emotions? Looking at your life from the perspective of being empowered changes everything. Being empowered means that there is a way to resolve any challenge. It doesn't mean that you can control others, but that you can either work through the issue with some form of cooperation or you can circumvent it altogether. Going around a problem doesn't mean avoiding it. When you own your connection to the Divine, you have the courage to face what ails you and let the wisest part of yourself respond.

> Affirmation: I am at peace, I am powerful, and I am at one with my Universe.

The Illusion of Suffering: People do a lot of things to avoid pain. What would you do if you knew that every time you cried, you got healthier on every level? When we experience any type of pain, it eventually leads us to express that suffering through our heart. If we're open to the process, the emotion builds until it pushes the heart chakra to expand, allowing the emotion to flood through. This is what is happening energetically and emotionally when we experience a *broken* heart. This process helps every part of our experience. Endorphins are released helping us to feel better, mentally clear, and to remove energy blocks from the physical body: creating opportunity to regain balance.

> Affirmation: I exercise my strength and compassion every time I cry; it keeps me safe and open to all the good things in life.

The Illusion of Death: When we are rooted in the physical world our focus would imply that death is real. What would it mean to you to know that we live on in consciousness? How would you address death and dying then? More importantly, how would you look at living? Our emotions are the gateways to these other dimensions of spiritual life. When the physical body dies, the consciousness, soul, or spirit lives on—sometimes in the emotional dimensions that we can experience and communicate through. Eventually, all souls will ascend to the Oversoul, only to prepare for reincarnation here in this earthly plane, or another plane of existence. Dying is an emotional transition we make to understand the spiritual dimensions.

> Affirmation: I have nothing to fear in death and embrace my life fully.

Spiritual Patterns and Your Soul

Everything in the Universe has a frequency, rhythm, and pattern. It's how our intuition recognizes the energy with which we resonate, the energy of our experiences, and the energy of the things we long for; they all have a signature that our unconscious mind seeks. When we find one of those things on our psychic radar, our response can be emotional discomfort, frustration, or even grief—depending on our state of readiness to receive the object of our attraction.

It is through this inner vision that we transcend the illusion of disability, mobility, and handicap. I'm not sure if it is the human use of fear for survival over the millennia that has left people associating what is considered *normal,* the standard to achieve. Unfortunately, anything not falling into the norm has been made out to be strange, weird, or inappropriate—leaving any of us unaverage folk to feel outnumbered or left out. But if you're one of the unaverage out there, you know the others are just hiding the things that make them truly distinctive. It is time to get back to recognizing that when one skill is not possessed, another unique and special one takes its place—making each of us a powerful and valuable part of our family and community.

In my family, I've been the butt of many jokes and sarcasm over the years but haven't minded. As I understood, it was the way they could communicate their subconscious recognition of the things that made me different—and it was always funny. My grandmother telling my mom one time that, "They really take to her..." (She was speaking of an African American service man who'd been fixing an appliance at her apartment and noticed my picture and said I was pretty. Racism, not funny; the fact that grandma made a connection to something outside her frame of reference, funny.) My Uncle Jim one time exclaiming, "Who *are* you?!" He was referring to the difference in my hands from the family's and implying I was left by aliens on mom's doorstep, to which we all laughed uproariously.

I was never offended by such remarks nor were they delivered with a mean spirit; they brought me comfort and connection to my family. As I grew, I learned that all of us, in our own way, at some point, feel like an outsider. In times of turmoil or great change, if we've lost a limb or a skill, it is this illusion of separation that drives our focus away from the abilities we already possess to the loss at hand. Of course, denial, anger, and grief can always be a part of the process of transition; however, self-pity is the unconscious focus on the illusion of being separate.

As we spoke of in earlier chapters, the presence of self-pity indicates something inside you needing your attention and care. Giving yourself that care will help transcend any unnecessary karmic patterns, creating space to understand the condition or shift in condition, and its karmic purpose. Anytime you move towards understanding your purpose, you connect to the vibration of energy that will support your efforts and offer a flow of ease to everything on your path.

Transforming Fear on All Levels

Many of us fear death or any other cycle completion because we fear the unknown of what comes next—the new beginning. We also fear the sign of a needed transition: pain. We stay in unfortunate relationship dynamics too long. We don't make efforts to connect with others, and we don't try new things or quit them before we've achieved success. All because we fear death: the illusion of a permanent ending.

The soul seeks to create balance and understand the impact of its force through creativity. Ultimately, it's not about the circumstances we have in life but the choices we make and the character we show in response to them. Spiritually speaking, living in any condition has immense value.

I hear many people say things like *this is my last life on the karmic wheel*, or *I'm an old soul or a new soul, therefore...*, whichever definition serves their need in the conversation or in life. In my experience and understanding, the reality is we are all old souls. This is a unique time on the planet, and everyone here currently carries a deep spiritual wisdom, even the people we deem as ignorant, selfish, or immature. This is the end of three great cycles for which we must all participate and bring our light. Choose knowledge and understanding. Choose inclusion instead of exclusion and embrace your own divine accountability.

> "...WE SEEM TO DEAL WITH REALLY DEVASTATING INFORMATION IN ONE OF TWO POSSIBLE WAYS: EITHER WE MINIMIZE IT TO THE POINT OF INSIGNIFICANCE OR WE IGNORE IT ALTOGETHER. THE PHENOMENON IS CALLED "NORMALCY-BIAS" AND IT TENDS TO BE STRONGEST AMONG PEOPLE WHO HAVE NEVER BEFORE ENCOUNTERED THE EXTREMES FACING THEM."[8]
>
> – GREGG BRADEN

How would you approach your life if you knew there would always be an opportunity to start over? Consider how you would advance towards your goals if the following are true:

- **It's all about what you do next.** Consider, regardless of your circumstances right now, your patterns do not obligate you to continue them if they no longer serve you.

- **You chose the life you're living.** Right now, exactly the life you have is the life you want. What are you grateful for?

- **No one is judging you; they are judging themselves.** What others do and feel is not about you. It is about them. If you connect to it, consider that you may feel similar or resonate with some other aspect of the energy or behavior.

- **You need spiritual awareness, not religion.** Organized religion is not a necessity to cultivate your self-awareness and relationship to Divinity. You are welcome to follow any path you desire as the ritual and personal path to kinship with the Creator. Consider those paths that are inclusive of all, without condition, as a true opportunity to challenge and build your faith as God, Yahweh, Allah, Brahman, and Wakan Tanka intended.

- **You can change your relationship to anything.** People spend a lot of time making efforts to stop relationships or end uncomfortable feeling dynamics in their lives, but it has always been my experience that the more you resist something the more valuable the information will be to you if you will face it and stay the course. How does your approach change if, instead of getting rid of something, you accept it as it is and modify your relationship to it?

- **Your challenges are your opportunities to show off your greatness.** Sometimes, our true greatness does not come from those things we think we should be, or want to be good at, but rather the things we naturally do with ease. Paying attention to what naturally comes easy and finding more opportunities to do that thing will surely lead to your success. It was my twelve years of working as a server in many restaurants that cultivated my solid people skills and compassion. (I was not a great waitress.)

- **People do the best they can with what they have.** It's okay to accept others as they are, showing compassion for their use of the skills they have. The real skill comes in not letting what they do, change what you do. Always do your best and be as honest and kind as you can.

- **What others do is not about you, it is for you.** Whatever response you get or behavior you witness from others is an opportunity to transition your habit of a limiting or fearful response. The more we allow flow and relaxation into our bodies, we open to faster frequencies of emotion that allow for more compassionate and innovative responses to the outside world, fostering support for everyone.

- **You are a success at everything you do; your result is your success.** I'm not a fan of the illusion of failure, or that we can veer off our path. I believe that every road we find ourselves on is where we should be, even if we lack the understanding of why and what will come of it. Being bad at one thing always reveals being good at something else.

- **Your open heart protects you.** When we refer to an open heart, we are talking about recognizing others with compassion, acceptance, and truth. When we are in danger physically, mentally, emotionally, or spiritually, the relaxation that comes from openly embracing what's happening allows for the most innovative response to the situation at hand. It doesn't override fear but allows for the fear to create clarity.

- **What matters is this moment right now.** When we are unreconciled with any part of our past or current life events and energy patterns—they are, in fact, our now. Be willing to drill down on what you're feeling; let it take you on a mental journey back in time and space to its origins. Finding forgiveness in that place begins the process of healing and integration of all that has happened in between, fusing the best of the two worlds together as one.

Try this exercise:

Take a few moments to think of a personal challenge happening in your life right now. Write it out on a piece of paper, and then contemplate how your perception or approach would change by applying these Universal Truths.

Cutting Spiritual Cords

A spiritual cord is an energy connection that we've established with someone. We can initiate this line of energy across time and space through our emotions and thoughts, or they can be set up through our physical-world relationships (platonic and sexual). We don't always cord into everyone we meet, but when we do, we can think of them continuously and feel their feelings. These energy cords become uncomfortable as our relationship to the person changes.

People come to me all the time wishing to remove these energy cords, and while we can shift the energy, it is the state of their personal condition and relationship to the person in question that determines how they move forward. It's a common misunderstanding that removing the spiritual cord ends the relationship, but that is not necessarily so; it can pave the way for each individual to change the karmic pattern that brought them together in the first place.

If you feel you have spiritual cords to people you no longer associate with or are just curious about who's corded into you, do the following.

Try this exercise:

Sit quietly with a pen and paper; take several deep breaths and focus on being showered with a bright white light coming from above you. Ask yourself who has a spiritual cord connected to you. Write down anyone who comes to mind, without judgment. You can do the exercise with your eyes open or shut, whichever helps you to focus. Once you've established a list of names, write on the paper: Ho'oponopono. I receive my energy back with love, and I send yours back to you with gratitude. Then, burn the paper in a fireplace or outside in a burning-pot or firepit.

The goal of this exercise is for you to have a deeper understanding of those with whom you share your energy and to release emotional and energetic bonds that are overwhelming or inappropriate. It is possible that spiritual cords with our loved ones will be reestablished if there is purpose for them. Releasing a spiritual cord does not make the relationship change or go away, it merely helps you change the way you relate to it.

Releasing the Past: St. Vincent's Guest House, New Orleans

On one of my many work trips to Louisiana, the night I arrived in New Orleans, my friend Faith and I stopped for a cup of coffee. Gazing out across Magazine Street from the coffeeshop, I began to feel sick—like someone punched me in the gut. The building standing there got my attention and wouldn't seem to let it go.

"Nettie Biddle?" I asked Faith. "Do you know someone named Nettie Biddle?"

"No," she responded. "Who's Nettie Biddle?"

"I'm not sure, but I think she lived in that building across the street. Her name was Kinetta Biddle: Nettie for short. I am really not feeling well."

"Are you okay?" Faith asked.

"I am feeling really nauseous and cold. My head hurts, and my eyes hurt like they're jaundiced."

This wasn't the first time Faith and I had been together when I'd experienced extreme empathy from a ghost in the area. Faith got out her phone and did an internet search for the symptoms I was experiencing.

"Is one of your symptoms jaundice?" She asked.

"Yes." I replied.

"It says those are symptoms of yellow fever." Faith blurted.

And just as quickly as she said it, my experience of those symptoms went away.

We asked our coffee server about the ominous looking building across the street. He told us it was called St. Vincent's Guest House, but it used to be an orphanage where over fifty children died during a yellow fever outbreak. Faith and I looked at each other, both our jaws dropping.

"Oh yeah, we're going there next." We laughed and hurriedly finished our coffee.

As we walked through the large, black, iron-spiked entrance gate, I could feel the density of the energy hitting my face. We walked up the stairs and were greeted by a woman in her sixties, the manager of what was now a single-room-occupancy hotel. She had a magnificent weathered face, with deep creases at the brow, and a two-pack-a-day rasp in her voice.

She laughed like Santa Claus. "How are you girls doing tonight?"

"Great! How about you?" I responded. "I just got in from out of town, and this building really caught my eye. What is it?"

"Well it used to be St. Vincent's Infant Asylum, built in 1862, but it's been St. Vincent's Guesthouse since the '90s," she said.

"Would you mind if we looked around?"

"Well, we're not supposed to, but you girls look okay." Once more, she gave us that big laugh. "Would you like to see a room? I can show you a room." She retorted.

"Yeah! Let's go," Faith responded.

The woman gave us a key to a room, and we were off. The place was a unique jumbled mess of history and unfortunate renovations. It housed all types—who happened to be congregating in the common area as we passed through. A seventy-five-year-old man sitting with a twenty-three-year-old punk-rock artist stopped us for a chat—just before a fight broke out between two drunken forty-something men across the courtyard.

Faith and I continued, visiting as many rooms as were available to us. Nettie Biddle was a nurse here. She took care of the children, and I think she is still taking care of the ones who died during the epidemic. Faith disappeared into a room at the top of the stairs while I sat for a moment to pray for Nettie and the children, clearing the imprint of their energy, completely freeing them to move from this place. Nettie thanked me, and they were gone.

Next thing I know, Faith was tapping my shoulder.

"Are you ready to go?" She asked.

'I think I am." I replied.

And on we went to check-in to the haunted Le Pavillon Hotel. We didn't want to miss the peanut butter and jelly sandwiches and hot chocolate they served from 10 p.m. to midnight. We arrived just in time to grab a sandwich and sit in the lobby to process all that had happened in the short journey from the Louis Armstrong International Airport to the Pavillon. We had traversed almost two centuries in less than three hours, and we were a little tuckered.

As we sat in the beautiful marble-floored lobby, complete with gold-leaf trim and marble columns—sipping hot chocolate—Faith asked, "Do you think that people who suffer or who die a horrible death are receiving retribution for bad things they've done in other lives?"

"Well, I think everything is an opportunity for spiritual and emotional growth." Shaking my head, I added, "There's no retribution for past activity, just the effects of the actions someone has taken and the, sometimes, very long process of reconciling them. I think of it this way: for me personally, the life I am living today is a product of having been abused, enslaved, and addicted in multiple lifetimes. Freedom, on all levels, is now very important to me.

"I have slayed the demons that are my duty to slay, and I no longer anesthetize myself. I participate in society, but I keep enough distance not to become a product of it, by setting firm boundaries for those around me. I have learned compassion for all people as a by-product of my spiritual heritage; because I've been murdered and killed others in previous lifetimes, I refuse to allow violence in my heart and environment. All of this is my karma."

Ultimately, we transform our relationship to everything we fear, until we no longer fear it. Then we are charged with the task of reclaiming every ghost, discordant experience or action, vile word, or resistance to death we've left in some spiritual dimension within the Akashic matrix. Once our accounts are even, we continue on...

> If You Can't Commit to Something Fully, Leave it for Another Time.

What is Spiritual Commitment

Staying present in the moment is another way to say commitment. Taking all your passion, focus, and force to use in the moment for what you're engaged in, creates efficiency and allows for success. We gain confidence from our daily experiences—from everything we complete. You know what doesn't matter at all? How big the goal is. Our spiritual and emotional memory retains what we've accomplished and our relationship to it, supporting our self-esteem and confidence.

Let's say you want to start a meditation practice. Start small, three minutes a day (or every other day, or once a month...). What is valuable is that you do what you say you will. Every time you complete a task your thoughts and actions become more powerful and begin to fill with confidence. The bonus is the meditation—every time you sit quietly for three minutes your mind, body, and spirit align. The more often all the levels of your energy are in alignment, the more at ease, confident, and joyful you feel. The perfect setup for approaching anything in life with fervor.

The next time you set a goal, be critically honest with yourself. Remember, you can set a new goal every minute of every day, but you can't get back all that time you spent feeling bad about yourself for not completing a mission because it was too big for your present set of circumstances. The alchemy of a miracle is many small, often hidden, successes one doesn't notice until the miracle is upon you.

"Nunya adidoe, asi metu ne o"
Knowledge is a baobab tree. No one person can embrace it all alone.[9]

— Ewe proverb

Faith Leads to Divinity

When conceptualizing the Divine: a view of the omnipotent, all knowing, all-inclusive oneness of all things is at least profound and at most unattainable by our humanity. Faith is the courier of our awareness: beginning with ourselves on all levels; then, regarding the awareness of others; and next, the awareness of our environment; and finally, the awareness of the grand matrix of spiritual dimensions that eventually vibrate at a frequency far beyond our human ability to truly conceptualize its entirety, let alone receive it. So, when we consider and contemplate the Creator, what we're really doing is cultivating our blossoming faith.

Our ability to trust the world we live in comes from knowing as much as possible about it. The more we know what to expect or feel prepared for the unexpected, our confidence can drive our decisions. Faith is what fills the gap between what we know and what we don't; our faith is connected to our gut feelings, intuition, and psychic channels. Faith is not walking blindly into what we don't know, it is opening ourselves to the spiritual channels of information at our disposal and trusting ourselves to receive and interpret that information.

My friend Rachael told me the story of her great grandmother and her daughter, both born with what were considered harbingers of their psychic connection to the spirit world. Her great grandmother was born in the late 1800s, when people held enormous fear of those who had spiritual gifts; they were considered witches, heretics, and demonically possessed. Great grandmother was born with a layer of skin covering her entire face, called a veil or cowl. Females born with this were often murdered in infancy because the public fear of sorcery was so strong. Luckily, her life was spared, and within months of the birth, the veil dropped off.

Rachael's daughter was born with something called an angel's kiss or a stork bite: a light red birthmark resembling angel wings in the center of her forehead, over her third eye chakra. It was an insignia also known to be a sign of great spiritual strength. Both women are deeply in tune with the cosmos and have had to embrace and cultivate faith in their gifts and trust for their interpretation of the wisdom they receive, in spite of the judgment of others around them.

The Magic of Radical Acceptance

No matter who you are, you must embrace the radical acceptance of your everyday life. This means to love the life you have right now. Not the one you hope to have at some other time and space, but exactly as it is in this moment. When you can be rooted with love in the life you are living, you are empowered to make choices that cause movement and action forward.

Radical acceptance doesn't mean you are content, or even happy, those are emotional lenses through which we choose to see our lives. Embracing life as it is now empowers you to pick and choose what is or isn't working, creating a way forward on the most effortless path.

Loving the Life and Love You Have Right Now

They say that you always have the life you want; however, this truth means something different for everyone. If you happen to be someone who continually attracts what you don't want—it's time to take a deeper look.

Real attraction comes from three things: trust, connection, and desire. But first, in order to address those elements, we need to look at what is our most valued currency in life. Is it safety and financial security, affection and emotional connection, or intelligence and humor? Take a moment and put these in your order of most importance.

You have the life you want because of the currency you choose and your true desire. There are a thousand combinations. I worked with someone once whose true currency was affection and emotional connection, but the fear she carried about being poor was stronger. She attracted a very wealthy man who did all the right things in the courtship process, most of them financial. But as she invested deeper into the relationship because of the apparent financial stability, she found out the person wasn't capable of real emotional intimacy and connection. Their sexual relationship wasn't sustainable, nor the relationship.

When it turns out that you have the love and life you *like*, it's because your currency and desire match, and you're able to allow yourself to accept and balance your needs with your desires. That leads us to the three golden nuggets of attraction.

Trust: Trust is when, at a core level, you trust your inner source—yourself. Sexual freedom and complete attraction happen when you aren't looking for things or people to fulfill your needs. Seeking a partner or job based on what you need, supports an inner theory that you can't fulfill your own requirements. Therefore, when disappointment comes—and it will—your attraction for your job or partner will be stifled for a time until you adjust your perspective. Trust also means trusting your potential sexual partner to be the kind of sexual partner that makes you feel comfortable. Consider the partners you're attracting are exactly what you feel comfortable with, and then take an inventory. For example: if you're attracting partners that are insensitive and harsh, consider, on some level, *that* is what makes you comfortable and begin to look at deeper spiritual or emotional patterning as to why.

Connection: Connection happens when you are open to another person energetically or emotionally and are able to allow the vulnerability that is required for an exchange. Vulnerability here means receptivity. You can be receptive to your partner's energy, emotion, or needs. It's possible to be open to another's energy or emotion unconsciously: I met a man and our initial attraction was off the charts. I couldn't sleep for days. The feelings I had weren't rational—they were subliminal. Keep in mind that I wasn't dating this man; we were acquaintances, and the connection we shared was in part because of my empathy towards him.

Desire: Desire is twofold. There is the hormonal desire generated by your procreative instincts. Most women have increased desire when they ovulate, and most men can sense a woman's ovulation cycle. I've not noticed it being any different for same sex partners. As for most people, awareness of the hormonal cycles is subliminal, and people often respond to how a person is responding to them, if they are open. The second element of desire is connection through resonance. When you witness, overtly or subliminally, a person who represents what you think you need, want, or with whom you align. Who out there has been attracted to the funny one? Only to find out that their humor is anchored in some sort of trauma that possibly makes a relationship unsustainable, as it's easy to use humor to mask deeper painful feelings. These are the two questions to ask yourself: What do you think you want, and what state or condition are you in? The answers will show you what you are attracting.

Make no mistake about it, we are all in a state of flux when it comes to trust, connection, and desire. They are core spiritual, emotional, and physical life lessons that everyone experiences. Know that they are elements to cultivate within yourself; there is no pass-fail here. You can't break them or do them wrong. You must always stay in the quiet ebb and flow of your awareness and command of them. Be patient with yourself and look at the subtle information that the Creator gives you about yourself through whom you attract.

Doing Spiritual Work

At the end of every spiritual cycle, we will experience a period of letting go of old dynamics and acclimating to new patterns that are evolving. The process requires apathy to create balance. Apathy is a form of detachment, and the degree and time it remains in one's life depends on the length and intensity of the life cycle. While engaging in this apathetic phase, sometimes people wake up and see all they've valued as nothing more than illusions. Suddenly, life becomes meaningless. In this period we release the definitions we place on things so that we may expand or change their value. This period can range from weeks to years. We choose happiness and the meaning we give life by recognizing our most powerful tool: flow.

People who are discovering the spiritual realms and their personal power are looking to take control in some way. Finding a way to do that is paramount. The idea of a door closing and another opening is effective here. For example, accept where you are and take a vacation from the meaning you've given things. Embrace the meaninglessness; it's freeing. It's a Universal Truth that a void in our thinking can't last. It eventually gets filled with new ideas.

When someone decides to do spiritual work, the goal of a session is to create healing and look at current spiritual factors of the circumstances causing conflict. For healing, we must address the current details and the spiritual patterns that promote them.

How Personal Transformation Changes Your Relationships

Under all circumstances, wanting to be a better person is admirable. It's something we all strive for, but what happens to your relationships when you make those long sought-after changes? Personal transformation and our partnerships can be a challenge to navigate as you better understand what drives you. The explanation of why you connect the way you do with your partner will make sense, even if it's not always pleasurable.

Enlightenment is a process of *lightening* up. Meaning your burden, confusion, and selfishness are giving way to joy, clarity, and presence. Sometimes we enter relationships that are based on the burdens we carry and the very pattern we are looking to release ourselves from. The partnerships and choices that are centered around your deepest wounds can disappear as quickly as the process of healing those wounds appear.

Burden to Joy: A burden is the weight of your ungrieved spirit seeking acknowledgement and transformation. The more you compassionately embrace its presence, it can transform into grief. This process creates a lightness unlike any other experience you will have.

A person new to the process of spiritual work often perceives others in their life with repulsion or judgment. As their sensitivities open, they witness their movement and lightness in reference to perceived negativity or misery of others. Phrases like higher or lower vibration, positive or negative attitude, or old or new soul are all common in this phase of development. What is true: a relationship created in this place is all about inner conflict and outer struggle.

Confusion to Clarity: It is through our emotions that we decipher and relate to our world. Confusion is the next logical phase of lightening up. Confusion means that you are fluctuating between dominance and submission to your higher self. This is often played out in your partnerships with others. At times, you perceive or desire the illusion of control, and in different situations, you give over to their dominance.

Partnership to Independence: This phase of lightening up helps you consciously recognize how you see your world through the way you see yourself. Victimization is a popular sentiment in this process, so a relationship here can often be volatile and steeped in conflict. Sometimes, it's over as quickly as it starts. The true spiritual purpose of these relationships is to promote the release of ungrieved pain on every level. On the upside, they are an efficient way of healing.

Selfishness to Presence: Self-awareness is not a gift; it is earned over lifetimes with hard won battles of self-mastery. The process of becoming present means recognizing that your anger is a tool you use falsely: to be present in the moment when you are not. The more you don't react and become truly present to what is happening, the easier you will see whatever you may need in the moment and readily have access to it. Following is something to contemplate.

> **In a Relationship:** Peacefulness to a victim is boring.
> - If that phrase made you angry: you are contending with your burdens but will soon experience a powerful transformation.
> - If that phrase only slightly irritated you or caused you sadness. You are squarely in your confusion here, and your goal is to surrender to the current emotional movement. Don't try to understand right now, just feel.
> - If you giggled a little at this phrase *because you know that's right*. You have surrendered to being at peace with your past and feel anchored in your present.
>
> No matter which response you have, you will attract partners that mirror the same thing back to you.

We are all travelers through the phases of enlightenment at any given time and in relationship to different circumstances. A truly enlightened person knows that it is not the absence of burden that gives us wisdom: it is the joy with which we pummel each one, that does.

How to Get Inspired

Well, as my mother always said, *If you're bored, you're boring*. As a child, learning to self-soothe and access deeper levels of knowledge can be a challenge, but as an adult it can be painful. The doldrums aren't around all the time and often arrive as a marker of the end of a cycle. While the following information will be helpful, it's important to be clear that using feelings of apathy as an excuse for unproductive choices only attempts to cover the real problems that ail you. Outgrowing people, places, or things is a part of life and is cultivated over time through many small choices you make every day. Ultimately, your lack of self-awareness won't be enough justification for people in your life to overlook your actions, or lack thereof. Nor should it be for you. The decision to change a relationship or situation should be deliberate and celebrated.

Bored with Yourself?

If you recognize you are bored with yourself, you have quadrupled the possibilities of getting interesting. Love is not something you fall in or out of, like life; it is something you choose. The way we love is based on how we relate to our Creator. If we are open and believe there is enough for everyone, it changes how freely we can give and receive love to and from others and how freely we engage in life; it is this flow of energy that keeps us connected and open to new opportunities.

> **Do these things and see what shakes loose:**
> - In your mind, go back in time and write down the top three things you witnessed about love and life in your first 20 years. Now, decide what dynamics you want to continue on into the future, and which should go. Cross out or circle them.
> - List three hobbies you've always wanted to become involved in. Choose one and take the first step.
> - List three things that you could do for someone else in need, either directly or anonymously. Choose one and do it. It's my experience that when you're honest and kind with yourself, and compassionate towards others, your perspective in life changes.

Bored with Your Partner?

One of the most common reasons people turn away from each other is unfulfilled expectations. Expectations of what a good partner should be or do, how the relationship is negotiated, or what it looks like when someone really loves you. It's always best (as you take your partners inventory) to spend time looking at why you react the way you do to your partner. Spiritually speaking, it is the love we give that creates the love response from the universe, not the love we receive.

> **Try this:**
> - Write down the top three things that frustrate you about your partner and take a moment to sit in contemplation of each thing.
> - Next, sit and close your eyes. Focus on your partner and how they feel.
> - Now, think of one of the items on your list and experience their feelings about it. Why do they do it? How does that affect your perspective?

Until there can be common ground and understanding there won't ever be harmony. Remember, you are the only person you control, and you have full permission to make as many changes as you want.

Bored with Sex?

Sexual boredom can be connected to laziness but is usually a sign of some other emotional or physical transition happening in the mind, body or spirit. This is connected to your emotional union as a couple. Get all the connecting that's at play here?

> **Make a new connection with your partner:**
> - First, get rid of any resentments you may be harboring for your partner. Sit with them, write out all your resentments on a piece of paper, as plainly as possible, and then write at the bottom of the page, *I'm sorry*, *I forgive you*, *thank you*, and *I love you*.
> - Don't share them now. You're welcome to share what you've written at another time but hold off in this moment. Remember, forgiving someone doesn't mean that what they did or didn't do was okay, it means that you are willing to let go of your suffering about it.
> - Now, sit back to back on a blanket on the floor with one another and focus on your breathing, then focus on theirs—recognizing the rhythm of breath that you have together. It is completely appropriate to get handsy with each other at this point. Of course, we all know that this isn't the complete answer to all the profound stressors of our lives, but it's a great start. Also, consider that when connection happens, so may tears. All is good.

Bored with Your Daily Life?

If you're tired of the same monotonous schedule, the same tired arguments, or are just plain tired, you're not alone. Our society today offers many stressors, from job security to national and world news. The desire for safety is the core reason we like schedules; we want to feel safe and controlling the few things we can is our attempt at getting it. Spiritually speaking, opening to the flow of the Creator is the answer to feeling safe.

Here are ways to do that:

- You may be tired or unwell, so remedy that first. Get on a health regimen, get a massage, and do what you need to in order to have a whole day of sleep in peace and quiet.

- Schedule in something you like (or a surprise) every week. It can be big or small, and engaging your family and friends to participate will make it fun. Some ideas could be: a note written and hidden, a surprise house cleaning, a new book and an hour to read it, or dinner out.

- Do something nice to appreciate yourself. My favorite is the gratitude board: a simple blackboard hung where appropriate. Every morning write something that you are grateful for in life. Bringing a shift in focus to what you have and acting towards giving yourself what you need can change everything.

Bored with Your Relationship?

If you're bored with your relationship, one or both of you probably hasn't spent quality time focusing on it, making room for petty negative behaviors to crawl in. I am certain, neither you nor your partner are using your superpowers as they were intended. Everyone has them: being kind, stable, invigorating, courageous, visionary, consistent, loving, et cetera. But in a negatively focused relationship, those same superpowers can be quite damaging. So, the first step is to stop the damage.

Sit with your partner and write out what you think their top five superpowers are. Now, write out the negative values of those superpowers. It is most likely those dynamics that are bringing you down.

For example, here are a few traits with their unwanted counter parts:

- Kind vs. Pushover
- Stable vs. Uninterested
- Invigorating vs. Irritating
- Courageous vs. a Bully
- Visionary vs. Not Present

Chances are that you fell in love with the positive traits, and now, many choices later, you are calling out the negatives in each other. Taking time to remember why you liked each other in the first place and placing focus on it can go a long way to getting the rhythm back in your relationship.

We are in the condition we are for all sorts of reasons: from simple to incredibly traumatic and complex. But while love heals all, it is our choices that fix all. Don't wait for the bad habits to set in, affecting your choices. Be honest with yourself and others. Know that all things can change with acceptance and forgiveness. Most of all, remember: you are beautiful, you are interesting, and you are powerful.

The Slayer's Altar and Ritual: Making Your Home a Sacred Space

What You Will Need:

- Seven-day candle: color of your choice
- Paper and pen
- A glass of water or a dish of tobacco for an offering
- Sage, rosemary, pine leaves, frankincense, or cedar for clearing the energy in your home by burning in every room
- Cleaning products
- Help

What we do with all the stuff we own can generate or stifle energy flow in our homes and in our life. The placement of your objects and your connection to nature and environment can support and regulate the flow of that energy impacting everything you do every day. The vibe of a new cycle heralds the winds of change to blow at the end of every major season or event, bringing new opportunity. These are perfect times to clear out unwanted items, clean, and make shifts in order, color, and design—all with intention.

It's a good idea to know what you want in life, or at least what you don't want. The three most important principal's for opening your mind, heart, and home for change are cleaning and clearing, preparing to receive, and harmoniously having the object of your desire. Our longings are manifested in many ways, subtle and overt. The more we recognize the subtle frequencies of the Universe, we embrace our role in the deliberate ways we engage in the giving and receiving that creates our lives.

Our human consciousness needs to be generous, more than we need to receive. The mind trick here is that receiving is a natural response to giving anything. So, being mindful of what you bring to others in their lives and learning to receive graciously (among other things: help) is the skillset to be acquired here. The more you give of yourself freely, the more it finds its way back to you. Here are a few changes to make in your home to increase the flow of exchange:

Clutter Free Zone

The most important thing to do when you want change in your life is to create space for it. Getting rid of clutter, cleaning out drawers, and having as much surface space in all rooms of your home is vital. Once you have cleared space, had a garage sale, or taken a few loads to the thrift shop—now it's time to clean. I mean really scrub those spaces: from floors to baseboards to windows and sills. Start with the bathroom and kitchen. Those two rooms of the house are where energy is piped in and released out several times a day. Keeping the lid down on the toilet is optimum. You'll really want to scrub the walls, appliances, and fixtures; take my word for it, there is nothing sexier than a clean corner of the bathroom floor.

Satellite for Receptivity

A person's preparedness to give and receive is always evident in their home if you look. Is the home crowded with stuff, or is it clean and clear of overwhelming objects? Do you feel welcome? Are the themes of décor inviting and inclusive to everyone? Are the colors inspiring or calming? All these elements are valuable to you and those you choose to be in partnership with on any level.

Take your inventory:

- How much extra space do you have?
- How clean is your environment?
- Do you have past memorabilia up everywhere in your home or is it concentrated to one area?
- Are the walls blank, if so, why?
- What are the themes of the art in your home, does it reflect you today?
- On a scale of 1–10 (10 being ready), how prepared are you to receive new energy?
- What are the themes of décor in your home, and what do they say about you?
- Is your home welcoming to others?

There are a couple of things you want to pay attention to, like making sure there are no sharp corners or jagged edges (for example, a table edge or wall corner). If there are, they are easily remedied by hanging a multi-faceted crystal, a wind chime, or by covering it with cloth. Creating a flowing environment without jagged, harsh, or blocked energy keeps you in a creative, innovative, and faithful place with yourself and the Divine, making the process to move through any challenges an adventure rather than a problem. It helps keep your mind and heart open to new ways to help yourself and others.

Living in Harmony

If you have the relationship you want with yourself, you will easily draw to you the life and love you seek. Creating that harmony and self-acceptance is your goal before all others. The center of the house radiates harmony to all other places in the home and all your life situations. It's an ideal place for a home or family altar where everyone can place their goals, hopes, and dreams. Each person in our home impacts the experience for everyone, so becoming a part of the solution to their challenges, and letting them be a part of yours, helps the energy of the entire home stay in flow.

Creating Your Altar

Choose a central place for your altar and collect all the items mentioned above. Place your candle and offering on the altar with the notes you've taken for your inventory (along with any other notes you may still have from exercises throughout the book). Now, take a moment to get clear on the intention of this altar by collecting any items that represent to you what you are inviting into your life. Remember, we aren't worshipping the items, we are awakening that energy in ourselves in order to recognize it in the outer world. All symbols are ancient archetypes that relate to the elements making up our Universe: heaven, earth, water, fire, wood, and metal.

The practice of working with the energy in your home is meant to cultivate your awareness. Helping you get to know your nature and the nature of flow in the Universe, and how the two interact. How you relate to the Creator is more expansive than the elements of your Universe and brings your personal spiritual beliefs into this process. Most of all, the point is to pay attention and care for your environment and yourself, finding new and conscientious ways to express and receive love in all ways in your life.

Epilogue

The following is a channeled message from a being with whom I have lived many incarnations on Earth. Because he is in spirit and I am in a physical body we've communicated telepathically most days for as long as I can remember. His most recent incarnation was in the 1800's as Chief Running Bear of the Oglala Sioux—when he called me Little Bear. Although he is considered my spirit-guide in this lifetime, he is my family. His steadiness, honesty, humor, and truth have been invaluable to me and the work I do; he is a testament of insurmountable courage and wisdom—for which I am deeply grateful.

Aho Mitakuye Oyasin

"When I speak to the people I tell them that they are more than they believe and more than they are told they are by others. You cannot wait for others to create solutions to the problems you face, you must choose the smallest one and get started on it. While we may never fully trust the white communities, the most valuable thing that the white man took from us was our self-trust. Our personal knowledge of our individual power and capabilities.

"As I witness from this spiritual vantage what has become of the world and my people—and by that I mean all the people—I discover: they do not trust themselves and therefore betray themselves, every day. They do not trust because they are not honest. The Creator has given us a design beyond what each of us can personally know, and that design has brought us to this place and no other. You cannot control the honesty of another man, but you can transcend his dishonesty by not allowing it to move you from your destiny.

"The Creator teaches us how to love ourselves and love one another through hating ourselves and one another. The presence of one begets the presence of the other, both are illusions to overcome. Eventually, the hate you feel breaks way to love because hate is too heavy a burden to carry. It is this love that will open you up to goodness. It is the path to follow, and we will all follow it eventually. It is my hope that you will heed this message and open your heart, deeply, to yourselves and each other. Surrender your heart to the Creator—the One Love that flows through us all—and know that there can be no other way at this time.

– Aho
Chief Running Bear of the Oglala Sioux

Notes

The following endnotes reflect quotations that are used with permissions via the doctrine of fair use, presented here along with other resources as well.

PART 1
1. James Comey, "James Comey: How Trump Co-opts Leaders Like Bill Barr," The New York Times, Nytimes.com, May 1st, 2019, https://www.nytimes.com/2019/05/01/opinion/william-barr-testimony.html.
2. Stephanie Lam, "Researchers Find Miracles in Yogi's Fasting," Sunlightenment.com, last modified May 2014, http://sunlightenment.com/researchers-find-miracles-in-yogi%E2%80%99s-fasting/.
3. Kahlil Gibran, "Kahlil Gibran Quotes," Quotes.net, n.d., retrieved December 1, 2019, https://www.quotes.net/quote/2822.

PART 2
1. Bertha Calloway, "Bertha Calloway Quotes," Quotes.net, n.d., retrieved December 1, 2019, https://www.quotes.net/quote/19789.
2. Tracee Dunblazier, *Heal Your Soul History: Activate the True Power of Your Shadow (The Demon Slayer's Handbook, Volume 2)* (GoTracee Publishing LLC, April 1, 2017), p. 126.
3. Esther Huertas, quoted by Rosa Torruellas in *Affirming Cultural Citizenship in the Puerto Rican Community*, Centro de Estudios Puertorriqueños, Hunter College of the City University of New York, 1991, p. 65.
4. FS Stinson, et al., "Prevalence, correlates, disability, and comorbidity of DSM-IV narcissistic personality disorder: results from the wave 2 national epidemiologic survey on alcohol and related conditions." US National Library of Medicine, National Institutes of Health, July 2008, http://www.ncbi.nlm.nih.gov/pubmed/18447663.

PART 3
1. Deepak Chopra, *The Soul of Leadership: Unlocking Your Potential for Greatness* (Harmony, 2010), Kindle Edition, Introduction.

PART 4
1. World Health Organization, *Preventing Suicide: A Resource for Police, Firefighters and Other First Line Responders*, (Department of Mental Health and Substance Abuse, World Health Organization, 2009), https://www.who.int/mental_health/prevention/suicide/resource_firstresponders.pdf.
2. Nassim Nicholas Taleb, *The Black Swan: The Impact of the Highly Improbable*, 2nd ed. (Random House Trade Paperbacks, 2010).
3. Bruce Lee, *Bruce Lee: A Warrior's Journey*, directed by John Little and Bruce Lee (United States, Hong Kong: Warner Home Video, 2000), Documentary.
4. Claire Hansen, "116th Congress by Party, Race, Gender, and Religion," US News, January 3, 2019, https://www.usnews.com/news/politics/slideshows/116th-congress-by-party-race-gender-and-religion?slide=2.

5 Dan Hardy, "How race and class relate to standardized tests," The Notebook.org, Philadelphia Public School, November 24, 2015, https://thenotebook.org/articles/2015/11/24/how-race-and-class-relate-to-standardized-tests/.

6 Ann Killion, "Why does the U.S. women's soccer team get paid less than the men?" San Francisco Chronicle, last modified July 7, 2019, https://www.sfchronicle.com/sports/annkillion/article/Why-does-the-U-S-Women-s-Soccer-team-get-paid-13689380.php.

7 Elia Winters, from personal chat forum response, September 22, 2019, https://eliawinters.com.

8 Lizzo, "Lizzo: 'I Feel like a Master,'" *Producer: John D'Amelio*, Editor: Ed Givnish, CBS News, CBS Interactive, Inc., October 6, 2019, https://www.cbsnews.com/news/lizzo-i-feel-like-a-master/.

9 Robin DiAngelo, *White Fragility: Why It's So Hard for White People to Talk About Racism*, reprint edition (Beacon Press, June 26, 2018), p. 131.

10 Tracee Dunblazier, *Heal Your Soul History*, p. 132.

11 David Jay Minderhout and Andrea T. Frantz, *Invisible Indians: Native Americans in Pennsylvania*, 1st ed. (Cambria Press, 2008).

12 Confucius, quoted by Mr. Selfdevelopment in "9 Powerful Life Lessons from Confucius," Pick the Brain: Grow Yourself, PicktheBrain.com, August 3, 2010, https://www.pickthebrain.com/blog/9-powerful-life-lessons-from-confucius/.

13 National Institute of Mental Health, "Suicide," National Institute of Health, last modified April 2009, https://www.nimh.nih.gov/health/statistics/suicide.shtml.

PART 5

1 Luc Bodin, Nathalie Bodin Lamboy, and Jean Graciet, *The Book of Ho'oponopono: The Hawaiian Practice of Forgiveness and Healing* (Inner Traditions/Bear & Company, 2016), Kindle Edition, Chap 1.

2 Tracee Dunblazier, *Heal Your Soul History*, p. 5.

3 Dr. Susan Albers, "Emotional Intelligence 2.0 : Learning the Art of Self-Awareness," Huffington Post, last modified May 27, 2012, http://www.huffingtonpost.com/dr-susan-albers/emotional-intelligence_b_1377591.html.

4 Evan Marc Katz, "Why Do So Many People Lie In Online Dating?" Evan Marc Katz: Understand Men. Find Love. Evan Marc Katz.com, retrieved September 1, 2019, http://www.evanmarckatz.com/blog/online-dating-tips-advice/why-do-so-many-people-lie-in-online-dating/.

5 James Patterson and Peter Kim, *The Day America Told the Truth* (Prentice Hall Direct, 1991).

6 Kim B. Serota, Timothy R. Levine, and Franklin J. Boster, *The Prevalence of Lying in America: Three Studies of Self-Reported Lies* (East Lansing: Michigan State University, 2010), https://msu.edu/~levinet/Serota_etal2010.pdf.

7 Eckhart Tolle, *The Power of Now: A Guide to Spiritual Enlightenment* (New World Library, 2004). Reprinted with permission by New World Library, Novato, CA. www.newworldlibrary.com

8 Gregg Braden, *Deep Truth: Igniting the Memory of Our Origin, History, Destiny, and Fate* (Hay House, 2011), p. 78.

9 Dorothy Bea Akoto-Abutiate, *Proverbs and the African Tree of Life*, Studies in Systematic Theology 16 (Brill, 2014).

Bibliography

Akoto-Abutiate, Dorothy Bea. *Proverbs and the African Tree of Life*. Studies in Systematic Theology 16. Brill, 2014.

Albers, Dr. Susan. "Emotional Intelligence 2.0 : Learning the Art of Self-Awareness." Huffington Post. Last modified May 27, 2012. http://www.huffingtonpost.com/dr-susan-albers/emotional-intelligence_b_1377591.html.

Braden, Gregg. *Deep Truth: Igniting the Memory of Our Origin, History, Destiny, and Fate*. Hay House, 2011.

Bodin, Luc, Nathalie Bodin Lamboy, and Jean Graciet. *The Book of Ho'oponopono: The Hawaiian Practice of Forgiveness and Healing*. Inner Traditions/Bear & Company, 2016. Kindle Edition.

Calloway, Bertha. "Bertha Calloway Quotes." Quotes.net. (n.d.). Retrieved December 1, 2019. https://www.quotes.net/quote/19789.

Chopra, Deepak. *The Soul of Leadership: Unlocking Your Potential for Greatness*. Harmony, 2010. Kindle Edition.

Comey, James. "James Comey: How Trump Co-opts Leaders Like Bill Barr." The New York Times. Nytimes.com. May 1st, 2019. https://www.nytimes.com/2019/05/01/opinion/william-barr-testimony.html.

Confuscius. Quoted by Mr. Selfdevelopment. "9 Powerful Life Lessons from Confuscius." Pick the Brain: Grow Yourself. PicktheBrain.com. August 3, 2010. https://www.pickthebrain.com/blog/9-powerful-life-lessons-from-confucius/.

DiAngelo, Robin. *White Fragility: Why It's So Hard for White People to Talk About Racism*, Reprint edition. Beacon Press, June 26, 2018.

Dunblazier, Tracee. *Heal Your Soul History: Activate the True Power of Your Shadow (The Demon Slayer's Handbook, Volume 2)*. GoTracee Publishing LLC, April 1, 2017.

---. *Master Your Inner World: Embrace Your Power with Joy (The Demon Slayer's Handbook, Volume 1)*. GoTracee Publishing LLC, May 6, 2016.

Fried, Hédi. *Questions I am asked about the Holocaust*. US edition. Scribe US, April 2, 2019.

Gibran, Kahlil. "Kahlil Gibran Quotes." Quotes.net. (n.d.). Retrieved December 1, 2019. https://www.quotes.net/quote/2822.

Hansen, Claire. "116th Congress by Party, Race, Gender, and Religion." US News. January 3, 2019. https://www.usnews.com/news/politics/slideshows/116th-congress-by-party-race-gender-and-religion?slide=2.

Hardy, Dan. "How race and class relate to standardized tests." The Notebook.org. Philadelphia Public School. November 24, 2015. https://thenotebook.org/articles/2015/11/24/how-race-and-class-relate-to-standardized-tests/.

Huertas, Esther. Quoted by Rosa Torruellas. *Affirming Cultural Citizenship in the Puerto Rican Community*. Centro de Estudios Puertorriqueños, Hunter College of the City University of New York, 1991.

Katz, Evan Marc. "Why Do So Many People Lie In Online Dating?" Evan Marc Katz: Understand Men. Find Love. Evan Marc Katz.com. Retrieved September 1, 2019. http://www.evanmarckatz.com/blog/online-dating-tips-advice/why-do-so-many-people-lie-in-online-dating/.

Killion, Ann. "Why does the U.S. women's soccer team get paid less than the men?" San Francisco Chronicle. Last modified July 7, 2019. https://www.sfchronicle.com/sports/annkillion/article/Why-does-the-U-S-Women-s-Soccer-team-get-paid-13689380.php.

Lam, Stephanie. "Researchers Find Miracles in Yogi's Fasting." Sunlightenment.com. Last modified May 2014. http://sunlightenment.com/researchers-find-miracles-in-yogi%E2%80%99s-fasting/.

Lee, Bruce. *Bruce Lee: A Warrior's Journey*. Directed by John Little and Bruce Lee. United States, Hong Kong: Warner Home Video, 2000. Documentary.

Lizzo. "Lizzo: 'I Feel like a Master.'" *Producer: John D'Amelio. Editor: Ed Givnish*. CBS News. CBS Interactive, Inc. October 6, 2019. https://www.cbsnews.com/news/lizzo-i-feel-like-a-master/.

McCullough, David. *The Great Bridge: The Epic Story of the Building of the Brooklyn Bridge*. Reprint edition. Simon & Schuster, January 12, 1983.

Minderhout, David Jay, and Andrea T. Frantz. *Invisible Indians: Native Americans in Pennsylvania*. 1st ed. Cambria Press, 2008.

National Institute of Mental Health. "Suicide." National Institute Health. Last modified April 2009. https://www.nimh.nih.gov/health/statistics/suicide.shtml.

Patterson, James and Peter Kim. *The Day America Told the Truth*. Prentice Hall Direct, 1991.

Serota, Kim B., Timothy R. Levine, and Franklin J. Boster. *The Prevalence of Lying in America: Three Studies of Self-Reported Lies*. East Lansing: Michigan State University, 2010. https://msu.edu/~levinet/Serota_etal2010.pdf.

Stinson FS, Dawson DA, Goldstein RB, Chou SP, Huang B, Smith SM, Ruan WJ, Pulay AJ, Saha TD, Pickering RP, and Grant BF. "Prevalence, correlates, disability, and comorbidity of DSM-IV narcissistic personality disorder: results from the wave 2 national epidemiologic survey on alcohol and related conditions." US National Library of Medicine, National Institutes of Health, July 2008. http://www.ncbi.nlm.nih.gov/pubmed/18557663.

Taleb, Nassim Nicholas. *The Black Swan: The Impact of the Highly Improbable*. 2nd ed. Random House Trade Paperbacks, 2010.

Tolle, Eckhart. *The Power of Now: A Guide to Spiritual Enlightenment*. New World Library, 2004.

Winters, Elia. Personal chat forum response. Retrieved September 22, 2019. https://eliawinters.com.

Woodard, Stephanie. *American Apartheid: The Native American Struggle for Self-Determination and Inclusion*. Ig Publishing, September 18, 2018.

World Health Organization. *Preventing Suicide: A Resource for Police, Firefighters and Other First Line Responders*. Department of Mental Health and Substance Abuse, World Health Organization, 2009. https://www.who.int/mental_health/prevention/suicide/resource_firstresponders.pdf.

Other Works by the Author

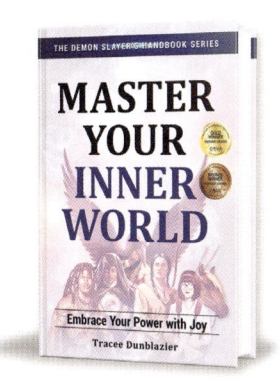

MASTER YOUR INNER WORLD: Embrace Your Power with Joy, *(Volume One, Demon Slayer's Handbook Series)*

Winner of the Coalition of Visionary Resources, Visionary Awards gold medal in Alternative Sciences and bronze medal in Shamanism, categories. Tracee covers many relevant topics such as: spirit guides and other dimensional entities, tools for healing, the spiritual purpose of anger, grief, and depression and how to transform strong emotions. You'll receive a new framework for healing from the soul to the body in a way that adjusts your perspective of the underworld and shows you the magnitude of your power in any situation. This book is a game changer for anyone who suffers. (Available in Spanish.)

"An encouraging playbook for would-be demon-slayers."—**Kirkus Reviews**

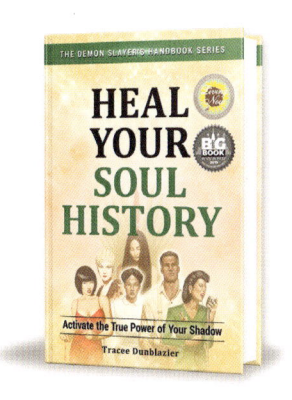

HEAL YOUR SOUL HISTORY: Activate the True Power of Your Shadow, *(Volume Two, Demon Slayer's Handbook Series)*

Winner of the Living Now Silver medal, the NYC Big Book Distinguished Favorite, and a COVR Visionary Award, this book will take you on a soul excavation and change how you look at your life and the lives of others from now on. Understanding the spiritual imprints of your unique soul and how they're impacting your life today, can help you gain power over the negative forces that hold you back and give you the opportunity to resolve deep-seated life patterns that shape your everyday relationships.

"An inspirational guide to using a soul's long history to combat present-day negative forces."—**Kirkus Reviews**

RAINBOW WARRIOR ACTIVATION DECK

Winner of the Living Now Gold medal, this brilliantly rendered and colorful 52 card deck set with a 124 page guidebook, created by national award-winning author and shaman—Tracee Dunblazier, and acclaimed intuitive artist– Justine Serebrin, is an inspiring solution for rising above the divergent forces all around us. Whether you're using it for meditation—reading for pleasure or profession, it's exactly the tool you need. This is the deck that grows with you.

"A knock-out of the park activation deck for use during meditation, as well as shadow and ascension work."

—**Melinda Carver,** Author & Columnist

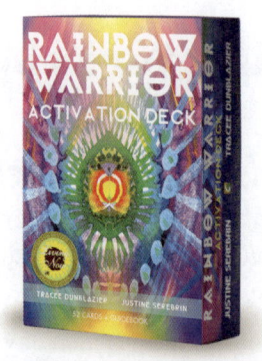

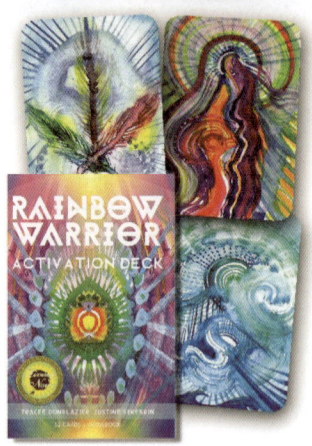

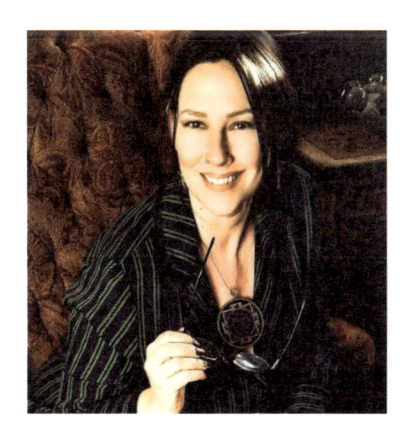

About the Author

Tracee Dunblazier GC-C, is a Los Angeles-based spiritual empath, shaman, and a six-time national award-winning author. As a multi-sensitive, Tracee's blend of intuitive information combined with different modalities, has provided the opportunity for thousands to achieve deep healing and create the success and peace they seek in their lives.

Empathic, delightfully vulnerable, and profoundly real—Dunblazier's two new keynotes: "Are You Haunted?" and "Conquer Your Karmic Relationships!" are enlightening presentations that will open your mind to what is happening right in front of you; the multiple energetic dimensions we all share. No matter where you sit on the spectrum of understanding, Tracee makes tangible the connection between mental wellness and spirituality. Many of us don't fully see what is holding us back from our dreams and aspirations—after these seminars; your eyes will be opened.

Her compassionate, humorous, down-to-earth style empowers her clients, readers, and listeners to address difficult topics with courage and clarity. Because of this, Tracee is consistently called upon by the media for expert commentary on spirituality and relationship dynamics.

In 2015, Tracee founded GoTracee Publishing LLC. It has since grown to be a nationally awarded hybrid-publisher that specializes in spiritual-healing narrative-nonfiction, and divination oracle decks—tools for meditation and self-discovery. Their best-selling Demon Slayer's Handbook Series and Rainbow Warrior Activation Deck offer light in dark places. They are game changers for those who suffer. GoTracee's publications expand the reader's understanding of spiritual transformation and offer the knowledge one needs to live their best life.

www.TraceeDunblazier.com

www.BeASlayer.com